THE
FOODBIBLE

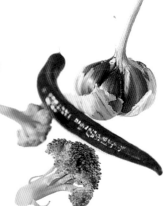

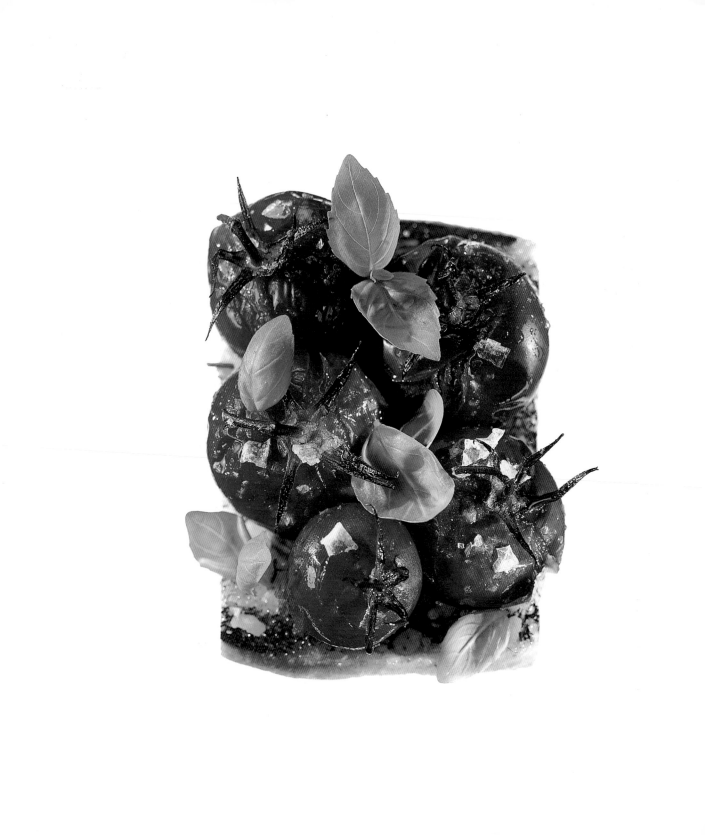

THE
FOOD
BIBLE

THE ULTIMATE GUIDE TO ALL THAT'S GOOD AND BAD IN THE FOOD WE EAT

JUDITH WILLS

QUADRILLE

To Gail Pollard with thanks for her invaluable assistance, knowledge and advice.

The recipes in the book are for 2 people unless otherwise stated. Both metric and imperial quantities are given. Use either all metric or all imperial, as the two are not necessarily interchangeable.

This new, fully revised and updated edition published in 2007 by
Quadrille Publishing Limited,
Alhambra House,
27–31 Charing Cross Road,
London WC2H OLS

Reprinted in 2007
10 9 8 7 6 5 4 3 2

Art Director Mary Evans
Publishing Director Anne Furniss
Editor and Project Manager Lewis Esson
Art Editor Vanessa Courtier
Nutritionist Gail Pollard BSc, SRD
Photography Martin Brigdale, Gus Filgate, Patrick MacLeavey
Home Economists Maxine Clarke, Zoe Sharp, Jane Stevenson, Nicole Szabason
Stylists Penny Markham, Luckie Smith, Helen Trent
Artwork Lynne Robinson
Production Candida Jackson, Vincent Smith
Typesetting Gina Hochstein, Peter Howard

First published in 1998 by by Quadrille Publishing Limited.

ISBN   978 184400 4430

Printed and bound in Singapore

Contents

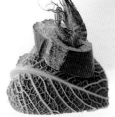
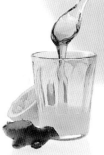

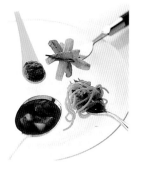
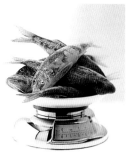
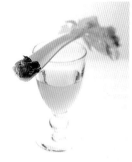
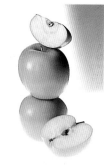

Introduction

What you eat and what you drink really are vital parts of what you are — and what you will become.

From before you are born all the way into old age, sustenance isn't just survival, it is your strength, your size, your short-term health, your long-term health, and — all other factors being equal — the length and quality of your life.

Every time you choose a meal, a snack, a food, a drink, you are making a decision that affects you and your body in a positive or a negative way.

You may feel that this is exaggerating the power of food. However, thanks to the efforts of people like Professor Philip James , who is Director of the Public Health Policy Group and who played a leading role in setting the parameters of the Government's Food Standards Agency — the role of diet in health and well-being is becoming more recognized.

Professor James believes that moderating diet can have a greater impact on public health than drugs, and he has stated that 'half the middle-aged people in Britain have overt nutritional disease'.

We now know that heart disease, high blood pressure, diabetes, and many other major and minor ailments and diseases, including cancers, are often, at least in part, linked to poor nutrition.

The UK has one of the highest rates of heart disease in the world. Two-thirds of the adults in the UK are overweight. Eighty per cent of adults with diabetes have the type that is often triggered by weight-gain and, therefore, diet. Experts also estimate that between a quarter and three-quarters of all cancer (the second biggest killer in the country) is diet-related.

Moreover, these diseases cost the UK health service billions of pounds every year. Heart disease costs £500 million in drugs alone. The British Heart Foundation says that cardiovascular disease is estimated to cost the UK economy just under £26 billion a year.

The fact is that food is not only vital fuel but also vital medicine, and the signs are that we as individuals and consumers are beginning to recognize this. The latest Food Standards Agency survey reveals that more people are checking the labels on foods, and that they are also eating more fruit and vegetables.

Supermarkets are taking notice at last. Justin King, Sainsbury's CE says, 'If we make our products more healthy, more people are buying them.' And as we buy healthier produce, sales of carbonated drinks, takeaway burgers and other high-fat, high-salt products are falling. It seems obvious, then, that we do want to make changes. I have compiled *The Food Bible* to help you make the right choices. Here is all the information you need for positive nutrition — food to keep you fit and well, strong and vital, all through your life.

The book also provides all the latest thinking and research on what foods you should eat, or avoid, when you have special needs or problems.

I feel qualified to write this book because, over the years, I have changed from caring little about food other than for its taste and ease of preparation, into someone who believes – passionately – that everybody deserves good food and good nutrition. I believe that good, healthy food is also delicious appealing food, and I hope to make everyone realize that eating for health doesn't mean compromise in those areas.

I hope that, with the help of *The Food Bible*, you will continue to take even more responsibility for your diet. In the long term, if we vote for good food through what we buy, then good food is what we will get.

Keep thinking 'five-star fuel' and remember, everybody deserves good food.

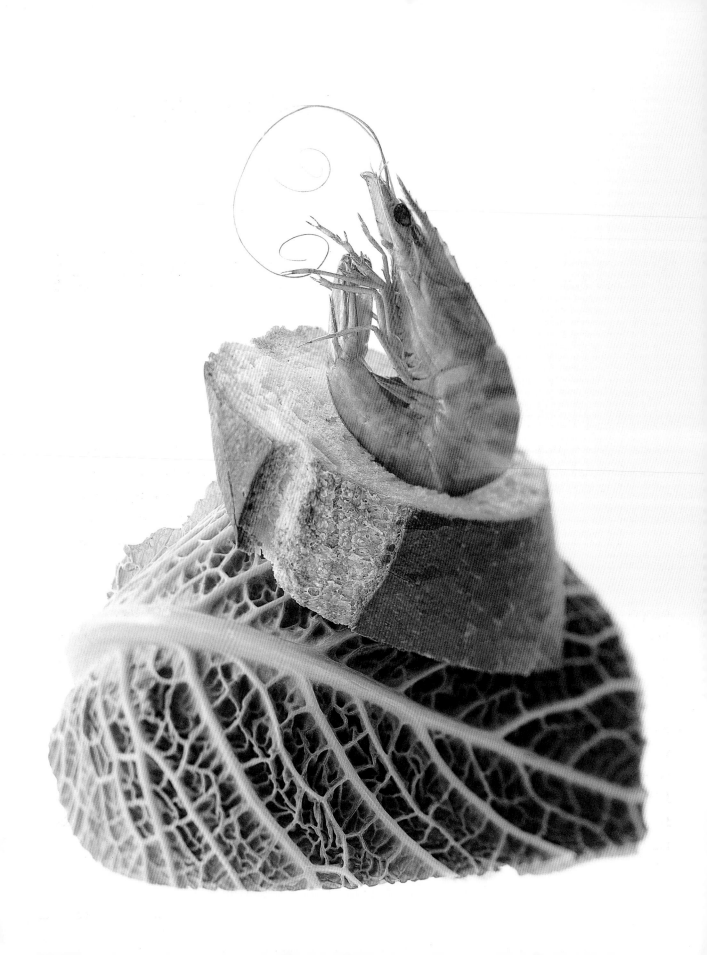

Food for a balanced diet

The experts are always telling you that you ought to eat a balanced diet. In fact, you've heard the message so often you probably know it by heart — eat less fat; more fruit and veg and fibre. But what exactly does that mean, and how do you know you're achieving the correct balance? Most of us, for example, still fall well short of eating enough healthy carbohydrates; and many of us who try to follow a diet very low in fat may be doing just as much harm to our health as those who eat a high-fat diet. Then there's the advice to eat 'five a day' of fruit and vegetables. What is a portion? And which fruits and veg can be included? Most people haven't got a clue.

And what about the other nutrients you hardly ever hear about? For instance, did you know that many of us eat far more protein than we really need, and that too much can be bad for you? Do you know that some fats are vital to our well-being and aren't all that easy to find in a typical diet? And did you know that many of us in the UK fall short of at least some of the vitamins and minerals our bodies need? Here is where you will find out all you need to know about 'a balanced diet', in a way that you can understand.

Pictured overleaf is a perfect day's eating for an average woman, containing all the carbohydrates, fat, protein, vitamins, minerals, fibre, etc. that are needed, in all the right quantities. Using this as our blueprint, we go on to show how you can achieve your own perfect diet. Your diet won't necessarily look the same, or indeed contain more than a couple of the same foods, because your needs, lifestyle and preferences may be different. That's the beauty of food — there is so much available in so much variety you can eat 'a balanced diet' without compromising your own needs. Section One sets out the foundation of your own diet for health and well-being, and shows how to give your body the fuel it needs for life.

THE BUILDING BLOCKS OF A HEALTHY DIET

To form our blueprint, the photographs on these pages show a perfect day's eating for an average woman, according to official DoH nutritional guidelines, containing all the carbohydrates, fat, protein, vitamins, minerals, fibre, etc, that are needed, in all the right quantities.

Taken together, the breakfast, lunch, main meal and snack (together with 200 ml /7 fl oz semi-skimmed milk and unlimited water to drink) give a total of 1,943 calories; 66.3 g total fat (30.7% of day's energy intake); 12.3 g saturated fat (5.7% of day's total energy intake); 19.4 g polyunsaturated fat (9% of day's energy intake); 28.6 g monounsaturated fat (13.25% of day's energy intake); 73.6 g protein (15.2% of day's energy intake); 280.4 g carbohydrate (54.1% of day's energy intake); 31 g fibre; contains only 1,285 mg sodium and gives 100% or more of the Reference Nutrient Intake for all the other major vitamins and minerals.

Breakfast
150 ml (¼ pt) orange juice, 60 g (2¼ oz) no-added-sugar-or-salt
luxury muesli, 100 g (3½ oz) fresh raspberries, 5 tbsp semi-skimmed milk,
50 g (2 oz) wholemeal bread, 5 g (¼ oz) low-fat spread, 10 g (½ oz) runny honey.

Lunch

175 g (7 oz) cooked weight brown rice combined into a salad with:
50 g (2 oz) cooked chickpeas, 7 g (⅓ oz) pine nuts, 25 g (1 oz)
cooked baby sweetcorn, 80 g (2¾ oz) tomato, 25 g (1 oz)
watercress, 25 g (1 oz) raw baby spinach, all tossed in
1 tbsp olive oil and balsamic vinegar or lemon juice or wine
vinegar.

Snacks

1 large banana (approx 175 g / 6 oz weighed with skin, 120 g / 5 oz without skin)
15 g (¾ oz) shelled almonds
50 g (2 oz) ready-to-eat dried apricots
one 13 g (½ oz) traditional oatcake

Evening meal

85 g (3 oz) salmon fillet, lightly grilled, 50 g (2 oz) sliced red
pepper, 50 g (2 oz) broccoli florets, 25 g (1 oz) spring onion, sliced, 25 g
(1 oz) mangetout stir-fried in 1 dsp (8 g) sesame oil, tossed in lime juice and black pepper, served with 100 g (4 oz) cooked weight whole-wheat noodles, 125 g (5 oz) cantaloupe (orange-fleshed) melon, 50 g (2 oz) wholemeal roll, 5 g (¼ oz) low-fat spread.

Energy-giving carbohydrates

Your body's most constant and basic requirement — apart, perhaps, from water — is energy. Energy to breathe, to move, to function, to power itself, for repair and growth. Like machines, we need an outside source of energy, but our fuel has to come from what we eat and drink.

That energy is measured in kilocalories (popularly just called calories). When you expend energy you 'burn up' calories, and when you eat you consume calories. The amount of energy or calories your body needs in a day depends on your size, age, proportion of muscle to fat, activity levels and many other factors.

However, guidelines — called Estimated Average Requirements (EARs) — have been laid down by the Department of Health, and they are set out in the table below. Those EARs for children, teenagers and the elderly appear in Section Three. (In these days of metrication, energy is also sometimes measured in kilojoules and 1 kilocalorie = 4.18 kilojoules.)

In order to maintain a reasonable and stable body weight, energy (food) intake and energy expenditure need to be balanced. Too little intake and too much expenditure can result in weight loss and being too thin, too much intake and too little expenditure can result in weight gain (from the surplus calories converting themselves into body fat) and eventual obesity. More about maintaining the correct energy balance appears later in Section Four, Food for Weight Control.

All food and drink containing calories can supply you with energy, in the form of carbohydrate, fat, protein or alcohol. Hardly any foods contain only one of these elements — the main exceptions being oils, which contain nothing but fat, and sugar, which contains nothing but carbohydrate. Most foods are a mixture of more than one element (along with combinations of the vitamins and minerals).

For example, bread is high in carbohydrate, but also contains protein and fat; whole milk contains carbohydrate, fat and protein, each in reasonable quantity; meat is a mixture of protein and fat; and so on.

The Food Charts at the end of the book give the protein, fat and carbohydrate content of about 400 items, along with the other elements important for good health. Reading the next few pages will help you interpret these charts.

Although all types of calorie — be they from carbohydrate, fat, protein or alcohol — supply you with energy, the majority of your energy supplies should come from carbohydrate. The wheel chart opposite shows you the proportions of each of the energy-giving nutrients that a healthy diet should contain, based on the DoH's figures, and including a 5% allowance for alcohol consumption (which provides energy in the majority of people's diets).

In fact, the DoH guidelines for carbohydrates are fairly conservative (and also suggest higher fat levels than several other international authorities, a situation which we will look at further over the next few pages). Many other countries have higher recommended carbohydrate levels (e.g. USA 55%, Sweden 60%) and the World Health Organization (WHO) says 55-75% of our total calorie intake should come from carbohydrates! Certainly, levels up to 60% of your total daily calorie intake are likely to be both good for your health and achievable, if fat and protein intake are adjusted downwards (we look at both of these options in more detail on pages 15-21).

There are two main sorts of carbohydrate — starches and sugars. At the moment, around 60% of the carbohydrates that we eat are starches, and about 40% are sugars. Starchy foods are plant-based foods, such as breakfast cereals, bread, potatoes, pulses, pasta and rice. Vegetables also contain starch in varying amounts; most fruits contain none, the main exception being bananas. The carbohydrates in these foods are called polysaccharides and are known as complex carbohydrates.

Sugars are either intrinsic, such as those found in fruits (the carbohydrates in almost all fruits are sugars) and vegetables (usually a mixture of both sugars and starches), which are part of the cellular structure of the food, or extrinsic (sometimes called 'free'), such as those found in table sugar, honey, fruit squashes, cakes, biscuits, confectionery and so on, and which are

AVERAGE DAILY ENERGY AND CARBOHYDRATE REQUIREMENTS FOR ADULTS

		Cals/day	Total Carbs/day*(g)	Maximum sugar/day(g)**
Women	19-50	1,940	258	52
	51-59	1,900	253	50
Men	19-59	2,550	340	68

* Total carbohydrate, including extrinsic sugars (see right), calculated at 50% of total calorie intake (1g carbohydrate = 3.75 calories).
** Non-milk extrinsic sugars calculated at 10% of total calorie intake (1g sugar = 3.75 calories); these figures to be part of total daily carbohydrate intake and represent maximum intake.

not bound into the cellular structure of the food but are 'refined', depleted of fibre, or added during manufacture. Milk contains an extrinsic sugar, lactose, which is not normally grouped with the other extrinsic sugars for nutrition purposes.

It is the complex carbohydrates and intrinsic sugars that should form the bulk of your healthy diet. The WHO suggests at least 50% of the calories in your diet should come from complex carbohydrates. These are the plant foods which not only supply your body with an easily converted form of energy but which also contain a whole range of other vital nutrients. They also have few health drawbacks and can therefore happily fill the energy gap left when we cut down on fats (see pages 15-19). Carbohydrates also 'spare' protein from being converted into energy, which can be important if protein needs are high or intakes poor.

The more unrefined the carbohydrate that you eat, the better for your health. Low-carbohydrate diets high in fats are linked with increased risk of many diseases, including heart disease, some cancers, especially bowel cancer, constipation and obesity.

Unrefined foods or marginally refined foods, such as brown rice, whole-grain bread, fresh vegetables and fruits, pulses, nuts and seeds, contain all or most of the original nutrients, including fibre, vitamins, minerals, and phytochemicals (see page 34) and tend to be low on the Glycaemic Index (see page 195). Refined carbohydrates, such as white rice, white pasta and white flour, contain less of these elements, although they are still worth eating.

Many common manufactured starchy products, such as mass-produced cakes, packet puddings and biscuits, have lost much of their natural fibres, vitamins and minerals and phytochemicals, and may also contain high levels of the less

healthy types of fat and extrinsic sugars, and are therefore worth cutting right down on in your diet.

Although a recent report from the World Health Organization recommends that these extrinsic sugars can be eaten in moderation as part of a healthy diet, they are the one type of carbohydrate for which the DoH has set an upper intake limit, at 10% (11% if you don't drink alcohol) of total daily calorie intake (see table opposite). One reason for this limit is that high consumption of non-milk extrinsic sugars is a major cause of tooth decay.

Another important issue is that a diet high in sugary, fatty foods, such as snack foods, sweets and cakes, may also be low in essential nutrients (as seen above), while contributing high amounts of calories. Many experts agree that the UK's ever-rising consumption of these types of foods is linked to our steadily rising levels of overweight and obesity (see Section Four, Food for Weight Control).

It is all too easy to consume much more extrinsic sugar than you would think. To reach that 10% total energy limit (52 g sugar), a woman would need to eat just one small slice of Victoria sponge (24 g sugar) and drink one standard can of cola (36 g sugar). As another example, she could have two coffees, each sweetened with 2 spoonfuls of sugar (20 g sugar), plus two chocolate digestive biscuits (20 g sugar), and half a pint of sweet cider (12 g sugar).

A GOOD BALANCE OF NUTRIENTS FOR ADULTS

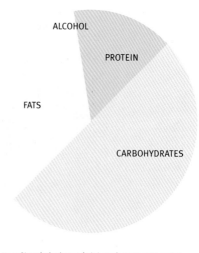

ALCOHOL

PROTEIN

FATS

CARBOHYDRATES

47-50% carbohydrates (minimum), up to 15% protein, 0-5% alcohol, 33-35% fat (maximum)

Foods for fibre

Plant foods of all types are our only source of dietary fibre — various compounds which are not easily absorbed by the digestive system. The type of fibre usually analysed for nutritional purposes is correctly called NSP or non-starch polysaccharides. NSP, such as cellulose and pectin, comes mainly from plant cell walls. It passes undigested through the small intestine into the bowel, where it is fermented by bacteria.

There are two kinds of NSP — insoluble and soluble. Most plant foods contain both types, but proportions vary.

Insoluble fibre is mainly cellulose and is found in all plants. Good sources are grains, especially wheat, corn and rice, vegetables and pulses. Insoluble fibre is important for avoiding constipation and haemorrhoids. Taken with sufficient fluids, a high-fibre diet increases stool bulk, speeds the passage of stools through the bowel, and may help to prevent bowel cancer, diverticulitis and irritable bowel syndrome. It also (with extra fluids) helps us to feel full.

There are various types of *soluble fibre*, such as *pectin* (good sources are citrus fruits and apples), *beta-glucans*, (oats, barley and rye) and *arabinose* (pulses). Several studies conclude that soluble fibre can help reduce LDL blood cholesterol levels (see Heart Disease, page 118 and overleaf). It also helps control blood sugar levels by slowing sugar absorption (see Section Four, Food for Weight Control) which may also help in diabetes.

Lignin is another fibrous compound found in plant cell walls, although not a NSP. It may be important for health (see Cancer, page 96) and is found mainly in flax seed, whole grains, berry fruits and some veg. Lignin and types of resistant starches and fibres in food are not included when calculating fibre content of food under the Englyst system used in the UK for many years. However, the AOAC method now favoured in the US and EU does include them, although of dubious health value. This system generally increases the apparent fibre content of many foods — some (e.g. many breakfast cereals) by around 200%. Currently, labels don't have to say which system they use.

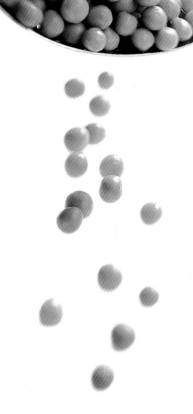

SELECTED GOOD SOURCES OF FIBRE (NSP)

Food/average portion size	Total NSP (g)	Soluble (g)
Haricot beans, 50g dry weight	8.5	4.0
Butter beans, 50g dry weight	8.0	3.2
Red kidney beans, 50g dry weight	7.8	3.5
Soya beans, 50g dry weight	7.8	3.4
Pot barley, 50g dry weight	7.4	2.0
All Bran, 30g serving	7.3	1.2
Wholemeal bread, 100g (3 slices)	5.8	1.6
Peas, frozen, 100g	5.1	1.6
Mango, 1 average	4.9	3.0
Papaya, 1 average	4.7	2.8
Parsnips, 100g	4.6	2.6
Shredded Wheat, 2	4.4	0.9
Wholewheat pasta, 50g dry weight	4.2	1.0
Brussels sprouts, 100g	4.1	2.2
Dried apricots, 50g	3.8	2.3
Dried figs, 50g	3.8	2.0
Blackcurrants, 100g	3.6	1.6
Pear, 1 dessert	3.5	1.1
Spring greens, 100g	3.4	1.7
Hazelnuts, shelled, 50g	3.3	1.3
Prunes, stoned, 50g	2.8	2.0
Orange, 1	2.7	1.8

(all figures based on the Englyst System)

How much fibre is enough?

In Western countries, most of us still don't get enough NSP in our diets, the average intake in the UK being approximately 12 g a day. The DoH recommends up to 24 g for both men and women, with 18 g as a good average, although for people prone to chronic constipation up to 32 g a day (with extra fluids) may be a good idea. Beyond 32 g a day there are no proven benefits and indeed there may be drawbacks, such as a possible malabsorption of minerals.

In any case, it is always best to get your fibre naturally, from high-fibre whole-foods, rather than from a bran supplement — the phytates (see page 29) in raw bran may prevent the absorption of vital minerals, including calcium and iron, and this may be of some significance especially for women and the elderly.

The chart opposite lists selected good sources of total NSP and soluble fibre. The Food Charts (pages 260-317) list NSP content for a wide range of foods.

The facts about fats

In dietary terms, fat has been the wicked witch of the late twentieth century. Every time we grab a fatty snack, we feel guilty. Yet we're still eating too much of the wrong kinds of fat — and probably too little of some of the healthy types. Here's what you need to know.

Fat is made up mainly of fatty acids and glycerol, along with some other compounds — fatty acids being by far the largest component (glycerol comprises roughly 3% of total fat energy intake: glycerol is naturally present as a building block of fats and you do not need to be concerned about intake).

The fatty acids can be divided into three main groups (if you ignore the man-made trans fats, see page 17): saturated, polyunsaturated and monounsaturated.

All fat-containing foods contain all three types of fatty acid, but in varying proportions. When people say, for instance, that 'butter is a saturated fat' that is not really true. Certainly the majority of the fat in butter is saturated (67%), but it also contains 25% monounsaturated fat and even a little polyunsaturated. Beef, another food that people typically think of as containing saturated fat, contains virtually as much monounsaturated fat as saturated, at 43%.

The Food Charts at the back of the book give percentages of all the fatty acids in about 400 foods. To help you balance the fats in your diet, the wheel chart below on the right gives ideal (average in the case of glycerols) percentages for each type of fat.

Currently about 39% of our total daily calorie intake is in the form of fats. Fat is mainly used by the body as energy — it provides more than twice as many calories per gram as either carbohydrate or protein (9 calories a gram). If fat surplus to energy needs is eaten, however, it stores itself in the body as adipose tissue (fat!). This can later be converted into energy if needed. A small amount of fat is also needed because it 'carries' the fat-soluble vitamins A, D and E (see pages 22–4).

Polyunsaturated fats are also needed to supply essential fatty acids (see overleaf).

Because a high-fat diet has been strongly linked with heart disease as well as some forms of cancer, obesity and other ills, however, the DoH advises us to cut fat intake down to 33% or less, and many other authorities advise going even lower (the USA and WHO recommend 30%). It's no good just saying, 'cut down on fat', because in terms of health all fats aren't equal, and a very low-fat diet may have health drawbacks.

HOW MUCH FAT SHOULD YOU EAT
(to total 33% **energy** intake)

	Total fat	% Sat	% Trans	% Poly	% Mono
% of total energy intake	33# max	10 max	2 max	6* min	12 min
Grams/day for women	71g	21.5g	4.3g	13g**	26g
Grams/day for men	93.5g	28.5g	5.6g	17g**	34g

includes 3% glycerols * (10% max) ** (21.5g max for women and 28.3g max for men)

IDEAL AMOUNTS OF DIFFERENT FATS IN THE DIET (as a % of total **fat** intake)

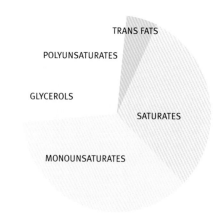

30% sat fat (max), 6% trans fats (max), 18% polyunsat fat (min), 36% monounsat fat (min), 9% glycerols (ave)

SELECTED FOODS HIGH IN SATURATED FATTY ACIDS
(all per 100 g weight)

	Saturated fatty acids (g)	Total fat (g)
Creamed coconut block	58.5	68
Suet, animal	56.0	100
Butter	53.5	80
Suet, vegetable	45.0	88
Lard	41.0	100
Hard margarine	35.0	80
Mascarpone cheese	30.5	46
Cream cheese	30.0	48
Double cream	30.0	48
Crème fraîche, full-fat	26.5	40
Stilton cheese	22.5	36
Cheddar cheese, full-fat	21.5	34
Chocolate	18.5	31
Fried bacon, lean and fat	16.0	41
Shortcrust pastry	10.0	28
Pork pie	10.0	27
Potato crisps	9.0	37
Minced beef	7.0	16
Lamb shoulder, roast	6.5	14

■ Saturated fat

This is the kind of fat that is usually solid at room temperature and is found in largest quantities in animal produce such as meat, cheese, cream, milk, eggs, butter and lard, and in milk chocolate and many manufactured pies, pastries, cakes and biscuits.

It has been proved that a diet high in saturated fats can raise levels of the 'bad' blood cholesterol, LDL, which is a major risk factor in heart disease, our biggest killer. A diet high in saturated fat may also be linked with other ailments and problems, including cancer and obesity. A diet high in saturated fat also 'competes' with the essential fats and may prevent them from doing their job within the body.

Currently our saturated fat intake is about 15% of our total calorie intake (39.5% of fat intake) and the DoH estimates that if we reduced our intake to about 10% (i.e. a cut of one-third) then risk of CHD (coronary heart disease, see page 118) would be 'reduced substantially'.

■ Polyunsaturated fat

The largest amounts of this type of fat are usually contained in the kinds of fat that are liquid at room temperature or cooler — vegetable oils, such as corn oil, safflower oil, sunflower oil and walnut oil are high in omega-6 (n-6) polyunsaturates, as are most nuts.

Polyunsaturated fats have the opposite effects of saturates by lowering LDL blood cholesterol, but experts believe that high levels of omega-6 polyunsaturated fat intake may nevertheless not be a good idea, especially used in cooking, because they may be easily oxidized in the body, producing free radicals which can damage body cells and may actually help cancers and other diseases to form. (A diet high in antioxidants will help counteract this effect). For that reason maximum levels have been set by the DoH at 10% of calorie intake, with 6% as a recommended average, though new EU proposals suggest 4–8%.

A certain amount of polyunsaturated fats ARE needed in our diets because they contain what are termed the *essential fatty acids* (EFAs) that our bodies need for normal health — *linoleic acid* (one of the n-6 group of PUFAs, often called omega-6s) and *alpha-linolenic acid*, one of the n-3 group of PUFAs, often called omega-3s. These are called essential because they are the only fats that our bodies actually need from food, as other fats can be manufactured in the body. Good sources of EFAs are shown in the boxes on page 19.

The essential fats are needed in small but balanced amounts — a minimum of about 2g for linoleic acid — according to the DoH and new Euro-proposed guidelines also suggest 2g for alpha-linolenic acid. An adequate and balanced intake of essential fatty acids may help in prevention or control of all kinds of ailments and conditions, such as heart disease, cancers, immune system deficiencies, arthritis, skin complaints and diseases of the nervous system.

One special type of n-6 PUFA is *gamma-linolenic acid* (GLA), which can be manufactured in the body from linoleic acid (but this process may occasionally be hindered) and is found in greatest quantities in evening primrose and starflower oils. This may be of particular help to women with PMS and

OMEGA-3 EDA AND DHA FATTY ACIDS IN FISH

(g/100g fish)	
Mackerel	1.8
Herring	1.8
Salmon	1.8
Tuna, fresh	1.4
Trout	1.0

menopausal symptoms and may help dyspraxia. Two other fatty acids of importance are the 'long chain' n-3s *eicosapentaenoic acid* (EPA) and *docosahexaenoic acid* (DHA), found in oily fish and fish oils. Two to three 100 g portions a week have been shown to be particularly beneficial in reducing the 'stickiness' of the blood and its tendency to clot, and therefore in helping to prevent CHD and stroke. They may also improve brain power and help beat depression. New Euro guidelines suggest 0.2 g (200 µg) of EPA and DHA a day, equivalent to one small portion of tuna a week. EPA and DHA can also be made in the body from alpha-linolenic acid. Linseed (flax seed) oil contains high levels of alpha-linolenic acid.

Polyunsaturated fats are also one of few rich sources of vitamin E.

■ Trans Fats

There is another type of fat related to these groups called the trans fats. Most of the trans fats in the diet are unsaturated fats which have been altered — hydrogenated — usually in food processing, and become hard at room temperature, such as when some margarines (which are a blend of oils) are manufactured. These hydrogenated fats then become more like saturated fats in the manner in which they act in the body.

Evidence is emerging that trans fats can actually be more damaging than saturates. For instance, in the case of heart disease it now appears, according to a very large USA trial, that trans fats not only raise levels of LDL blood cholesterol (the 'baddie') but also lower levels of the 'good' cholesterol, HDL, and can predispose to weight gain around the waist – the apple shape linked to heart disease.

Trans fats are the only types of fat to do this — natural saturated fats, such as butter or cheese, may raise LDL levels but also raise HDL levels. The DoH and Euro guidelines recommend our intake of trans fats is no more than 2% of total energy intake, but in view of the latest evidence it may be wise to consider trying to limit this further.

The amount of trans fats within manufactured foods is only sometimes listed on the nutrition label, but in general most hard margarines and cooking fats contain the highest concentrations. They will also be found

SELECTED RICH SOURCES OF POLYUNSATURATED FATTY ACIDS (PUFAS) (all per 100 g weight)

	Polyunsaturated fatty acids (g)	Total fat (g)
Safflower oil	74	100
Walnut oil	70	100
Sunflower oil	63	100
Corn oil	51	100
Blended vegetable oil	48	100
Walnuts	47	68.0
Sesame oil	44	100
Mayonnaise, commercial	44	75.5
Sunflower margarine	37	84.0
Brazil nuts	23	68.0
Low-fat spread, typical	10	40.0
Sardines, canned in oil, drained	5	13.5
Tuna, canned in oil, drained	5	9.0

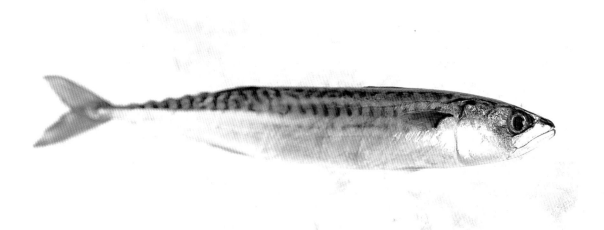

SELECTED RICH SOURCES OF MONOUNSATURATED FATTY ACIDS (MFAS)
(all per 100 g weight)

	Monounsaturated fatty acids (g)	Total fat (g)
Olive oil	73	100
Macadamia nuts (shelled)	61	78
Rapeseed oil	59	100
Hazelnuts (shelled)	50.5	64
Lard	44	100
Groundnut oil	44	100
Sesame oil	38	100
Blended vegetable oil	36	100
Almonds, shelled	35	56
Olive oil margarine (60% fat)	32.5	60
Corn oil	30	100
Brazil nuts (shelled)	26	68
Duck, roast, with skin	19	38
Bacon, fried, lean and fat	18.5	41
Hummus	18	29
Low-fat spread, typical	17.5	40
Double cream	14	48
Avocado	12	19.5
Mackerel fillet	8	16
Beef, minced	7	16

in quite significant quantities in many mass-produced baked goods, such as biscuits, cakes and puddings, in many soft margarines, and in take-away foods such as fish and chips. They are banned in organic food production.

In the Food Charts at the back of the book, trans fats are included in the Total Fat column.

Monounsaturated fat

This, the last of the types of fat, is also usually liquid at room temperature but may solidify when cooled (say, in the fridge), and is found in greatest quantities in olive, rapeseed and groundnut oils, as well as in olives themselves and many nuts and in avocados, but it is also present in fairly reasonable quantities in all fats, most dairy produce, eggs, fish, meat and many other foods.

BEST SOURCES OF EFA LINOLEIC ACID (g/100 g)

Safflower oil	73.9
Evening primrose oil	68.4
Grapeseed oil	67.8
Sunflower oil	63.2
Walnut oil	58.4
Hemp seed oil	57
Soya oil	51.5
Corn oil	50.4
Sesame oil	43.1
Margarine, soft polyunsaturated	33.8
Sunflower seeds	32.8
Groundnut oil	31
Walnuts	29.5
Sesame seeds	25.3
Pine nuts	24.9
Brazil nuts	22.9
Rapeseed oil	19.7
Pumpkin seeds	19.3
Linseed oil	15
Almonds	9.8
Cashew nuts	8.1
Olive oil	7.5
Pistachio nuts	7.1
Linseeds	5.7
Fat spread, 40% not polyunsaturated	5.1
Oatcakes	4.7
Fat spread, 20-25% not polyunsaturated	4.1
Soya flour, full-fat	3.6

BEST SOURCES OF EFA ALPHA-LINOLENIC ACID (g/100 g)

Linseed oil	53.1
Hemp seed oil	19
Linseeds	14
Walnut oil	11.5
Rapeseed oil	9.6
Evening primrose oil	8.2
Soya oil	7.3
Walnuts	5.6
Margarine, soft polyunsaturated	2.1
Soya flour, full-fat	1.7
Fat spread, 40% not polyunsaturated	1.3
Butter, unsalted	1.2
Rabbit, raw	1.0
Corn oil	0.9
Butter, slightly salted	0.9
Tuna, canned in oil, drained	0.9
Pine nuts	0.8
Groundnut oil	0.8
Fat spread, 20-25% not polyunsaturated	0.7
Olive oil	0.7
Cream, double	0.7
Lard	0.6
Sardines, canned in oil, drained	0.4
Grapeseed oil	0.4
Ghee, vegetable	0.3
Kipper	0.3
Sesame oil	0.3
Salmon	0.2

Monounsaturated fats were, at first, thought to have no effect on blood cholesterol levels, but it is now known that they actually have a better overall effect than polyunsaturated fats — by not only lowering the 'bad' LDL cholesterol but by maintaining or even slightly raising the levels of the 'good' HDL cholesterol.

There is also evidence that a diet rich in monounsaturates — the typical 'Mediterranean' diet — is linked with lower heart disease rates and also with increased longevity and lower risk of some cancers though this is still being debated. Oils high in monounsaturates are also often rich sources of the antioxidant vitamin E.

The DoH recommends that the remainder of the fatty acids in our diet not eaten as saturated or polyunsaturated or trans fats should be eaten as monounsaturated, i.e. 12% of the total. However, for the sake of your circulation, your heart and your health it would probably be wise to replace more of the saturated and trans fats in the diet with monounsaturates. i.e. aim to eat less than 10% of total energy as saturates and more than 12% as monounsaturates. To do this would mean eating more plant-based foods and much less animal-based and commercially produced foods (the advice given on pages 119-120 will help you to do this with ease).

▪ Cholesterol

Cholesterol is present in many foods of animal origin, including meat and dairy produce, eggs, fish (especially shellfish) and many fatty manufactured products. There are two types of cholesterol — low-density lipoprotein (LDL) and high-density lipoprotein (HDL). A surplus of LDL in the blood is a major factor in the 'furring' of the arteries and formation of the plaques that lead to atherosclerosis, heart disease and stroke; whereas HDL — often called 'good' cholesterol — actually helps to remove cholesterol from the tissues and delivers it to the liver for excretion.

Although high levels of LDL blood cholesterol are not good news, a certain amount of cholesterol is necessary for cell functioning, and about three-quarters of what we need is manufactured in the body, while one-quarter comes from the diet. Dietary cholesterol has a fairly small effect on blood cholesterol levels but for people with CHD or risk factors (see Heart Disease, page 118), or raised blood LDL cholesterol levels, it may be wise to avoid cholesterol-rich foods. Cholesterol-lowering margarines can help, but these may reduce the absorption of antioxidants by the system.

The WHO sets an upper limit for daily cholesterol intake from foods at 300 mg a day. This is roughly equivalent to, for example, one medium egg and 100 g of beef steak. The Food Charts at the back of the book list the cholesterol content of over 300 foods.

See also the Healthy Heart Diet on page 142.

Protein

Any child will tell you that protein is what we need to eat to build us up and keep us strong — and it is true. Adequate protein is essential. How much is enough, though, and can you get too much?

For a start, enough protein is definitely essential. It is essential for growth and development in children, for cell maintenance and repair (especially those muscles), for the regulation of all body functions, and for various other jobs that fat and carbohydrate just can't do. It is the 'clever' nutrient. While it is likely that many people get more than enough, some people are going short.

■ What is protein?

Protein is a component of very many foods, but it doesn't always take the same form. It is made up of *amino acids*, like building blocks. Proteins from different food sources contain different amino acids. Twenty-two of these amino acids are used in the body in different combinations to make the body's own proteins, such as muscle, and for all the other activities outlined above.

The amino acids can be divided into two broad types — non-essential amino acids and essential amino acids. *Non-*

PROTEIN RNIs FOR ADULTS (kg body weight x 0.75)	
Body weight	g/protein per day
51kg (8 stone)	38
57kg (9 stone)	43
63.5kg (10 stone)	48
70kg (11 stone)	52
76.5kg (12 stone)	57
83kg (13 stone)	62
89kg (14 stone)	67
95.5kg (15 stone)	72
102kg (16 stone)	77

essential amino acids can be made from an excess of other amino acids in the diet. *Essential amino acids* cannot be made like this and so must be provided in the diet. There are eight essential amino acids for adults — isoleucine, leucine, lysine, methionine, phenylalanine, threonine, tryptophan and valine.

■ How much should we be eating?

As we saw on the wheel chart on page 13, as a rough guide the DoH allows for up to 15% of the calories in our diet to be from protein. The WHO suggests 10-15%, a figure which is recognized by most nutrition professionals. A more accurate guide for individuals, according to the DoH, is to reckon 0.75 g of protein per day for every kg of your body weight, which does work out at nearer the 10% level for most people. This is also less than the amount we are currently eating on average (13.5% according to the 1996 National Food Survey), which means that many of us are actually getting more protein than we need. Cutting down a little will allow more calories to come from the complex carbohydrates, which are so important for health. The chart above shows suggested protein intake based on the 0.75 formula.

■ What happens if we eat too much?

Each gram of protein contains 4 calories. Any protein which we eat and which isn't needed for the tasks described above can be converted into glucose and used for energy. Bearing in mind that the traditional animal sources of protein are more expensive to buy than the cheaper carbohydrate sources of energy, your budget may also prefer that you don't waste money on protein you don't need!

Of course, if 13.5% is our current average protein intake, it follows that some people will be eating much more than that. A high-protein diet (especially one high in animal protein) has been linked with bone demineralization — more calcium is excreted in the urine (see Osteoporosis, page 130), so it may be particularly important for women to keep their protein intake to less than 15%. There is strong evidence that a high-protein diet — particularly one high in animal protein — has a detrimental long-term effect on kidney function. There is a small amount of evidence that high protein intakes may also be linked to higher blood pressure levels.

For these reasons, the DoH recommends that daily protein intakes over 1.5 g per kilo of body weight be avoided. To give an example, for a woman of 63.5 kg (10 stone) this works out at 95 g protein per day or just under 20% of total daily calories — showing that, while enough protein is essential, it doesn't need much extra on a regular basis to pose possible problems.

■ Which are good sources of protein?

Animal sources of protein, such as all animal fleshes, dairy produce, fish and eggs, contain all eight essential amino acids within themselves which is why they have been called 'first-class' proteins. All vegetable sources of protein — with the exception of soya beans — don't, which is why they have been called 'second-class' proteins. Some

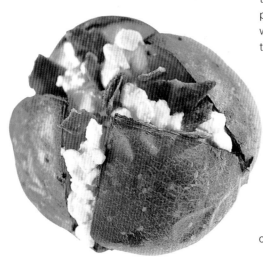

SELECTED GOOD SOURCES OF ANIMAL PROTEIN

Food	(g/average portion)	
	Protein	Total fat
Chicken breast portion without skin	42	2.9
Ostrich, 100g	39	3.4
Beef, roast, lean, 100g	32	5
Cod, 175g	31.5	1.2
Venison, 100g	22	1.6
Beefburger, quarter-pounder	21	19
Salmon fillet, 100g	20	11*
Prawns, peeled, 75g	17	0.6
Cheddar, half-fat, 50g	16	7.5
Eggs, 2 medium	14.2	12.2
Cottage cheese, 100g	14	4
Pork pie, 150g individual	14	38
Cheddar, full-fat, 50g	13	17
Stilton, 50g	11	18
Bacon, lean back, 2 small rashers (50g)	9.5	4
Natural fromage frais, 0% fat, 100g	7.7	0.2
Milk, skimmed, 200ml	6.6	0.2
Natural low-fat yoghurt, 100g	5	0.8

* Low in saturates

SELECTED GOOD SOURCES OF PLANT PROTEIN

Food	(g/average portion)	
	Protein	Total fat
Soya beans, 50g dry weight	18	9.3*
Peanuts, fresh, 50g	13	23*
Quorn chunks, 100g	12	3.5
Black-eye beans, 50g dry weight	12	0.8
Lentils, 50g dry weight	12	0.9
Red kidney beans, 50g dry weight	11	0.7
Cashews, 50g	8.9	24*
Baked potato, 225g cooked weight	8.7	0.5
Vegeburger, one 50g	8.3	5.6
Tofu, 100g	8	4.2
Pasta, wholemeal, 50g dry weight	6.7	1.3
Pasta, white, 50g dry weight	6	1.0
Soya milk, 200ml	6	3.8
Peas, frozen, 100g	5.6	0.7
Wholemeal bread, 60g (2 average slices)	5.5	1.5
Pot barley, 50g dry weight	5.3	1.0
Couscous, 50g dry weight	5.3	1.0

* Low in saturates

vegetable sources have certain amino acids but not others, and they need to be combined with the correct 'missing' amino acids in other forms of protein in order to be utilized in the body. For instance, the protein from pulses forms a complete protein when combined with grains or with nuts and seeds, e.g. rice with a dhal, or hummus with pitta bread or beans on toast. For more on protein in the diet of vegetarians and vegans, see pages 60–63.

As we've seen, a diet too high in saturated fats and trans fats is best avoided, and so protein sources containing too much of these types of fat are also best limited. Ironically, some of the more traditional sources ARE high in saturated fats — Cheddar cheese, for instance, is 25% protein but a whopping 75% fat, of which 63% is saturated. So, if choosing protein from animal sources, it is important to choose plenty of the lower-fat varieties. In general, fish is the best low-fat source of animal protein and standard dairy produce the highest in fat.

As we've also seen, we should be eating MORE complex carbohydrates for good health, and so eating more protein from plant sources is a good idea for most of us. However, many people don't realize that all kinds of plant foods do contain protein. All pulses are a particularly good source. Many of the high-starch foods, like potatoes, bread, rice and pasta — because they are eaten in bulk — are quite good sources. They are also, naturally combined with other protein foods and so provide 'complete protein'. For example, one average baked potato (225 g cooked weight) will provide about 8.7 g of protein, which is 11.5% of the calories in the potato and approximately one-sixth an average woman's daily needs, while giving less than 1.5% fat, of which only a trace is saturated.

Unlike animal proteins, plant proteins are not totally digested in the body and nutritionists usually allow a conversion factor of 85%, i.e. 85 g of animal protein is equal to 100 g of plant protein. A person who relies mostly on plant protein, therefore, may want to eat slightly more than the minimum levels given.

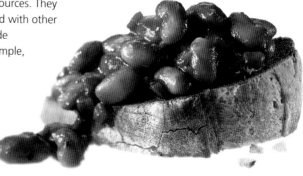

Vital vitamins

Vitamins are the 'unseen' components of a healthy diet — the tiny particles without which we wouldn't survive. We are discovering more information about their importance in the diet all the time...

Vitamins are organic substances which are indispensable for the everyday functioning of our bodies, for our good health and proper development. Each has a different role to play and most have to be provided in what we eat and drink. We need only very small amounts of the vitamins — normally just a few milligrams (1,000 mg = 1 gram) or even micrograms (1,000 μg [micrograms] = 1 milligram) a day. Vitamins A, D, E and K are fat-soluble vitamins and can thus be stored in the body. Vitamins C and the B group are water-soluble vitamins and can't be stored — excess is excreted in the urine — and so they need to be consumed on a regular basis. Each of the eleven vitamins is discussed separately in the pages ahead.

✳ Recommended amounts are given for each vitamin for adults. The UK DoH offers Reference Nutrient Intakes (RNIs) which were set in 1991 and which they say will be enough for 97% of people in any group. For comparison, we include the EC's RDAs (recommended daily amounts) which are used in EC countries for food labelling, and the USA RDAs for ages 19–50, many of which have very recently been updated. (Recommended amounts for children, pregnancy and the elderly appear in Section Three.)

✳ A short explanation of the role of each vitamin is given, followed by general sources, symptoms of deficiency and excess.

✳ 'Best sources' charts list selected top sources for each per 100 g of food item. Other

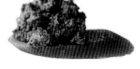

items may provide more of the vitamins per 100 g, but may have been omitted because they are not normally eaten in large enough quantities to make a real contribution — e.g. parsley contains a creditable 673 μg vitamin A retinol equivalent per 100 g, but a normal portion is about 2 g.

✳ If you want to know whether a particular food which isn't listed here contains a certain vitamin, the Food Charts at the back of the book list the significant vitamin content of about 400 foods.

✳ Many people use vitamin pill supplements — often in the belief that if enough is good, more is even better. Although this may sometimes be true for some people and of some of the vitamins and minerals, it is by no means always a good idea to take more than the RDA. Indeed, most vitamins and minerals can be toxic in excess. The use of supplements is discussed in more detail in Section Two on page 146.

■ Vitamin A

RETINOL AND RETINOL EQUIVALENTS
UK RNI 600 μg (female), 700 μg (male) **EC** RDA 800 μg **USA** RDA 700 μg (female), 900 μg (male)
Vitamin A (retinol) is essential for healthy vision, eyes, skin and growth. Symptoms of deficiency include poor night vision, gradual loss of sight and reduced resistance to infection. Excess vitamin A is stored in the liver and can be

SELECTED BEST SOURCES OF VITAMIN A (ug per 100 g)	
Lambs' liver	17,300
Chicken liver	9,700
Liver pâté	7,400
Cod liver oil	1,800
Butter	887
Double cream	654
Stilton cheese, blue	386
Cheddar cheese, average	363
Brie	320
Eggs	190

poisonous, causing liver and bone damage, headache, double vision and other side-effects. Excess retinol consumption is linked with certain birth defects and foods high in retinol, such as liver, should be avoided by pregnant women (see Pregnancy section on pages 172-5). The DoH recommends that regular intakes should not exceed 7,500 μg in women and 9,000 μg in men.

Retinol is found only in foods from animal sources, such as liver, milk, butter, cheese, eggs and oily fish, but the body can convert carotenes — particularly beta-carotene, the pigment found in greatest quantities in orange-fleshed and dark green vegetables and fruits — into retinol. Beta-carotene is also an important nutrient in its own right. Adequate intake of beta-carotene has been linked with low risk of certain

SELECTED BEST SOURCES OF BETA-CAROTENE (ug per 100 g)

	Beta-carotene Equivalents	Retinol
Carrots, old	8,118	1,353
Sweet potato (orange-fleshed), baked	5,130	855
Swiss chard	4,596	766
Chilli peppers	4,110	685
Red peppers (capsicum)	3,840	640
Spinach	3,840	640
Butternut squash	3,270	545
Curly kale	3,144	524
Spring greens	2,628	438
Frozen mixed vegetables	2,520	420
Cantaloupe melon	1,998	333
Mango	1,800	300
Tomato purée	1,300	217
Savoy cabbage	990	165
Dark-leaved lettuce, e.g. butterhead	910	151
Tomatoes	640	107
Broccoli	575	96

SELECTED BEST SOURCES OF VITAMIN D (ug per 100 g)

Cod liver oil	210
Kipper fillet, baked	25
Red salmon, canned in brine, drained	23.1
Cod roe, fried in oil	17
Herring fillet, grilled	16.1
Pilchards, canned in tomato sauce	14
Sardines, grilled	12.3
Rainbow trout, grilled	11
Salmon, grilled	9.6
Smoked mackerel fillet	8
Margarine	7.9
Tuna, fresh	7.2
Sardines canned in oil, drained	5
Tuna canned in brine, drained	4
Smoked mackerel pâté	3.3
Tuna canned in oil, drained	3
Bran Flakes, Fruit 'n Fibre, Cornflakes	2.1
Eggs	1.8

cancers and it is an antioxidant (see page 24). For this reason, beta-carotene sources have been listed separately. 6µg beta-carotene = 1µg retinol, which is called a 'retinol equivalent'.

The US National Cancer Institute has recommended a daily amount of 6,000µg beta-carotene, an amount which is not that difficult to obtain from five or more good portions of fruits and vegetables a day. The beta-carotene list here is not comprehensive; for more good sources, see the Food Charts at the end of the book. Beta-carotene is not toxic, although fairly high intakes of over 30mg per day may make the skin orange-tinged, and high doses of beta-carotene supplements (not carotene-rich foods) may increase the risk of cancer in smokers.

■ Vitamin D
CHOLECALCIFEROL
UK RNI *no recommendation for non-pregnant adults under 65* **EC** RDA 5 µg **USA** RDA 5 µg
Vitamin D intake is important for the absorption of calcium and phosphorus in the body, helping to form bones and carry out other mineralization. One research trial has found that vitamin D can halt the progress of osteoarthritis.

Deficiency of vitamin D can lead to rickets in children and weakness and pain in adults. In excess, vitamin D can produce kidney damage by causing excess calcium to be deposited in the organs. Levels of 50 µg a day have been known to have this effect, so it is wise to regard the RDAs as a maximum as well as a minimum.

There is no UK RNI for adults under 65 leading a normal lifestyle, as vitamin D is the only vitamin which we don't need to take in via the diet — it can be manufactured by the action of sunlight on the skin, and as vitamin D is not present in significant amounts in many foods this is our most important source. For those confined indoors, and the elderly, the RNI is 10 µg/day. Other dietary sources are fortified margarines, dairy produce, oily fish and fortified breakfast cereals.

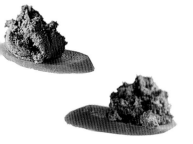
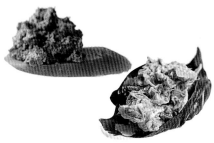

■ Vitamin E

TOCOPHEROLS

UK RNI 5 mg **EC** RDA 10 mg **USA** RDA 15 mg

The most active vitamin E compound is (d) alpha-tocopherol, which is a powerful antioxidant, protecting the cell membranes from oxidation damage and helping to prevent the build-up of plaques in the arteries, as well as 'thinning' the blood, thus helping to protect against heart disease and ageing. In one large UK trial published in 1997, vitamin E from 268 mg up to 537 mg per day reduced the risk of non-fatal heart attacks by a massive 77%.

Vitamin E has also been shown to increase the body's immune response and therefore may protect against disease and cancer. A new study has shown that smokers who took vitamin E supplements were nearly one-third less likely to get prostate cancer. It can also help reduce the pain of osteoarthritis. Vitamin E is important for maintaining healthy skin and for helping the healing process of all damaged tissue, including skin wounds, and one trial found that 600 mg per day supplements significantly improved levels of sperm activity in males with low fertility.

It is very rare for adults to show clinical symptoms of vitamin E deficiency. Occasionally, malabsorption can occur, though, leading to deficiency. Optimum levels for the full antioxidant effect are, however, thought by some experts actually to be much greater than the RDAs and so it may be wise to increase your intake of vitamin E-rich foods to offer optimum protection. A supplement may be of benefit (see page 146). In trials, supplements from 70 mg up to 540 mg per day have been used. Vitamin E excess rarely causes any problems, although people on anti-coagulant drugs, such as Warfarin, should avoid very high intakes, as vitamin E also acts to thin the blood.

The higher the diet is in polyunsaturated fats, which are quite vulnerable to oxidation in the body, the more vitamin E the diet should contain. Luckily foods that are rich in PUFAs also tend to be rich in vitamin E. The DoH estimates that, for people consuming the recommended 6% of total calories as PUFAs, 5-7 mg per day of vitamin E should be sufficient.

Best sources of vitamin E are vegetable oils, nuts, avocados and other vegetables and cereals.

See the chart above and the Food Charts at the end of the book.

SELECTED BEST SOURCES OF VITAMIN E (mg per 100 g)

Food	mg	Food	mg
Wheatgerm oil	136	Soya oil	16
Sunflower oil	49	Groundnut oil	15
Safflower oil	41	Pine nuts	13.5
Polyunsaturated spread	38	Popcorn, plain	11
Sunflower seeds	38	Marzipan, homemade	11
Hazelnuts, shelled	25	Peanuts, plain	10
Sun-dried tomatoes	24	Brazil nuts, shelled	7
Almonds	24	Low-fat spread	6.3
Rapeseed oil	22	Sweet potato, baked	6
Cod liver oil	20	Potato crisps	5.8
Mayonnaise	19	Peanuts and raisins	5.7
Corn oil	17	Tomato purée	5.4

ANTIOXIDANTS

The vitamins C, E and beta-carotene, along with the mineral selenium, and many of the phytochemicals discussed later, are antioxidants, which protect our bodies against the damaging effects of an excess of substances called 'free radicals'.

Everyone produces free radicals in the process of creating energy and this is quite normal. However, excess may be produced by various factors, such as stress, tobacco smoking, pollution, sunlight, radiation, illness, and so on. These surplus free radicals may cause cell damage and this may predispose to cancer and other illnesses, and is thought to be how the ageing process takes place. Free radicals can also oxidize polyunsaturated fats in the body which can cause further damage. The oxidation of LDL cholesterol may be a factor in the build-up of plaque in the arteries, a factor in CHD (see Heart Disease, page 118).

The antioxidants present in our diet help to neutralize the free radicals in our body and stop them producing their damaging effects. For instance, vitamin E protects polyunsaturated fats from oxidation; vitamin C helps the body's natural defences against the free radicals and interacts with vitamin E. Much more research still needs to be done for us to understand exactly how antioxidants work and their full range of effects.

A diet high in fresh fruits, vegetables and other plant foods will be naturally high in the antioxidant vitamins. Research to date seems to show that it is better to get your antioxidants as part of your natural diet rather than as supplements, particularly in the case of beta-carotene. The antioxidant minerals and phytochemicals are discussed in more detail in the pages ahead.

■ Vitamin K

The last of the fat-soluble vitamins, vitamin K is essential for the normal clotting of blood. It is widespread in food in small quantities, but best sources are dark green leafy vegetables and the skins of fruit and vegetables.

It can also be synthesized in the intestines, so deficiency in adults is extremely rare and for this reason no RNIs or RDAs have been set. Some new-born babies are deficient and so vitamin K is usually given at birth.

■ Vitamin C

ASCORBIC ACID

UK RNI 40 mg **EC** RDA 60 mg **USA** RDA 75 mg (female), 90 mg (male)

Another important antioxidant vitamin, vitamin C has a protective role for the body, helping to maintain a healthy immune system. It is necessary for building healthy connective tissue, bones and teeth, and helps the healing of wounds and fractures. It also helps in the absorption of iron. Extra vitamin C may be needed at certain times, for instance when the body is under stress (e.g. illness, high workload) and for certain people (e.g. smokers, heavy drinkers, people working in heavily polluted atmospheres). The USA has recommended an extra 35 mg a day for smokers. An upper 'tolerable limit' has been set by the USA of 2 g vitamin C a day.

As an antioxidant (see the box opposite), vitamin C appears to help cut the risk of CHD. Low levels of vitamin C are associated both with high blood pressure and with increased risk of heart attack; however, one large trial concluded that, once vitamin C intake is adequate, high-dose supplements will probably not be associated with lessened risk. Other trials have shown that vitamin C can dilate the arteries and help blood-flow in heart patients.

Vitamin C may also help to reduce the length and severity of colds if taken in doses up to 200 mg, and it may also help reduce fatigue and help to mobilize body fat and weight loss in slimmers. New research indicates it may also reduce the risk of osteoarthritis.

A deficiency of vitamin C results in poor wound healing, bleeding gums, lowered resistance to infection, nosebleeds, and long term can result in scurvy, although this is rarely seen today.

An excess of the vitamin can give a laxative effect, including diarrhoea and gastric upset. It has often been said that high intakes may also increase the production of oxalic acid and, hence, kidney stones in susceptible individuals, but this has not been substantiated.

Vitamin C is found mainly in fruits and vegetables, and is easily lost in storage, processing, preparation and cooking (see page 208). For example, fresh peas contain approximately 24 mg vitamin C per 100 g; canned garden peas only 1 mg. The only plants which contain no vitamin C are unsprouted grains and dried pulses.

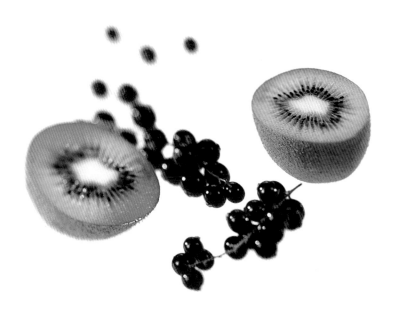

SELECTED BEST SOURCES OF VITAMIN C (mg per 100 g)

Rosehip syrup	295	Brussels sprouts, lightly boiled	60
Guava	230	Kiwi fruit	59
Chilli peppers, red	225	Cabbage, red	55
Peppers, red (capsicum)	140	Mange-tout peas	54
Blackcurrants, stewed	130	Oranges	54
Peppers, yellow (capsicum)	130	Broccoli, green or purple,	
Peppers, green (capsicum)	120	lightly boiled	44
Chilli peppers, green	120	Sweetcorn, baby, lightly boiled	39
Spring greens, lightly boiled	77	Nectarines	37
Strawberries	77	Mangoes	37
Kale, lightly boiled	71	Grapefruit	36
Papaya	60	Green salad	36

The B Vitamins

The B vitamins are a group of six water-soluble vitamins which work together in the body and are essential for growth and the proper development of a healthy nervous system; for body maintenance and food digestion and the metabolism. Each, however, has its own role to play.

As they can't be stored in the body, it is important that adequate amounts of the B vitamins are eaten on a regular basis. Certain people will need more of the B group than others — for example, smoking, alcohol, illness and stress deplete the body's levels.

The vitamins in the B group, like vitamin C, are depleted through the storage, processing, preparation and cooking of food (see pages 208-9 for notes on how best to retain the water-soluble vitamins in food).

In general, it isn't advisable to take high doses of just one of the B vitamins, unless with medical advice, as the group work synergistically together.

Vitamin B1

THIAMIN

UK RNI 0.8 mg (females), 1.0 mg (males)
EC RDA 1.4 mg **USA** RDA 1.1 mg (females), 1.2mg (males)

Vitamin B1 is needed to release the energy from carbohydrate foods and helps to ensure that the brain and nerves have adequate glucose for their needs. A lack of B1 can lead to the deficiency disease beri beri. Heavy drinkers may be short of B1. An excess isn't harmful as it is excreted. B1 is found in a variety of foods, especially pork, bacon and nuts.

Vitamin B2

RIBOFLAVIN

UK RNI 1.1 mg (females), 1.3 mg (males)
EC RDA 1.6 mg **USA** RDA 1.1 mg (females) 1.3 mg (males)

This B vitamin is involved in the release of energy, too, but more from fat and protein than carbohydrate. Adequate

SELECTED BEST SOURCES OF B VITAMINS

Vitamin B1 (mg per 100 g)

Quorn chunks	36.6	Special K	1.3
Yeast extract	4.1	Bacon rashers, back, grilled	1.2
Vegeburger, grilled	2.4	Peanuts, plain	1.1
Vegetable pâté	2.1	Pork, lean fillet	1.0
Ready Brek, made up	1.8	Bran Flakes, Fruit 'n Fibre	1.0
Sunflower seeds	1.6	Wholewheat spaghetti, dry	1.0

Vitamin B2 (mg per 100 g)

Yeast extract	11.9	Vegetable pâté	1.3
Lambs' liver	4.6	Liver pâté	1.2
Shreddies	2.2	Venison, roast	0.7
Special K	1.8	Goats'-milk cheese	0.6
Grapenuts	1.5	Cheddar cheese	0.5
Weetabix	1.5	Eggs	0.5
Nori seaweed, dried	1.3	Tomato sauce for pasta	0.5
Bran flakes, oat bran flakes	1.3		

Vitamin B3 (mg per 100 g)

Yeast extract	73	Peanuts, plain	19
Start cereal	24	Pork fillet, lean	18
Special K	23	Fruit 'n Fibre, Corn Flakes	17
Chicken breast, no skin	22	Ovaltine powder	17
Lambs' liver	21	Tuna, fresh	17
Tuna canned in oil, drained	21	Shiitake mushrooms, dried	15
Grapenuts	20	Swordfish, grilled	14
Turkey, light meat, roast	20	Mackerel, grilled	13

Vitamin B6 (mg per 100 g)

Wheatgerm	3.3	Squid	0.7
Turbot, grilled	2.5	Walnuts, shelled	0.7
Fruit 'n Fibre	1.8	Beef steak, lean	0.7
All Bran	1.3	Chicken breast, no skin, grilled	0.6
Lentils, dry	0.9	Hazelnuts, shelled	0.6
Salmon, grilled	0.8	Swordfish, grilled	0.6
Turkey, light meat	0.8	Baked potato	0.5

Vitamin B12 (µg per 100g)

Lambs' liver	54	Scallops, steamed	9
Seaweed, nori, dried	27.5	Prawns, cooked	8
Mussels, steamed, shelled weight	22	Skate, grilled	8
Oysters, shelled weight	17	Salmon, steamed	6
Sardines, canned in oil, drained	15	Tuna, canned in oil, drained	5
Herring, grilled	15	Eggs	2.5
Anchovies, canned, drained	11	Lean beef	2
Rabbit meat	10	Cheddar cheese	1.1

vitamin B2 is needed to maintain healthy skin and mucous membrane (e.g. inside the mouth and nose) and if deficiency occurs symptoms may include a sore mouth. Excess B2 is excreted in the urine, so there is no safe upper limit recommended. B2 is found in many foods; particularly rich sources are offal, dairy produce and fortified breakfast cereals.

■ Vitamin B3

NIACIN

UK RNI 13mg (females), 17 mg (males)

EC RDA 18 mg **USA** RDA 14 mg (females), 16 mg (males)

Vitamin B3 is also involved in the release of energy from food and can be manufactured from the amino acid tryptophan within the body, but the DoH has still offered RNIs to ensure adequate niacin. A deficiency results in the disease pellagra, which initially affects the skin and can be very serious if left untreated. Excess B3 (over 3 g a day) can cause liver damage, dilation of the blood vessels and kidney damage. Niacin is found in meat, fish and fortified breakfast cereals, as well as a variety of other foods.

■ Vitamin B6

PYRIDOXINE

UK RNI 1.2 mg (females), 1.4 mg (males)

EC RDA 2 mg **USA** RDA 1.3 mg

B6 is important for the metabolization of protein, is also involved in the production of B3 from tryptophan and is necessary for healthy blood. In recent years vitamin B6 has been used by nutritionists to help ease PMS, often in conjunction with evening primrose oil, but in 1997 the UK government banned over-the-counter sales of supplements containing more than 10 mg of B6 (levels up to 50 mg are allowed under medical supervision) as high levels can cause nerve damage. The DoH reports that damage can occur at levels over 50 mg per day. Obvious symptoms of deficiency of B6 are rare, but the latest research into causes of heart disease indicates that a deficiency of B6, along with deficiencies of folic acid and B12, may cause high levels of the amino acid homocysteine in the body, now believed to be an important cause of CHD. Richest sources of B6 are meats, fish, eggs, whole grains, fortified cereals and some veg.

■ Vitamin B12

UK RNI 1.5 µg (male and female)

EC RDA 1 µg **USA** RDA 2.4 µg

Vitamin B12 is necessary for the formation of blood cells and nerves, and a deficiency leads to the form of anaemia called pernicious anaemia and can also lead to nerve damage. It is now also known that low intake of B12, along with low intakes of B6 and folic acid, can lead to high levels of homocysteine, which is linked with CHD (see vitamin B6 above).

Vegans often take supplements of B12, as it is only found naturally in animal produce and seaweed. A little can be synthesized in the body by bacteria. High intakes appear to have no toxic effects. Excellent sources of B12 are offal and meat; dairy produce also contains some.

■ Folate

FOLIC ACID

UK RNI 200 μg (males and females)

EC RDA 200 μg **USA** RDA 400 μg

Folic acid is necessary for the formation of blood cells and for proper development of infants. It is routinely given to pregnant women as a supplement, at 400 mg a day, to help prevent birth defects such as spina bifida. Deficiency can lead to megaloblastic anaemia and, along with deficiencies of B6 and B12, can cause high levels of homocysteine, which is linked to CHD (see Vitamin B6 on page 27). 12% of UK men and 47% of women are deficient in folate. In the UK, flour is due to be fortified with this important vitamin by law and some brands are already fortified.

There are no known toxic effects of high levels, but they may hinder zinc absorption, though this shouldn't pose a problem in normally nourished non-pregnant adults. Folic acid is found in offal, leafy green vegetables, whole grains, nuts, pulses and fortified breakfast cereals, amongst many types of foods.

SELECTED BEST SOURCES OF FOLATE (μg per 100 g)

Yeast extract	1,150
Chicken livers	995
Black-eye beans, dry weight	630
Soya beans, dry weight	370
Grapenuts	350
Soya flour	345
Wheatgerm	331
Special K	330
Cornflakes (and most other commercial breakfast cereals)	250
Lambs' liver	205
Chickpeas, dry weight	180
Asparagus, lightly boiled	155
Baby sweetcorn, lightly boiled	152
Purple sprouting broccoli, lightly boiled	140
Swiss-style muesli	140
Red kidney beans, dry weight	130
Brussels sprouts, lightly boiled	110

Minerals

Minerals are inorganic substances, and various vital body processes — as well as normal development — are reliant on adequate intakes of them. Altogether 15 minerals have been classed as essential in the diet. The major minerals, needed in larger quantities, are calcium, magnesium, potassium, sodium and phosphorus. Iron and zinc, although needed in milligrams rather than grams (1,000 mg = 1 gram) are also usually classed as major minerals. The 'trace elements', needed in much smaller (but equally essential) quantities, are selenium, copper, fluoride, iodine, manganese, chromium and cobalt.

In general, the three main functions of minerals are as constituents of bones and teeth (particularly calcium, magnesium and phosphorus); as salts regulating body fluids (sodium, potassium and chloride); and as components of enzymes and hormones, regulating or helping all the functions of the body, including the nervous system, blood supply and energy release (most minerals).

A deficiency of certain minerals may result in all kinds of health problems, such as anaemia (iron), osteoporosis (calcium) and weak immune system (zinc). Research over the last few years is also finding strong evidence that optimum intake of certain minerals can help to prevent heart disease — for example, calcium, magnesium and the antioxidant mineral selenium.

Minerals are present in most foods and drinks, in varying quantities. A varied healthy diet, providing adequate calories, should ensure intake is at least the minimum recommended by the DoH, but this isn't always the case. One reason is that levels of minerals in even an apparently healthy diet may vary. For example, some minerals in both plants and animal produce are dependent upon the soil in which the plants are grown or on which the animals graze, and mineral content of soil varies in different parts of the country. Another reason is that minerals are not always easily absorbed by the body (calcium needs vitamin D, for example, and absorption of several minerals can be hindered by certain acids in other foods). A third reason is that some people may need more than the minimum recommended levels at certain times; for example, women with heavy periods may need extra iron, and so on. In the pages ahead we look at the main minerals that may be lacking in our diet.

For more information on minerals and the body's requirements throughout every stage of life, see Section Three. For notes on recommended daily amounts and the pitfalls of supplementation, see the introduction to Vitamins on page 22. The Food Charts at the back of the book list significant mineral content of about 400 foods.

■ Calcium

UK RNI 700 mg (males and females)

EC RDA 800 mg **USA** RDA 1,000 mg

Calcium, as the major constituent of bone and tooth mineral, is the mineral needed in greatest quantities. The average human body contains about 1 kilo of calcium and around a gram a day is needed to maintain that level.

Adequate calcium intake is vital throughout life. In infants and through to adulthood, it is vital to ensure peak bone mass is reached. In women it is important to help prevent osteoporosis in later life. Calcium is also important for the smooth functioning of the muscles, including the heart, for blood clotting, for nerve function and other activities. There is some evidence that low calcium levels may be linked with CHD, as hardness of tap water is related to lower CHD. Symptoms of deficiency include muscle cramps and weakness. Rickets is a disease caused by calcium (or calcium absorbtion) deficiency.

Only about 40% of the calcium that we eat is absorbed. Adequate vitamin D is needed for this process (see Vitamins, page 23) and absorption can also be affected by certain foods. Essential fatty acids may help absorption, and exercise helps maintain bone mass. Foods high in insoluble fibre, such as wheat bran and whole grains, can hinder absorption (if taken at the same time), due to the phytates they contain (although this effect may be temporary), and so can oxalates, found in spinach, rhubarb, chard, chocolate and beetroot, and the tannin in tea and coffee. If you drink tea or coffee, leave a gap between your meal and your drink. A diet containing high levels of protein (120 g a day or more) may cause bone demineralization and calcium to be excreted in the urine.

For all these reasons, many nutritionists believe that the UK RNIs are too low. Calcium works closely in the body with magnesium, and a high calcium intake may require additional magnesium. Calcium needs of special groups of people (e.g. pregnant women, children and the elderly) are discussed in Section Three. Calcium in a vegetarian diet is discussed on page 63.

Rich sources of calcium include cheese, yoghurt and milk, dark green leafy vegetables, white bread and flour (fortified). Canned fish (such as sardines and salmon) can be a rich source, but only if the bones are eaten.

SELECTED BEST SOURCES OF CALCIUM (mg per 100 g)

Food	mg	Food	mg
Poppy seeds	1,580	Muesli	200
Parmesan cheese	1,200	Low-fat natural yoghurt	190
Gruyère cheese	950	Goats'-milk soft cheese	190
Kombu seaweed, dried	900	Haricot beans, dry weight	180
Whitebait in flour, fried	860	Spinach	170
Cheddar, reduced-fat	840	Brazil nuts, shelled	170
Edam	770	Chickpeas, dry weight	160
Cheddar, full-fat	740	Naan bread	160
Sesame seeds	670	Kale, lightly boiled	150
Mozzarella, full-fat	590	Greek yoghurt, sheep's	150
Sardines canned in brine, drained; including bones	540	White bread, French	130
Brie	540	Dairy vanilla ice-cream	130
Tofu, steamed	510	Semi-skimmed milk	120
Danish blue	500	Skimmed milk	120
Sardines, canned in oil, drained, including bones	500	Tilapia fish	120
		White bread	120
Nori seaweed, dried	430	Whole milk	115
Feta cheese	360	Prawns, cooked and shelled	110
White chocolate	270	Purple sprouting broccoli, lightly boiled	110
Almonds, shelled	240	Spring greens, lightly boiled	75
Soya beans, dry weight	240	White cabbage	49
Figs, ready-to-eat	230	Broccoli, lightly boiled	40
Milk chocolate	220		

SELECTED BEST SOURCES OF IRON (mg per 100 g)

Food	mg	Food	mg
Curry powder	58.3	Peaches, dried, no-soak	6.8
Ground ginger	46.3	Haricot beans, dry weight	6.7
Nori seaweed, dried	19.6	Fruit 'n Fibre, plus most	
Special K	13.3	other commercial cereals	6.7
Ready Brek	13.2	Red kidney beans, dry weight	6.4
Black pudding	12.3	Cashew nuts, plain	6.2
All Bran	12.0	Pot barley, dry weight	6.0
Lentils, green or brown,		Couscous, dry weight	5.0
dry weight	11.1	Bulgar wheat, dry weight	4.9
Cocoa powder	10.5	Apricots, dried, no-soak	3.4
Sesame seeds	10.4	Beef, lean	2.1
Pumpkin seeds	10.0	Kale, lightly boiled	2.0
Soya beans, dry weight	9.7	Eggs	1.9
Chicken liver	9.2	Lamb, lean	1.6
Soya mince (TVP)	9.0	Bacon, lean grilled	1.6
Lentils, red, dry weight	7.6	Brown rice, dry weight	1.4
Lambs' liver	7.5	Baked beans in tomato sauce	1.4
Liver pâté	7.4	Spring greens, lightly boiled	1.4
Weetabix	7.4	Broccoli, lightly boiled	1.0

■ Iron

UK RNI 14.8 mg (females), 8.7 mg (males)
EC RDA 14 mg **USA** RDA 18 mg (females),
8 mg (males)

Iron's main function is to carry oxygen from the lungs to all the cells of the body. Half the body's store is used to make haemoglobin, which acts as the carrier. Iron can also increase resistance to infection and help the healing process. Lack of adequate iron (or iron absorption) leads to anaemia, with symptoms including tiredness, pallor, weakness and lack of energy. Women, in particular, need to ensure their diet is high enough in iron as it is lost in the blood through menstruation. It is thought that many women are iron-deficient.

Iron is supplied in the diet by both animal foods and plants. Iron from meat sources is better absorbed than that from plant sources, but if body stores of iron are depleted, or when needs are great, then absorption from plants increases.

Absorption is affected by other factors, including intake of phytates, oxalates and tannins (see Calcium, page 29), and also by calcium itself, which can bind with iron in plant sources, though it is thought that in these circumstances the body adapts to absorb extra as needed.

Vitamin C aids iron absorption — certain foods, such as dark leafy greens, contain both iron and vitamin C. Other iron-rich foods should be eaten if possible with foods rich in vitamin C (e.g. a glass of orange juice with lentil soup).

Excess iron can cause stomach upsets, constipation, and kidney damage. Good iron sources are offal and red meats, dark green vegetables, pulses and whole grains, nuts and seeds and fortified breakfast cereals. Many dried herbs are excellent sources, but are not often used in sufficient quantity to make much contribution to the diet. Ground spices can do so, though — e.g. one teaspoon of ground ginger gives nearly 1mg of iron, and curry powder slightly more.

■ Zinc

UK RNI 7 mg (females), 9.5 mg (males)
EC RDA 15 mg **USA** RDA 8 mg (females),
11 mg (males)

Zinc is present throughout the body tissues and helps the activities of a wide variety of enzymes. It is essential for normal growth and development; for a healthy reproductive system and fertility; and for healthy foetal development. It helps to keep skin healthy, helps wound healing, regulates the sense of taste, and is important for immune system strength. It also helps destroy surplus free radicals in the body (see Antioxidants, page 24).

A deficiency of zinc during pregnancy and infancy can cause retarded growth and sexual development. A deficiency in adulthood can cause increased risk of infections, skin and hair problems, slow wound healing, impaired sense of taste and smell, low sperm count, night blindness and other problems. There is also some evidence that low zinc coupled with high copper levels is linked to violent behaviour.

Zinc levels may be affected by smoking and alcohol. It is found in

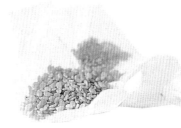

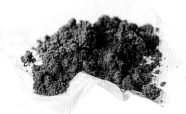

SELECTED BEST SOURCES OF ZINC (mg per 100 g)

Wheatgerm	17.0
Calves' liver	14.2
Poppy seeds	8.5
Oysters, raw, weight including shells	8.3
Quorn	7.5
Cocoa powder	6.9
All Bran	6.7
Pumpkin seeds	6.6
Pine nuts	6.5
Seaweed, nori, dried	6.4
Beefsteak	6.0
Cashew nuts, plain	5.9
Crab, canned in brine, drained	5.7
Corned beef	5.5
Fresh crab, meat only	5.5
Sesame seeds	5.3
Parmesan cheese	5.3
Pecan nuts, shelled	5.3
Lamb leg, roasted, lean	5.2
Sunflower seeds	5.1

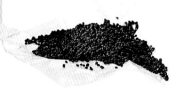

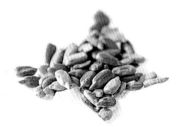

greatest quantities in meat and dairy produce. It is also found in good amounts in whole-grain cereals and pulses, but — like calcium and iron — its absorption may be hindered by eating foods rich in phytates, oxalates and tannins (see page 29). Both calcium and iron can also interfere with absorption, though it is thought that this is only of relevance at doses supplied in supplements.

People at risk from zinc deficiency may then be smokers and heavy drinkers, some vegetarians, people with long-term illness, and anyone who eats a poor or meagre diet. Excess zinc (over 50 mg a day) can hinder copper absorption and possibly iron.

■ Selenium

UK RNI 60 µg (females), 75 µg (males)
EC RDA none **USA** RDA 55 µg

Selenium is an important trace element — it is an antioxidant (see page 24) and, as such, helps to protect us from heart disease, some cancers and premature ageing. In one large recent American study, selenium supplementation at 200 µg per day was associated with a 50% drop in deaths from cancers of the lung, prostate and colon. Deficiency may increase the risk of these diseases.

Working with vitamin E, it helps control the production of hormone-like substances called prostaglandins, and is important for normal growth, fertility, thyroid action, healthy skin and hair, and more. One study showed that women with low levels of selenium had increased risk of miscarriage; and other tests show that selenium levels are often low in people with rheumatoid arthritis and that selenium supplements may reduce pain and inflammation. Yet another recent study has linked low selenium in HIV sufferers with a twenty-fold increased risk of dying of HIV-related causes.

Because selenium comes from plants or plant-eating animals, the amount we eat relates to that in the soil — some areas, including the UK, have low levels; the USA level is high. One recent study found that UK intake is an average of only 34 µg per day — about half that required. Unlike other minerals, the amounts in the food we eat can't be guaranteed (depending on where it comes from), but brazil nuts are a very rich source and fish, seeds and offal should all be good sources. Levels listed here are a guide only.

Selenium is, however, toxic in excess, producing nerve disorder and hair- and nail-loss. Up to 1,000 µg per day should be safe, but the DoH has set an upper limit for males of 450 µg per day as a precaution. For notes on supplementation, see page 146.

SELECTED BEST SOURCES OF SELENIUM (ug per 100 g)

Brazil nuts, shelled	1,530	Wheat flour, wholemeal	53
Mixed nuts and raisins	170	Sardines, canned in oil, drained	49
Lambs' kidneys,	160	Sunflower seeds	49
Dried mushrooms	110	Swordfish	45
Lentils, green or brown, dry weight	105	Mussels, cooked	43
Tuna, canned in oil, drained	90	Lambs' liver	42
		Sardines, grilled	38
Tuna, canned in brine, drained	78	Wholemeal bread	35
Squid	66	Cod	33
Lemon sole	60	Salmon	31
Tuna, fresh	57	Cashew nuts, plain	29
Mullet, red, grilled	54	Prawns, cooked	23
		Pork, lean, roast	21
		Walnuts, shelled	19

■ Magnesium

UK RNI 270 mg (female), 300 mg (male)
EC RDA 300 mg **USA** RDA 310/320 mg
(female 19–30/31–50), 400/420 mg
(male 19–30/31–50)

Magnesium is present throughout our bodies. It works with calcium to maintain healthy bones, it helps release energy and to absorb nutrients, as well as regulating temperature, nerves and muscle function. Adequate levels are important to maintain a healthy heart, and lower levels of CHD have been noted in hard-water (calcium- and magnesium-rich) areas. There is evidence magnesium can help relieve PMS and may be involved in preventing osteoporosis.

If magnesium is deficient, symptoms include muscle weakness and abnormal heart rhythms, tiredness, appetite loss, fits and cramps. Absorption can be hindered by heavy alcohol consumption.

Magnesium-rich foods include whole grains, nuts and seeds, and green vegetables. Tap water can also be a good source if you live in a hard-water area.

■ Potassium

UK RNI 3.5 g (3,500 mg) (males and females) **EC** RDA none **USA** Adequate intake 4.7 g

Potassium works with sodium to regulate body fluids and is essential for correct functioning of the cells. It regulates nerves, heart-beat and blood pressure. If the diet is high in sodium more potassium will be needed to help prevent fluid retention. In trials, young men who had a low potassium intake (390mg per day) were less able to excrete excess sodium — and their blood pressure was higher — than when they took the RNI. High blood pressure can be lowered by a diet low in sodium and high in potassium.

Potassium is found in a wide range of foods, and clinical deficiency is unusual, but diets low in fresh fruit and vegetables (good sources) and high in salty snacks may create a potassium/sodium imbalance. Also, people taking diuretics or laxatives, or on some types of drug (e.g. steroids), may excrete too much potassium. Severe deficiency can result in serious heart problems – even heart attack. Excess is unlikely in a normal diet, but very high levels of supplementation would be toxic. Low-sodium, potassium-rich foods include dried fruits, pulses, nuts, potatoes, bananas, garlic, onions, and many other fruits and vegetables.

■ Phosphorus

UK RNI 550 mg (males and females)
EC RDA 800 mg **USA** RDA 700 mg

About 1 kilo of body weight is phosphorus and most is in the skeleton. It is an essential part of all body cells, helping in the release of energy and regulating protein activity. As it is a major constituent of all plant and animal cells, and added to many commercial foods, deficiency in the diet is not likely and, on average, we eat about twice the UK RNI.

High intakes of phosphorus without adequate calcium may upset the body's phosphorus/calcium balance and cause bone demineralization, and so may be a factor in osteoporosis. Luckily, many foods high in phosphorus are also high in calcium — milk and cheese are rich natural sources of both. Other foods high in phosphorus include meats, fish and eggs. For women with risk factors for osteoporosis, it may be wise to keep a watch on phosphorus intake, but not by cutting back on a nutritious diet.

■ Sodium

UK Lower RNI 575 mg (males and females) **UK** Upper RNI 1,600 mg/day (males and females) **USA** Daily maximum 2.3 g

Sodium is unlike all the other minerals necessary to humans in that it is the only one we have come to recognize as a particular taste (as part of salt, sodium chloride), adding it to foods in the home and buying large amounts of added-salt processed products. Sodium also occurs naturally — usually in much lower amounts — in foods, including meat, fish, vegetables, and even fruit.

Sodium, with potassium and chloride, helps to regulate the body's fluid balance

SELECTED BEST SOURCES OF MAGNESIUM (mg per 100 g)	
Cocoa powder	520
Brazil nuts, shelled	410
Sunflower seeds	390
Sesame seeds	370
Instant coffee (dry weight)	330
Pine nuts	270
Cashew nuts, plain	270
Soya mince granules	270
Soya beans, dry weight	250
Liquorice	170
Hazelnuts and walnuts, shelled	160
Shredded Wheat	130

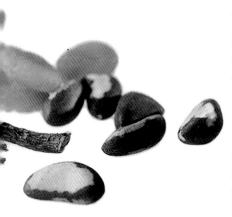

and is present in all body fluids, especially outside the cells, such as blood. Sodium is also necessary for nerve and muscle activity, but most of us eat far more than we need — we average over 3.5 g per day. As salt, or sodium chloride, is 40% sodium and 60% chloride, that represents over 9 g of salt. The DoH says that levels as low as 69mg of sodium per day can be sufficient, but has set a lower RNI of 575 mg per day (1.5 g of salt) and an upper limit of 1,600mg per day (4 g salt, or less than a level teaspoonful).

High intake of sodium is linked with high blood pressure and heart disease. Not everyone is susceptible to raised blood pressure through high sodium intake, but it is estimated that 10-25% of the population are, and one recent report concludes that at least 34,000 lives a year in the UK could be saved by halving the salt in our diets. The 2003 Government report on Salt and Health recommended 'a target reduction in average intake of salt by the population (aged over 11 years) to 6g a day' as an achievable target – still 2g higher than the RNI.

Excess sodium in the diet is also linked with fluid retention and kidney stones, as well as possibly with bone health. A diet high in sodium increases need for potassium.

Sodium deficiency in the UK is not common, but may happen during heavy and/or prolonged exercise, due to loss in the sweat, and in high temperatures. Signs of sodium deficiency are cramps, weakness, fatigue, nausea and thirst.

Main sources of sodium in the diet are salt used in cooking and at the table (approximately 20% of the sodium we eat), stock cubes, canned and packet soups, bottled, canned and jarred sauces, cured and smoked foods, pickles, savoury snacks such as crisps, prawns, hard and processed cheeses, spreading fats, and breakfast cereals (which account for another 25% of daily salt eaten). Many other processed foods contain fairly high amounts of salt, though — baked beans, canned spaghetti, sweet biscuits, even bread is higher in salt than you might realize, at 175 mg an average slice.

To reach your day's maximum RNI of 1,600 mg sodium or 4 g salt, you would need to eat no more than, say, one average portion of bacon, an average Cheddar cheese sandwich and a dab of pickle plus a portion of Cornflakes. Or just half a stock cube and 15 ml soy sauce in your stir-fry could take you to the limit. People wanting to cut down their salt

intake should limit the amount of processed foods they eat, choosing reduced-salt versions if available. Less salt should be added at table and in cooking (salt substitutes are available).

■ Other minerals

A *fluoride* deficiency will encourage tooth decay, but these days deficiency symptoms are rare as most of our dietary fluoride comes from fluoridated tap water and toothpaste, as well as tea.

Iodine is required for the functioning of the thyroid gland and deficiency can cause goitre, but in the UK average intakes are well above the RNI of 140 µg per day at 255 µg per day. Iodine is found most abundantly in milk and seafood.

Chromium is important for helping to control glucose levels in the blood, including insulin function, and may help to control blood cholesterol. There is no RNI, but safe levels have been concluded at over 25 µg per day. Meat and offal, eggs and seafood, cheese and whole grains are good sources.

Deficiencies of the trace elements *copper, sulphur* and *manganese* are rare, although a diet very high in zinc may inhibit absorption of copper.

SELECTED FOODS AND THEIR SODIUM CONTENT (mg per 100 g)

Food	mg	Food	mg
Salt	39,300	Tomato ketchup	1,630
Chicken stock cubes	16,300	Sweet pickle	1,610
Salted dried cod	7,530	Prawns, cooked	1,590
Soy sauce, light or dark	7,120	Twiglets	1,340
Minestrone soup, dry pack	6,400	Processed cheese slices	1,320
Soya mince granules, dry	4,420	Danish blue cheese	1,260
Chilli pickle, oily	4,050	Smoked cod	1,200
Tomato soup, dried	3,100	Cornflakes	1,100
Bacon rashers, back, grilled	2,700	Edam cheese	1,020
Black bean sauce	2,150	Canned cook-in sauce	940
Parma ham	2,000	Tortilla chips	860
Tendersweet bacon, back, grilled	1,990	Potato crisps	840
Smoked salmon	1,880	Canned creamed tomato soup	830
Salami	1,800	Margarine, average	800
Pretzels	1,720	Butter, average (not low-salt)	750

Phytochemicals — the 21st-century food pharmacy

The food scientists are now discovering that, for your health's sake, it may be even more important to eat a diet rich in fruits, vegetable and other plant foods than it is to cut down on the saturated fat, junk foods or calories. Here we look at the whole new world of the phytochemicals and how they can protect your health.

Just as vitamins were discovered in the first half of the 20th century, scientists are now uncovering a wealth of new health-protecting compounds in plant foods. These compounds are not nutrients as such, but have been described as 'biologically active non-nutrients'. The scientists have called them phytochemicals (from 'phyto' meaning plant).

There are literally thousands of different phytochemicals and they can be present in plants in quite high amounts — maybe several per cent. They include the substances responsible for giving the plant its colour, flavour, odour — its particular unique characteristics, you could say.

A lot of research has been done in the past few years to try to discover the health-giving properties of these compounds and it now seems that they have much to offer in the fight against many types of cancer, heart disease and various health problems.

Many are antioxidants, others help to block or suppress harmful cell reactions, for instance. Many help the body in more than one way — and more is being discovered about the phytochemicals all the time. One thing is for certain — if you want to protect your health, you MUST eat up your fruits and vegetables, just like your mother always used to tell you to do.

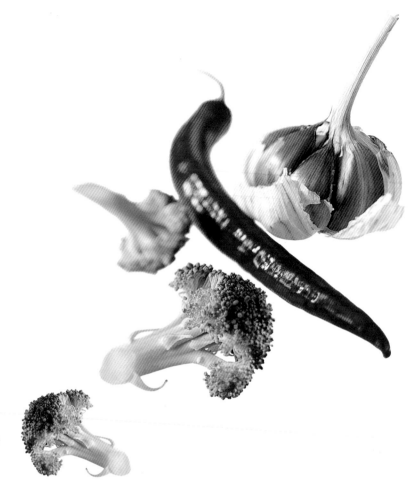

■ Carotenoids

Probably the first phytochemical to be linked with health was beta-carotene, the orange pigment in carrots, sweet potatoes and other plants, which can convert to vitamin A and which was cited as one of the first antioxidants, along with vitamins C and E. In fact, the carotenoid group of compounds in foods numbers about 600, many of which are also potent antioxidants. Here are just some of them.

Lycopene is the red pigment found mainly in tomatoes, red grapefruit and watermelon. Cooked tomatoes, including those in ketchup and bottled pasta sauces, are a particularly active source. It has been found that adequate intake of lycopene can reduce incidence of heart attacks by 50%, by antioxidant activity and possibly by lowering LDL blood cholesterol levels. It may also help prevent prostate, lung, stomach and several other types of cancers.

More carotenoids with promising anti-carcinogenic properties are lutein, found in dark green leafy vegetables, blackcurrants and potatoes; beta-cryptoxanthin, found in mangoes; capsanthin, in red peppers; phytoene, in squash and pumpkin; and canthaxanthin, in mushrooms.

■ Bioflavonoids

These are a group of no less than 6,000 (or so!) polyphenolic compounds which many years ago were classed as 'vitamin P' and then more or less dismissed as of no significance. Now we know better.

The flavonoids usually appear to be most potent in fruits or in sweet vegetables, probably because the sugars help the flavonoids to be absorbed. Providing the orange and yellow colours in citrus fruits (for example), the flavonoids are antioxidants and also help the absorption of vitamin C. The main discovery to date is that they seem to help prevent cancers, but different flavonoids have different roles.

Taxifolin and rutin are two important flavonoids in citrus fruits, including oranges and grapefruits. Ellagic acid, found in greatest amounts in strawberries, blackberries, cherries and grapes, blocks the action of cancer-inducing cells.

There is a sub-group of flavonoids called flavonols, of which one of the most researched, and probably the most abundant in foods, is quercetin — an antioxidant found in black tea and red wine as well as in onions, tomatoes, apples, potatoes, grapes and broad beans. Studies have linked high quercetin intake with lower risk of CHD. Quercetin may also help to prevent eye cataracts and hay fever as it has antihistamine properties. The polyphenols in persimmon (sharon fruit) help the body metabolize fat and can fight blocked arteries.

Green tea (the unfermented form of black tea) contains catechins, the antioxidant effects of which may include the slowing down of the ageing process as well as protecting the circulatory system from damage.

Glucosinolates

These phytochemicals, which were once thought to be toxic to humans and act as natural pesticides, are found mainly in cruciferous and green vegetables; among the best sources seem to be broccoli, Brussels sprouts, cabbage, kale and cauliflower. The stronger the taste, the higher the potency of the chemicals, research indicates.

Broccoli is a particularly rich source of glucosinolates, which break down into a substance called sulphoraphane that appears to have a strong anti-cancer effect by stimulating our natural defences; so much so that food scientists are attempting genetically to inject it into other vegetables so that their benefit is spread wider.

Another glucosinolate is sinigrin, found in large quantities in sprouts, which has a different anti-cancer effect by suppressing the growth of pre-cancerous cells.

Watercress is rich in isothiocyanate, which can break down and render harmless one of the main cancer-causing agents in tobacco smoke.

Organosulphides

Garlic, onions and the other members of the allium family — leeks and chives — are the main providers of these sulphides which seem to stimulate the immune system, are antioxidant and appear to fight many cancers, particularly stomach cancer, ulcers and heart disease.

Garlic is rich in allicin, which is antibiotic and antiviral. Its content of diallyl disulphide appears to shrink cancerous tumours, and other phytochemicals it contains may help prevent pre-cancerous cells from forming, as well as helping to lower LDL blood cholesterol, raise HDL blood cholesterol and helping in the prevention of blood clots.

Phytoestrogens

These are a group of phytochemicals with a structure similar to oestrogen, the female hormone that protects against heart disease and osteoporosis.

There are two main types of phytoestrogens in our diet: isoflavones – part of the flavonoid group – are found in pulses, particularly soya beans, and lignans, present in linseeds and most cereals, fruit and vegetables.

They have been much touted as a cure or preventative for conditions such as breast and other hormone-dependent cancers, heart disease, osteoporosis and menopausal symptoms.

However the Food Standards Agency's May 2003 report Phytoestrogens and Health found that much of the evidence for the beneficial effects of phytoestrogens was inconclusive and/or of limited value.

Their only positive findings were a 'small protective effect in the lumbar spine' (related to osteoporosis), a conclusion that non-fermented soya may lower the risk of colon cancer, and a 'considerable body of evidence' that soya can have beneficial effects on LDL and total cholesterol (but it may not be the isoflavones in the soya that produce this effect). Other work since this report has found no link between soya and heart health.

The report found that caution should be used in feeding babies soya formula, due to potential risks. Women with breast cancer should avoid a high-soya diet, and a high-phytoestrogen diet may interfere with thyroxine therapy for hypothyroidism.

See also: Supplements, Heart Disease, Cancer and Antioxidants.

Alcohol

Approximately 90% of men and 80% of women in the UK drink alcohol. The amount we consume has doubled since the 1960s. This isn't all bad news — IF the drinking guidelines are followed.

According to MAFF statistics, on average our national alcohol consumption accounts for at least 6.9% of our total energy intake for men and 2.8% for women, which is about 5% of total energy for the population and represents just over one unit of alcohol a day each. Other reports say we drink more than this — Alcohol Concern cites 16 units a week for men and 5 for women as average.

Approximately 27% of men and 15% of women drink over safe limits.

So what is alcohol? It is a drug and an intoxicant with the power to kill — three-quarters of a bottle of whisky (24 units of alcohol) drunk rapidly would produce coma and death in many people. It is also a source of energy, containing 7 calories a gram, which is more than protein or carbohydrate but less than fat.

Some alcoholic drinks do contain a few nutrients (beer contains some B vitamins, red wine contains some iron, but spirits are totally nutrient-free); unlike fats, proteins and carbohydrates, however, alcohol is not an essential part of our diet.

At high levels of intake it has many drawbacks, both major and minor, including the short-term effects of intoxication, risk of accident, increased risk of some cancers, liver and pancreas damage, weight gain and/or nutritional deficiencies, heart damage, and so on (see Alcohol Abuse, page 86).

At low levels of intake, however, alcohol doesn't appear to pose health problems for most people; and there is evidence that moderate drinkers have less incidence of CHD than people who don't drink at all. They will also live longer, with less risk of Alzheimer's, impaired cognitive function, and cancer.

These benefits appear to be linked partly with polyphenolic phytochemicals found in alcohol (see page 35) — flavonoids such as resveratrol in red wine, for example, and antioxidants in dark beers.

International studies have concluded that about 20–30 g alcohol a day will reduce 'all cause' deaths by 30%, death from CHD by 25-35% and cancer by 20%.

Most international researchers (though not all) agree that red wine is probably the 'healthiest' alcoholic drink to take because of the concentration and type of polyphenols in the grape skins. But recent research demonstrates that the ethanol in all alcohol in moderation incurs protective effects. For CHD, it works by reducing the levels of 'bad' blood cholesterol LDL, increasing the 'good' kind, HDL, and by reducing the 'stickiness' of the blood platelets and levels of fibrinogen (clotting factor).

However, what do you do if you don't WANT to drink? Well, tests show that red grape juice contains similar polyphenols to red wine, but of course, the ethanol is lacking.

What are safe limits?

Until 1995 the UK accepted safe limits for alcohol were 14 units a week for women and 21 for men. In December 1995, however, the DoH published an interdepartmental government report called 'The Sensible Drinking Message' and its main advice, summarized, is as follows:

* 1-2 units of alcohol a day gives a significant health benefit in reducing CHD for men over 40 and for post-menopausal women.
* It is better to drink the units regularly rather than save them up and binge.
* Men who drink 3-4 units a day and women who drink 2-3 units a day do not face significant health risks. Women's lower recommendation is because they generally have a smaller liver (which processes the alcohol) and less of the alcohol-processing enzyme ADH in their stomach so they metabolize alcohol less well than men.
* Consistently drinking four or more units a day for men or three or more for women is not advisable, due to increasing health risks associated with higher levels of alcohol intake. Individual reactions to alcohol vary, so this can only be a benchmark.

The key to drinking for health seems to be 'little and often'. Taking one drink with a meal may confer optimum benefit.

Apart from your sex, other factors can affect how well or badly you tolerate alcohol. Short people and overweight people tolerate it less well. Alcohol on an 'empty stomach' will make you drunk quicker as it is absorbed into the bloodstream more quickly. Long term, it ·may also cause stomach upsets such as gastritis or ulcers. Alcohol with 'fizz' also goes into the bloodstream quicker, whether it is champagne or a gin and lemonade. If you are run-down, weak, ill, tired or stressed, your alcohol tolerance may also be affected.

Women in pregnancy

A March 2006 report by the Royal College of Obstetricians and Gynaecologists set out to update previous information on drinking alcohol in pregnancy. It finds:

   * Binge drinking in early pregnancy may be particularly harmful. (Binge drinking for women is 5+ drinks in one session.)

   * Alcohol affects female fertility.

   * Alcohol is associated with increased miscarriage. One study reports an increase in first trimester miscarriage with drinking more than 5 units a week.

* Major structural malformations (in the foetus) are seen three times as often in heavy drinkers.

* At levels in excess of 10 units per week there is an increase in preterm birth.

* There is clear dose response relationship between alcohol consumption in the second half of pregnancy and fetal growth.

* Children exposed to alcohol in the uterus may suffer from serious cognitive effects and behavioural problems.

   According to the DoH, while the safest approach may be to avoid any alcohol during pregnancy, there is no evidence of harm from low levels of intake, defined as no more than 1–2 units of alcohol once or twice a week. In the USA since 1981, however, the advice has been to avoid all alcohol during pregnancy, and the UK Medical Council on Alcohol advises women to avoid it during the first trimester.

Alcohol units — a guide

A unit of alcohol contains 8 g of pure alcohol – one single measure of spirits or 300 ml (half pint) of standard beer or lager, or a glass of wine. With wine, and to a lesser extent with beer, however, there can be problems in working out exactly how many units you are getting.

   Many people think they are drinking one unit when they have a 'glass of wine', or reckon that half a bottle is three units, but sadly this is not often the case — a glass of wine can easily be 1½ units or even more, and half a bottle of wine can be 5 units or more.

   Why? Well, what is a 'glass' of wine? A standard glass is 125 ml, the kind pubs usually use. It is quite small, and you get six glasses to the 75 cl bottle of wine. Restaurants and private homes usually use much bigger glasses, so a glass then might easily be two or more units.

The bigger problem is that the standard wine unit is based on a 125 ml glass of wine, containing only 8% alcohol by volume. This is a very low level for a wine. Average alcohol by volume is nearer 11–12%, though there are exceptions. Some wines can go as high as 14–15% alcohol by volume.

   A 125 ml glass of 12% wine — 50% stronger than 8% wine — will, then, represent 1½ units, not 1, and a 12% bottle of wine will be 9 units not 6. If you're drinking out of a bigger glass than standard, and having high-strength wine, you can see how easy it would be actually to be drinking twice as many units as you might think you are.

   Beers also vary tremendously in alcohol by volume — one unit of beer is based on alcohol by volume of 3–4%. Some strong beers go up to 10%! Half a pint of such a beer would be over 2 units.

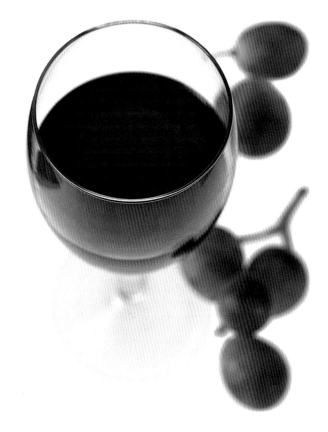

PUTTING IT ALL TOGETHER

Surprising though it may seem, putting together all the theoretical information into a practical eating plan for yourself isn't difficult. In the next few pages we look at different meals, your preferences, and how they can fit into a healthy lifestyle. There is no real need to worry about the exact nutritional content of every morsel of food you eat — trying to count grams of fat or the protein or carbohydrate in every meal, for example, would not only be time-consuming but, almost impossible. The fact is that almost any kind of meal can be adapted to form part of a healthy diet if you follow a few easy guidelines.

Use your eyes! Using the photograph opposite, you can see the proportions of the different types of food that will ensure your healthy meals.

Carbohydrates

To get your fifty per cent or so of carbohydrates you need to ensure that at every meal you have a good portion of (preferably unrefined) starchy carbohydrate food such as rice, pasta, potatoes, or bread — the bottom layer of the illustration opposite.

At most meals you also need about two portions of fruit and/or vegetables in good-sized portions (next layer up).

Proteins

Most meals should include a low- or moderate-fat protein (the third layer of the illustration opposite). That means choosing fish, game, poultry, pulses and extra-lean meats. Portions of these can be quite small.

Remember, if you choose pulses they also have an excellent starch content and will count towards your carbohydrate intake. High-fat proteins, such as hard cheese, dairy products and fatty meats, should be eaten in even smaller portions and less frequently.

Fats

As you've seen, fat is present in a great many foods and, as all fat is a calorie-dense food, it is easy to eat too much without realizing. Choosing plenty of complex carbohydrate, vegetables and fruit and adding low-fat protein to this will ensure that you keep the fat content of your meal low. That means you can add small quantities of the fats YOU choose — ideally, healthy plant oils most of the time, such as olive or corn oil, perhaps some vegetable fat spread, and a little butter now and then when it helps the taste of the dish. Don't forget that some carbohydrates, such as certain breads, contain more fat than you think.

A FEW USEFUL TIPS

* Some types of meals lend themselves particularly well to the high-carb, medium-protein, lower-fat balancing act. You will find it easy with Italian pasta meals, with eastern Mediterranean meals based on bulgar, other grains and pulses. Indian and far Eastern meals using rice and noodles are ideal too.

* When planning meals and snacks, keep thinking 'carbohydrate foods' first. Then consider what protein foods you need to add. The traditional way of planning meals in the affluent West has been to think 'protein' first and then add carbs and vegetables as an afterthought. The other way around will ensure a much better balance.

* Split your meals up fairly evenly throughout the day in terms of both calorie content and times at which you eat them. This ensures more even blood sugar levels, avoidance of hunger and a happier digestive system.

* If you feel hungry, eat. But eat a good-quality food, not a high-fat, high-sugar snack.

* Remember that our calorie needs vary from person to person, and depend on many factors (see Section Four, Food for Weight Control), so use the meal portion sizes and nutrient guidelines here as just that — guidelines.

Drinks and snacks

Use what you drink as another chance to get nutrients — vitamin C from juices, calcium from low-fat milk or fortified soya milk, even phytochemicals from tea — but don't forget that one of the best drinks of all is water, tap or bottled. Look on snacks as a good excuse for extra nutrients, rather than feel guilty.

Sugars and alcohol

As by far the largest part of your daily calorie needs have now been taken up, you will only have a little room left for the sugars and for alcohol... add these to your diet in moderation, if at all. As a general guideline, take a maximum of 10% of your total day's food intake in the form of sugary, fatty or alcoholic extras and treats that add little in the way of important nutrients to your diet.

The importance of variety

Balancing most of your meals this way forms the basis of a healthy diet for life.There is, however, one other very important tip, which will also ensure that most people will get adequate amounts of all the necessary vitamins, minerals and phytochemicals. The message is 'variety'. Eat as wide a variety of foods as you can — different sources of carbohydrate, varying types of protein, lots of different vegetables, salads and fruits. Not only does this prevent boredom, it also ensures that you get all the micronutrients you need.

This is because even foods of the same group are not all good sources of the same things. For example, protein-rich cod is a good source of some B vitamins and selenium, but contains little calcium; while low-fat cheese is a good calcium source – and so on.

The last guideline of good nutrition is this: don't believe that by cutting out things from your diet, you are necessarily doing your body a favour. Variety and balance are the most important elements, and within this framework there can be room for all kinds of food. Restriction isn't always a good thing. Good nutrition isn't just about cutting down items perceived to be 'bad'. Don't cut nutritious foods from your diet or restrict yourself unnecessarily unless you have a particular health complaint which needs such a restricted diet (see Section Two).

'Five a day' — interpreting the fruit and vegetable guidelines

Departments of health throughout the Western world are advising us to eat at least five portions a day of fruits and vegetables for good health. Based on all the research to date, that is sensible advice no one should ignore. In fact, we should aim for 'five' as a minimum.

However, many people are confused as to what exactly the five portions means. For example, does it include potatoes? How big is a portion? Do the five portions all have to be different? And does everything have to be fresh? Here are the answers.

1 Total weight of all five portions should be at least 400g (14 oz) of edible fruit or vegetable. Aim for an average of 80g per portion.

2 Vary your choices as much as possible. Different fruits and vegetables have differing nutritional qualities — e.g. avocados are high in fat and vitamin E, while carrots are high in beta-carotene and low in fat. So try to eat five different fruits and vegetables each day.

3 Items can be cooked, but it is best to cook them without too much added fat or sugar (though vegetables cooked with a little oil are fine). Try to get one raw salad a day.

4 Potatoes, sweet potatoes and yams are excluded as they are starchy carbohydrates and should be counted towards the day's complex carbohydrate intake. However, other root vegetables such as swede, turnip, parsnip and carrot can be included in the five a day.

5 Pulses like kidney beans, lentils and soya beans can be included (and that covers baked beans), but as they are also a protein source and contain good amounts of starchy carbohydrate, the Food Standards Agency says that, however much you eat, pulses can only count as one portion a day. Unlike most other vegetables, pulses also contain no vitamin C unless sprouted.

6 Fruit and vegetable juice or smoothies can be included, but however much you drink, it only counts as one portion a day, as the fibre is lost and the fruit sugars in juice are more likely to produce tooth decay in high quantities. Fruit juice is best freshly squeezed rather than bought long-life. Fruit squashes are excluded.

7 Dried fruit can be counted, but the rest of the day's five should come from other fruits and vegetables as, although dried fruit is usually high in fibre and can contain useful minerals and vitamins, it contains no vitamin C, is energy-dense and high in sugar.

8 Frozen and canned fruits and vegetables are included. Frozen items have a similar nutritional profile to their fresh counterparts — and sometimes can actually contain more vitamin C if picked and frozen immediately (see Food from Farm to Table, page 80). Canned produce is usually not so useful as fresh, and produce chosen should be canned without sugar or salt and preferably thought of as an occasional replacement for fresh or frozen items.

9 Nuts and seeds are excluded.

10 Composite (recipe) foods can be included as long as they include enough fruit or vegetables to constitute a portion (see the box below). A home-made apple pie will probably count, as will the vegetables in a casserole or pie. (Mixed fruits or vegetables reaching the required weight for one portion will count as one portion.) Many processed foods are unlikely to meet the portion size requirement. Items such as packet pasta sauces and soups should not count. Commercially made salads, such as coleslaw, will count if portion size is met, but you need to be aware that their fat content may be high.

11 All other fruits and vegetables not mentioned above will count (as long as portion size guidelines opposite are followed).

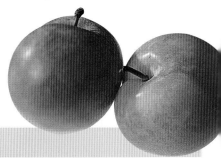

EASY WAYS TO GET YOUR 'FIVE A DAY'

Here are some examples of how easy it is to incorporate five a day into your menus:

Example 1:
* Portion of fruit juice at breakfast time
* Handful of dried fruits mid-morning
* Bowlful of salad with bread and cheese at lunch-time
* Portion of root vegetables and portion of green vegetables with roast chicken in the evening

Example 2:
* Portion of berry fruits with breakfast yoghurt
* Glass of fruit juice with baked beans on toast at lunch-time
* Double serving of mixed stir-fried Mediterranean vegetables (200 g/7 oz) in evening with baked fish

Example 3:
* Glass of fruit juice on waking
* 1 apple and 1 banana chopped into breakfast muesli
* Home-made carrot soup for lunch
* Large bowlful of salad with venison steak for evening meal

■ Portion sizes

Portion size of your 'five a day' is important. A couple of lettuce leaves or the two or three slices of tomato in a sandwich won't be enough to count — most salad items eaten raw weigh very little because of their high water content and you need a really good bowlful of them. All the portion sizes are minimums— larger portions may be preferable, depending on your size, age, appetite and own needs.

The table below gives portion-size guidelines per person, and throughout this book, unless otherwise stated, a 'portion' is as listed here.

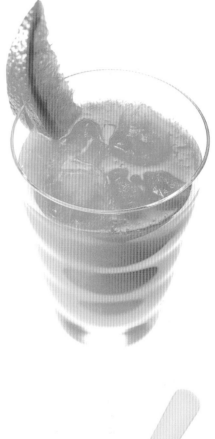

Food	Portion size	Example
✱ Very large fruits	One good slice (80 g)	Melon
✱ Large fruits	One fruit	Orange, apple, banana
✱ Small to medium fruit	Two fruits	Kiwis, plums
✱ Very small fruits	1 cupful or 80 g	Berries, cherries
✱ Cooked fruits/fruit salads	3 heaped tablespoons/80 g	Stewed apples, fresh fruit salad
✱ Dried fruits	1 heaped tablespoon	Apricots, raisins
(dry ready-to-eat weight — stewed dried fruits count as cooked fruits)		
✱ Fruit or vegetable juice or smoothie	150ml	Orange juice, tomato juice
✱ Green leafy vegetables	4 heaped tablespoons/80 g	Cabbage, broccoli
✱ Root vegetables	3 heaped tablespoons/80 g	Carrots, swede
✱ Small vegetables	3 heaped tablespoons/80 g	Peas, sweetcorn
✱ Other vegetables	3 heaped tablespoons/80 g	Onions, courgettes, tomatoes
✱ Pulses	3 heaped tablespoons (cooked)/80 g	Baked beans, lentils
✱ Salad	1 dessert bowlful	Lettuce, tomato, cucumber

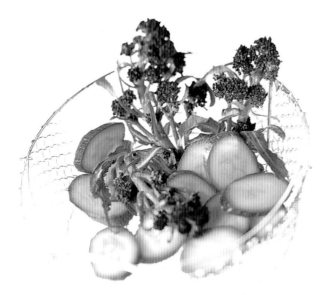

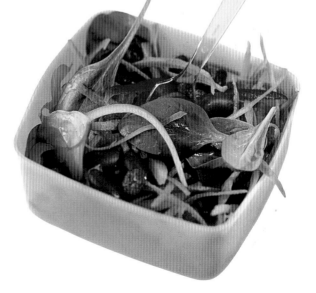

Power breakfasts

Some reports say that up to a quarter of us don't eat breakfast at all — yet it is a very important meal. Here's how to get it right.

Breakfast... it says what it is. A meal that breaks the fast your body has endured, probably for at least 12 hours, since your evening meal on the previous day. Looked at that way, it is surprising that so many of us don't bother with breakfast at all, but prefer to cram all our food intake into a few short hours every day, from lunch-time until a big burst in the evening.

■ Why do I need breakfast?

There are at least three good reasons why having a healthy and balanced breakfast is important for you and your well-being.

One: after a long period without eating, your blood sugar levels will be dangerously low. As you attempt to go through the morning without eating you may suffer various symptoms such as headache, shakiness, weakness, lack of concentration and even reduced brain power, research suggests. Performance of any kind of strenuous physical activity could also be quite significantly impaired in these circumstances.

QUICK BREAKFAST

A typical quick breakfast, but not ideal

30 g cornflakes, 125ml semi-skimmed milk, 30 g slice of white toast with 5 g soft margarine and 2 tsp marmalade.
299 calories, 6.8 g total fat, 2.7 g saturated fat, 9g protein, 53.75 g carbohydrate.

This breakfast of cereal and toast is the kind that millions of people eat every day and one which most people would consider healthy. Yes, it is low in fat and saturated fat and contains just about the right amount of protein, a good amount of calcium (and other vitamins and minerals, because cornflakes are fortified) and plenty of carbohydrate. Yet it has several drawbacks.

It is very short on complex carbohydrate and fibre, containing only 0.75 g in the whole breakfast, which is just 4% of a day's average adequate intake, and would have you feeling hungry again much sooner than the healthy breakfasts. There is no fresh fruit or juice or vitamin C, and the amount of energy it provides would be quite low for most people.

Even quicker, and a better bet for most ★ ★ ★ ★ ★

75 g no-added-sugar-or-salt muesli, 125ml skimmed milk, 110 g fresh raspberries, 125ml orange juice.
388 calories, 6.2 g total fat, 1.4 g saturated fat, 14.25 g protein, 73.25 g carbohydrate.

This breakfast is better than the first one on several counts. It, too, is low in total fat and even lower in saturated fat, but contains more essential fatty acids in the muesli. It is very high in carbohydrate (at 71% of the meal), most of which is complex carbohydrate, high in fibre at 6.5g and low on the Glycaemic Index, which means that it will keep hunger at bay well into the morning and help regulate blood sugar. Protein content is higher than the breakfast on the left, at nearly 15% of the meal — an ideal amount for early in the day. The breakfast gives two portions of fruit towards the day's five portions of fruit and vegetables, and contains more than the recommended daily needs of vitamin C (at 84 mg) as well as providing calcium, iron and vitamin E. It provides more energy, which is good. Males, teenagers and active people could add bread or serve extra muesli.

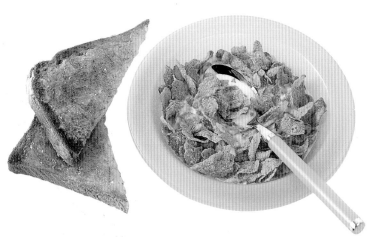

Two: breakfast is an ideal opportunity to get certain nutrients into your diet that you may not find space for later in the day — fresh or dried fruits and fruit juice, for example, can help you attain the 'five a day' and boost your vitamin C levels.

Yoghurt or milk can provide important calcium, especially for women — many people only take these foods at breakfast, and things like porridge and muesli can be a good opportunity to eat fibre and oats, which can help lower LDL blood cholesterol.

Breakfast also provides calories, of course — important for children and teens, physically active adults and anyone who has a problem maintaining body fat (thin people). Even for overweight people trying to lose fat, breakfast is still vital — see the next point and Section Four.

Three: if you miss breakfast you will probably suddenly feel very hungry mid- to late-morning and crave something sweet, such as a doughnut. This, in effect, is your body telling you that you didn't give it breakfast and it needs glucose — fast! Highly refined sweet food will provide that within minutes, so you eat the sugary snack — which also often happens to contain a lot of fat and few nutrients. In other words, you swap a balanced nutritious meal for a less balanced, less nutritious snack.

COOKED BREAKFAST

Traditional cooked breakfast

1 medium egg fried in 2 tsp oil, 100 g raw weight back bacon, fat left on, lightly grilled, 40 g mushrooms fried in 1 tbsp, vegetable oil, 1 chipolata sausage, 30 g white bread spread with 5g butter, 2 tsp ketchup.
682 calories, 53.7 g total fat, 14 g saturated fat, 29.7 g protein, 21 g carbohydrate.

71% of the calories in this breakfast come from fat and 18.5% from saturated fat — that's about twice the recommended level for both. Both figures could have been even higher if the bacon had been streaky and fried in lard, not grilled. However, this is still far too high for a normal meal. Although the protein content isn't too bad and there is plenty of iron and B vitamins here, basically the balance of the meal is all wrong. Carbohydrate represents only 11.5% of the calories in the meal, when we should be aiming for an average of at least 50%. There is less than a gram of fibre here — only about 5% of a day's requirement. The meal is high in salt and also contains no vitamin C. The high fat content is reflected in the fairly high calorie content, as fat is twice as calorific as either carbohydrate or protein.

The healthier version ★★★★

1 medium egg, fried in 1 tsp oil, 100 g raw weight back bacon, extra lean, grilled to crisp, 80 g low-salt, low-sugar baked beans, one 50 g tomato, grilled, one 100 g hunk of wholemeal rustic bread spread with 3 g 60%-fat olive oil spread, 2 tsp ketchup.
550 calories, 22g total fat, 5.8 g saturated fat, 34.7 g protein, 57.2 g carbohydrate (without optional orange juice).

Fat content is reduced considerably, mainly by using leaner bacon and cooking it crisper, by replacing the sausage with a virtually fat-free protein source in baked beans, by omitting the fried mushrooms, which soak up lots of fat, and by brushing a non-stick pan with oil on which to fry the egg. You actually have more food on your plate by weight. The plate's fibre content is up to 9.3 g, and only just over 35% as fat (under 10% saturated) — a much better balance, though still a bit low in carbohydrates, so other meals in the day should reflect that. There is plenty of protein and a variety of vitamins and minerals. The vitamin C content is a little low still, but having saved many calories on the original version, an optional glass of citrus juice could be added to provide this.

■ What is a healthy breakfast?

A good breakfast should contribute to your day's diet enough calories, some protein, a reasonable amount of complex carbohydrate, a little fat and a variety of vitamins and minerals. Within that broad outline there is plenty of scope, as the ten healthy breakfasts on the right show.

Most people don't allow enough calories for their breakfast. A quarter of your day's calorie intake — that would be around 500 for women and 650 for men — would be a good amount to aim for most days. Exactly what proportion of carbohydrate, protein and fat those calories should consist of is a matter of debate amongst researchers. Some have shown that a high-carbohydrate, low-fat breakfast makes you more alert and assertive and that a high-fat meal slows down the brain; others that it is a high-protein breakfast that helps brain power and that too much carbohydrate slows you down.

The key seems to be a sensible balance of all three main nutrients. A breakfast including at least one-third of your day's protein needs is certainly a good idea; whether or not protein helps you power through your morning's work, it certainly helps to stave off hunger pangs, because it takes longer to be digested than carbohydrate. And, of course, if you get little protein at breakfast-time you will need to make up that shortfall later in the day. Try to pick at least one calcium-rich protein food, such as milk or yoghurt on most days.

The breakfast should also include a small amount of fat which, like protein, helps to keep hunger at bay and regulate blood sugar levels. This is a good opportunity to give your essential fatty acid intake a boost, perhaps with nuts and seeds added to a cereal. A pure vegetable oil spread on any bread would add a little more fat. By using skimmed milk and low-fat yoghurts, saturated fat intake can be kept to a minimum.

Breakfast should provide a good mix of both starch and sugars. Sugar is best provided in the form of fruit or fruit juice, which will soon (within 20 minutes or so) break down into glucose and raise the blood sugar levels, as well as providing your first vitamin C of the day. Starch is ideally provided in bread and/or cereals, and for morning-long sustenance at least some of this should be as unrefined as possible, for example, whole-grain cereals and whole-grain breads. There is nothing wrong with a slice of white bread spread with some jam, but on its own it will quickly have you hungry again as the refined flour and sugary jam are quickly digested. Moreover, a breakfast high in refined carbohydrate won't boost your fibre.

A balanced breakfast will provide a good range of vitamins and minerals and make an important contribution to your day's intake.

■ So is it good-bye to the Sunday brunch?

Lovers of bacon and eggs may by now be feeling slightly depressed, but there is no need. Although the traditional cooked breakfast is extremely high in fat (see previous page), there is no need to give it up completely. A cooked breakfast can fit quite easily into your diet once a week or so. Even 'reworked', such a breakfast is still not perfect — containing a bit too little carbohydrate and too much protein, — but it is very easy to balance that out during the rest of the day by having a lowish-protein lunch and a very-high-carbohydrate evening meal, for example.

A cooked breakfast, higher in calories than you may normally eat, is actually a very good idea if you have an active physical day ahead — say a long brisk Sunday walk. Such a breakfast a few hours before a traditional Sunday lunch, however, would not be a good idea. Remember — good nutrition is mainly about common sense and balance.

■ Top ten quick and healthy breakfasts

1 150 ml (¼ pint) low-fat bio yoghurt with 1 small banana chopped in, ½ grapefruit or glass of grapefruit juice, large slice of wholemeal bread with a little olive oil spread and honey.

2 150 ml (¼ pint) low-fat bio yoghurt topped with 50 g (2 oz) no-added-sugar luxury muesli and a portion of strawberries, small slice of bread with olive oil spread and yeast extract.

3 Two Weetabix with a dessertspoon of chopped walnuts and skimmed milk to cover, handful of dried ready-to-eat apricots, 1 slice of bread, olive oil spread and honey, glass of orange juice.

4 Two Shredded Wheat with 1 dessertspoon sunflower or pumpkin seeds and skimmed milk to cover, 1 pear, small slice of wholemeal bread with olive oil spread and marmalade.

5 A tub of natural low-fat fromage frais with a level teaspoon of brown sugar and a slice of cantaloupe melon, chopped, plus a dessertspoon of chopped toasted almonds, 1 slice of bread, olive oil spread and yeast extract.

6 A large bowl of porridge made with rolled oats and half semi-skimmed milk to water, 2 teaspoons honey, 1 dessertspoon sultanas, 1 glass of orange juice.

7 175 g (6 oz) low-sugar, low-salt baked beans on 1 large slice wholemeal toast with a little olive oil spread, 1 orange or glass of orange juice, second slice of bread with spread and marmalade.

8 All Bran with 1 apple chopped in and skimmed milk, ½ grapefruit ,1 slice of bread with olive oil spread and honey.

9 1 large banana mashed with 1 kiwi fruit and1teaspoon of lemon juice on 1large slice of wholemeal bread with olive oil spread, glass of semi-skimmed milk.

10 Milkshake: blend 200 ml (7 fl oz) semi-skimmed milk with 1 small banana, 3 tablespoons of orange juice, 2 teaspoons of runny honey and 1 teaspoon of wheatgerm, drink chilled;1 large slice of wholemeal bread with yeast extract.

Desserts

Desserts can be a good opportunity to get vitamin C and/or calcium and/or fibre into your diet.

For vitamin C
* Fresh fruit, especially strawberries, kiwi, citrus, mango
* Fruit salad
* Summer pudding
* Fresh fruit compote, especially blackcurrants, berries
* Any of the desserts in this book

For calcium
(but remember ice-cream can be high in fat)
* Yoghurt
* Ice-cream
* Low-fat custard
* Low-fat rice pudding

For fibre
* Any of the fresh fruit desserts mentioned above
* Dried fruits
* Dried fruit compote
* Fruit crumble with oat, nut and whole-meal flour topping
* Baked apple with chopped nuts

Many people save truly indulgent desserts for when they go out or entertain (see Eating Out section, page 64). Gâteaux, flans, tarts and pies, as well as most rich chocolate desserts, are all heavy on calories and fat. Here, though, are some ideas for more indulgent and quick desserts which won't do too much damage to the overall balance of your diet and come within the '10% of total calories' criteria:
* Individual tubs of jelly
* Blancmange desserts topped with aerosol cream
* Individual crème caramel
* Individual fruit trifle or mousse

Drinks

USA guidelines say males should have 3.7 litres total fluids a day and women 2.7. This includes all fluid intake – water, tea, coffee, soft drinks, juices and the fluid that is in the food that we eat.

However plain water is one of the best drinks for most of us.

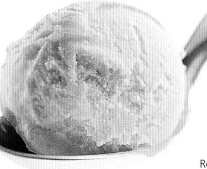

Recent research has shown that, on average, we spend — just at home — over £3 a week each on drinks. We look at the advantages and drawbacks of the most popular drinks. For more detailed information on particular drinks see the Food Charts on pages 260-317.

Milk
This is one of our main sources of calcium, as well as providing protein. Full-fat milk is high in saturated fat; semi-skimmed and fully skimmed are better alternatives for most people. Milk taken as a late-night hot drink can help sleep (see Insomnia, page 123). For people with a lactose intolerance or vegans, calcium-fortified soya milk is a good alternative.

Fruit juice
These are usually good sources of vitamin C, but they can contribute to tooth decay. They are higher in calories than most people realize, at around 80 calories for a 200 ml (7 fl oz) glassful. It is best to dilute them down with some water.

Tea and coffee
In moderate amounts, these are both good antioxidants, as well as being stimulating. In excess, they may no longer act as stimulants and can cause tiredness. They are virtually calorie-free, but don't take either with a meal as they can hinder absorption of some nutrients. They are mildly diuretic, but not enough to counteract their hydrating effects. Herbal teas are a good alternative (see page 255).

Squashes and carbonated drinks
These are usually sources of many additives and are often very sweet. They contain few nutrients unless they are added by the manufacturer. Low-calorie versions are similar, but with artificial sweetener. Sparkling mineral water with a dash of fruit juice would be preferable — and nicer?

Alcoholic drinks
Don't use these as thirst quenchers, and don't drink alcohol during the day. Save your allowance for your evening meal, when it can aid digestion and is less quickly absorbed into the bloodstream.

See also: Constipation, Hangover, Weight Control, Alcohol Abuse, Alcohol, Food Charts.

A new look at lunch

For most of us, lunch needs to be something quick and easy — even when we're not working, there's usually little time to spare. But it doesn't HAVE to be a cheese sandwich every day.

Even if you've had a good breakfast, you shouldn't skip lunch. If you do, you'll probably find that around 4-5pm you are so hungry you'll eat a pack of biscuits or something similarly high in fat and sugar.

Hunger isn't the only consideration, though. Lunch-time is an ideal time to pack in some powerful nutrients to help you to health… it's a good time to get your quota of fish or pulses; to eat plenty of salad and fruit; to get ahead on your vegetable intake with big bowls of soup.

Like breakfast, your lunch should be a sensible balance of carbohydrates and proteins, plus a little fat. Because your evening meal is going to be higher in carbohydrate and lower in protein (see overleaf), your lunch can contain a large proportion of your day's protein intake while being slightly lower in carbohydrate. Research shows that a high-carbohydrate lunch can result in sluggish performance in the afternoon.

Before deciding what you will have for your lunch, it's a good idea to plan out also what your evening meal will be, so that you don't 'double up' on certain things and miss out on others. For example, if you are going to have meat as part of your evening meal, avoid having meat at lunch-time and choose a vegetable protein instead, such as pulses, or have fish. If you're having pasta in the evening, don't also have pasta salad at lunch-time, and so on.

When choosing a lunch for speed, beware of the possible nutritional pitfalls.

SOME SUGGESTIONS FOR HEALTHY QUICK LUNCHES

* Double portion of Cannellini Bean and Basil Spread (page 213); 100 g ciabatta loaf; large salad of Continental leaves; 1 orange.
* 100 g (2 oz) rollmop herring; portion of cold new potatoes; mixed salad bowl with French dressing; Apple and Apricot Shake (page 254).
* Portion of Tuna, Avocado and Tomato Salad (page 223) with added cooked wholewheat pasta; 1 apple.
* 1 portion of Hummus (page 212) with 2 oatcakes; 1 banana; Watermelon Refresher (page 253).
* 1 portion of Lentil and Coriander Soup (page 218); rye bread; 1 orange.
* 1 portion of Country Pea Soup (page 219); wholemeal bread; dried figs, 1 banana.
* 1 warmed chapati; 1 portion Feta and Pepper Spread (page 212); selection of crudités; 1 apple; handful of dried apricots.

PACK A PUNCH

Before

Cheddar cheese and pickle sandwich (50 g cheese, 85 g white bread spread with 7g margarine, 2 tsp sweet pickle), 1 chocolate mini roll, 1 packet (30 g) of light crisps, 1 apple, 200ml diet cola. *772 calories, 36g total fat, 18.7 g saturated fat, 28.5 g protein, 86.5 g carbohydrate, 4.8g fibre.*

This typical lunch-box – despite the 'diet' cola, 'light' crisps and apple is not all that well balanced. It is high in saturates, trans fats and salt, and low in complex carbs and fibre, while not being a particularly good source of vitamins. The Cheddar is a good source of calcium, but a lower-fat hard cheese would also supply this. Incidentally, most 'light' crisps contain almost as many calories as ordinary crisps.

After ★ ★ ★ ★ ★

50 g lean cooked chicken (no skin) in 100 g French bread with 2 tsp curried tofu mayonnaise (page 246, with pinch of curry powder and 1 tsp mango chutney); 140 g mixed salad (tomato, cucumber, pepper, red onion, sweetcorn, celery); 25 g slice of malt loaf; 1 apple; 20 g mixed shelled nuts, 30 g ready-to-eat dried apricots, 200 ml orange juice. *731 calories; 15 g total fat, 3 g saturated fat, 32 g protein, 122g carbohydrate, 8.5 g fibre.*

Just as appetising and even more to eat, this lunch offers roughly the same calories, but is lower in saturated fat and artificial additives, and high in vitamin C, iron, fibre, EFAs and a good range of other vitamins and minerals.

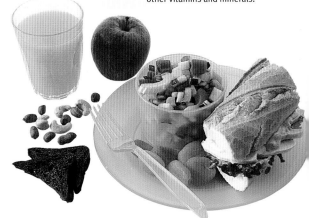

Many ready-made soups are high in salt and can be low on 'real' ingredients' — if you're going to choose ready-made, choose chilled rather than canned or packet soups. In fact, almost anything that needs reconstituting or comes out of a can should be limited to an occasional stand-by. However, there is nothing wrong with baked beans on toast — a high-fibre, low-fat and filling meal — but choose the low-salt, low-sugar kind.

Anything in pastry is probably very high in fat, saturated fat and calories, so limit items like pasties, pork pies and sausage rolls to very occasional use.

Many sandwiches are high in fat, but calorie-counted ones containing plenty of fresh salad can be fine, though this wouldn't be enough for an average person's lunch. When making your own sandwiches, garnish with lots of salad, go easy on the spread and, if choosing high-fat Cheddar cheese, grate it to go further.

Vary the types of bread you use, too — there is nothing wrong with decent white bread sometimes, although wholemeal will boost your day's fibre intake. With some fillings you will need no butter or other spread on your bread, but if you do, go for an unsaturated spread containing no or few hydrogenated (trans) fats.

Deli counter salads and pre-packed supermarket ones are often very high in fat — slaws, potato, pasta and rice salads are the worst culprits. The other problem with a 'salad' lunch is that often the true fresh salad part of the meal is nothing more than a couple of lettuce leaves, a few thin slices of tomato and a sprig of cress. This weighs next to nothing and will contain virtually no nutrients. To be a real working part of your healthy meal, salad has to come BIG.

Think 'masses of things' when you think salad. Add some nuts, seeds, cold cooked vegetable items like beans, chunky bits of carrot or pepper, dried or fresh fruits.

Pub and wine bar lunches are often high-fat affairs — a traditional ploughman's or quiche and salad are typical saturated-fat-laden fare. For tips on eating out at lunch-time see page 64.

Home-packed lunches can be a healthy alternative to a lunch-time cafeteria meal or take-away, but even so it is all too easy to put together a packed meal that's very high in salt, fat and sugar, and low in fibre and vitamins. They can also get boring, so if you eat — or could eat — a packed lunch regularly, invest in suitable plastic containers and vacuum flasks for salads, desserts and soups. Dressings and utensils can usually be kept at work.

LUNCH AT HOME

Before

295 g can of low-cal veg soup; 45 g white roll spread with 5g margarine; 50 g extra-lean ham; 25 g mortadella; 2 tbsp coleslaw; small green salad (lettuce, some cress, cucumber); 2 tsp light mayonnaise. *483 calories, 25.8 g total fat, 6.6 g saturated fat, 19.8 g protein, 38.4 g carbohydrate, 2.7g fibre.*

A typical quick lunch for the calorie-conscious, with extra-lean ham and light mayo. Yet, it contains a day's recommended max salt, at nearly 6 g (the soup is particularly high), nearly half its calories are from fat at 48% (mortadella and coleslaw the main culprits), and carb content is too low at under 30%. There is little complex carbs and fibre represents only 15% of a recommended day's intake.

After ★ ★ ★ ★ ★

1 wholemeal pitta, with 50 g extra-lean ham, 50 g canned chickpeas, 1 tomato, 50g Little Gem lettuce, 25 g watercress and 1 tbsp French dressing (made with olive oil); 1 diet fruit yoghurt, 1 kiwi fruit. *462 calories, 13 g total fat, 1.7 g saturated fat, 27.5 g protein, 60g carbohydrate, 9.6 g fibre.*

Similar meal with about the same calories, but only 26% from fat, now fatty mortadella and coleslaw are replaced with chickpeas and more fresh salad and fruit. Only 3.3% saturates left, plus useful amount of EFAs from olive oil dressing and chickpeas. 50% carbs, with protein at 24% — a good lunch balance. Salt is much lower at nearly 3g, because everything except ham and bread is low in sodium; chickpeas and pitta have added fibre to give 53% of day's needs.

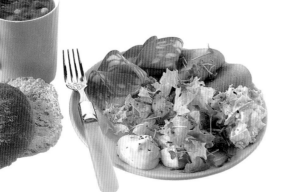

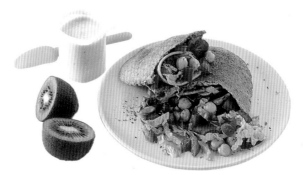

Evening meals

Though there may be a fragment of truth in the saying that we should breakfast like kings and dine like paupers, most of us look forward to our evening meal and treat it as the main food event of the day.

Although many people do, it's wise not to blow all your day's calories in the evening. The digestive system usually responds best to a 'little and often' approach — three similarly sized meals and two small snacks are ideal. However, most of us prefer our largest meal in the evening when there is time to relax. Certainly, there is no harm in allotting around 35-40% of your calories to the evening. However, do try to eat such a meal no later than two hours before bed.

Like breakfast and lunch, dinner should provide a mix of nutrients. But, this is the best time of the day to go to town with carbohydrates. These have a calming effect and may help the brain 'slow down', to relax and get a good night's sleep.

A meal rich in complex carbohydrates, particularly those low on the Glycaemic Index such as pulses and wholewheat pasta, will also sustain you through the night. And yet, so often, we prepare a supper based mainly on a high-protein food. Most of us still don't say 'let's have rice tonight', we say 'let's have a steak', and only as an afterthought do we consider accompaniments.

For healthy eating in the evening, the single most important rule you should bear in mind is to think of the protein element of your meal — especially animal or dairy protein - as a SMALL PART of the meal, the 'accompaniment', and think of starches and vegetables as the LARGE

TRADITIONAL MEAL MAKEOVER

Before

200 g roast chicken, including crispy skin, 3 roast potatoes (150 g); 70 g peas and carrots; 4 tbsp unskimmed gravy; 50 g ready-made parsley stuffing. *798 calories, 41.5 g total fat, 11.2 g saturated fat, 53.6 g protein, 55.5 g carbohydrate.*

This, by no means large, plateful contains just about the right proportion of a day's calories for a main meal at 41% (for women), 31% (for men), but contains 41.5 g of fat, which is 47% of the meal and 64% of the recommended daily max intake for females and nearly 50% for a man. Saturated fat and protein content are both very high, too, compared with the meal's low carb content, which provides just 26% of the calories. Also low in vegetables and has only 5g of fibre. If a woman ate this meal plus the cereal 'before' breakfast on page 42 and the salad 'before' lunch on page 47, and nothing else at all, she would already be 14% over the max recommended day's fat intake at a total of 74g, while her carb intake would have given her only 57% of her needs and her fibre intake would be merely 8.5g, or less than half a day's adequate intake.

After ★★★★★

125 g lean roast chicken (no skin); 225 g new potatoes in skins and 100 g butternut squash, brushed in 2 tsp olive oil and baked; 60 g peas; 100 g dark leafy greens; 50 g home-made rice, apricot and nut stuffing; 5 tsp pan juices made into sauce with a little wine and cornflour. *631.5 calories, 21 g total fat, 4 g saturated fat, 45.7 g protein, 68.5 g carbohydrate.*

How to eat more for fewer calories and fat! Removing skin from chicken, just brushing veg with oil and using skimmed pan juices for gravy reduces fat easily, although EFA content is higher. A smaller amount of chicken is compensated for by more vegetables, providing carbs, vitamin C, beta-carotene and iron. By eating this, plus 'after' breakfast and lunch, a woman would have consumed 1,480 calories or 76% of day's energy needs; used up only 62% of her total day's recommended max fat intake at 40.25g and only 33% of her max saturates intake at 7.1g. She would have attained 78% of her minimum carb needs at 201.5g and a total fibre intake of 28g and would have eaten 7 portions of fruit and veg. EFA and micronutrient requirements will have all been supplied.

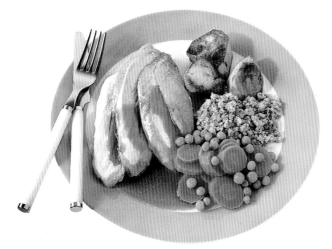

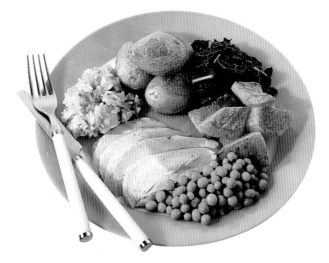

TIPS FOR HEALTHY EVENING EATING

✴ Limit meat to once or twice a week maximum.

✴ Have fish at least twice a week.

✴ Have a vegetarian or vegan night at least twice a week, not relying heavily on cheese.

✴ Have poultry or game once or twice a week.

✴ Remember that full-fat hard, blue and creamy cheeses are high in saturated fat and calories, and best used sparingly.

✴ Remember pastry is very high in fat, saturated fat and calories — keep for occasional use.

Filo is better than other pastries, as you add your own fat, so can use less, and can use olive oil.

✴ Only use as much fat when cooking as absolutely necessary.

If following a recipe, you can reduce the fat used in many of them without detriment.

✴ Check out how many portions of fruit and vegetables you've had in the day and use your evening meal to make up the total to at least five portions.

✴ Add a glass or two of wine some evenings if you like.

✴ If your main meal is large, instead of having a dessert, have a snack during the day instead or a late-night milk drink, so that you don't have too many calories all at one time your plate.

PART of the meal, the 'stars'. By cutting back on animal protein, you not only allow more room for the healthy carbs and vegetables but you also naturally cut back on fat and saturated fat.

You can fit even traditional meals, such as roasts — if not exactly, then at least partially — into this ideal simply by altering the balance on your plate — less meat or poultry, more vegetables. (See the example on the left.)

To reinforce the message that you don't need to worry about getting enough protein in your evening meal this way, let's look back at the breakfasts and lunches we've analysed in the previous pages. In the 'after' muesli and salad lunch there was 41.75 g of protein altogether. An average woman has a minimum daily need of about 50 g protein and a maximum daily need of about 73 g, so she will need only between 8 and 31 g more protein after that breakfast and that lunch to fall within a suitable intake range. An

average man's needs are about 64-95 g a day, so he will need only another 22-53 g.

As a mere 100 g (3½ oz) small portion of lean meat contains 35 g (1¼ oz) of pure protein, and as protein is present in many of the other foods on your plate, you can see that perhaps that half-pound steak (50 g/1½ oz pure protein) isn't such a good idea after all. Even after tweaking the roast meal opposite to a better balance, it still contains 45.7 g protein — bringing the day's intake to more than enough for a woman and enough for a man.

The meal now provides under 30% of its calories as fat and the carbohydrate content has gone up to over 40%. This last figure is still low as we're aiming for 50% as a minimum — but by choosing the right dessert and other daily snacks we can boost the day's carbohydrate intake even further.

A woman could make up her day's calorie intake with a carbohydrate-rich dessert (see page 45) and a snack or

treat (overleaf). Her protein needs have already been well met and she needs no more fat as the fat intakes are maximums not minimums.

NOTE: A man would need to increase portion sizes by about a third on all the 'made-over' meals to get enough calories and nutrients.

■ *Swop this* … 175 g (6 oz) lamb steak, new potatoes, small salad
For this … Large portion of whole-wheat noodles stir-fried with 90 g (3¼ oz) sliced lamb, 200 g (7 oz) mixed vegetables, sesame oil and light soy sauce.

■ *Swop this* … Battered fish and chips
For this … Large portion of brown rice with salmon and red pepper brochettes and tomato sauce.

■ *Swop this* …Cottage pie and peas
For this … Baked sweet potato or brown rice with small portion of chilli con carne, large salad.

■ *Swop this* … three-egg cheese omelette
For this … kedgeree with haddock and one hard-boiled egg, peas

DAY'S TALLY SO FAR

Before Cereal and toast breakfast, cold meats lunch, first roast chicken dinner
1,580 calories, 74 g total fat, 20.5 g saturated fat, 82.5 g protein, 148 g carbohydrate, 8.5 g fibre.

After Muesli breakfast, pitta and yoghurt lunch, second roast chicken dinner
1,480 calories, 40.25 g total fat, 7.1 g saturated fat, 87.5 g protein, 201.5 g carbohydrate, 28 g fibre.

Snacks and treats

If your regular meals are nutritionally well balanced, as we've seen in the last few pages, it is actually quite easy to make room for a daily dessert or extra snack without pushing your fat, calorie or sugar levels too high.

Here we look at ways to fit your favourites into your daily diet and offer suggestions for healthier alternatives to high-fat, high-sugar treats.

Most of us consume a fair proportion of our daily calories in the form of snacks, desserts, drinks and 'extras'. So, even if your actual 'meals' are fairly well balanced, it is easy to put your total diet out of balance with a poor choice in these extras. Too many high-calorie high-fat snacks can contribute towards weight gain as well as being likely to increase your intake of saturated fats and trans fats, and possibly sugar. Over-indulgence in such snacks can also fill you up and reduce your motivation to eat fresh and nutritious foods.

On the other hand, a carefully chosen day's eating will give you room to indulge in one or two favourite treats, such as a slice of cake, some biscuits, a chocolate bar or an alcoholic drink.

It is wise to allow no more than 10% of your total day's calorie intake for such items — that would be 194 calories for women and 255 for men. Alternatively, if the day's eating hasn't been ideal otherwise, one or two well-chosen healthy snacks can actually help to improve the day's total nutritional profile. Let us look at some examples of both sensible and not-so-sensible choices of these little 'extras'.

The boxes opposite give the calorie and fat content of some typical 'indulgence' foods, so you can fit them into your overall diet now and then if you like.

For comparison, there follow some suggestions for healthier snack alternatives.

EXAMPLE 1

This is a woman who has eaten the 'before' breakfast, lunch and evening meal on the past few pages, and has notched up 1,580 calories, leaving her 360 to 'play with' (1,940 calories a day is an average woman's intake for weight maintenance). However, she has already eaten 14% OVER her day's fat allowance at 74 g and is nearly at her saturated fat limit — and she's still low on carbohydrate (particularly complex) and fibre. She decides to opt for these extras:

200ml (7 fl oz) skimmed milk for her tea and coffee — 66 calories, virtually no fat.

One 100g (3½ oz) portion of vanilla ice-cream — 194 calories, 9.8 g fat, 6.3 g saturated fat.

1 plain scone — 174 calories, 7 g fat, 2.4 g saturated fat.

1 double whisky — 96 calories, fat-free.

Not exactly an excessive list, but one which finishes her day's eating profile like this:

2,110 calories - which is 9% more than she needs, so she may slowly gain weight on such a diet.

91g of total fat — which is 29% too much.

29g saturated fat — which is 24% too much.

208g of carbohydrate — which is 20% too little and is also far too low in complex carbs.

10.5g fibre — which is only just over half average needs.

One snack of fresh fruit and one of dried fruit would have been a better bet than the ice-cream and scone, while keeping the milk (for calcium) and the whisky, bringing the day's calorie and fat total to reasonable levels, increasing complex carbs and fibre, and raising her tally of fruits and veg for the day to four — still low, but better than the two she managed with her main meals.

EXAMPLE 2 ★★★★★

This woman eats the 'after' breakfast, lunch and main meal and has so far eaten: 1,480 calories, 40.25 g total fat, 7.1g saturated fat, 201.5 g carbohydrate and 28g fibre.

She has 460 calories left to use up, has plenty of room for manoeuvre on her fat intake, is already well on the way to getting her day's carbohydrate intake and has eaten masses of fibre, plus seven portions of fruits and vegetables. She opts to add:

200ml (7 fl oz) skimmed milk — 66 calories, virtually fat-free.

1 Flapjack (page 251) — 189 calories, 8.7 g fat, 1.8 g saturated fat.

1 portion of Citrus Granita (page 249) — 142 calories, virtually fat-free.

150 ml (¾ pint) glass of port — 79 calories, fat-free.

Her final profile for the day then is:

1,956 calories — almost exactly spot-on for average weight maintenance.

49 g total fat — only three-quarters of what she could have eaten according to health guidelines, representing 23% of her total day's calorie intake, but still plenty to give her all her essential fatty acids.

9 g saturated fat — less than half what she could have eaten according to health guidelines, representing 4.1% of her total day's calorie intake.

If this second woman had wanted to indulge in a chocolate bar or similar rather than the seemingly healthier citrus granita, she could have done so and still been within her day's allowance for fat and only marginally over her day's calorie target.

SNACK COMPARISONS

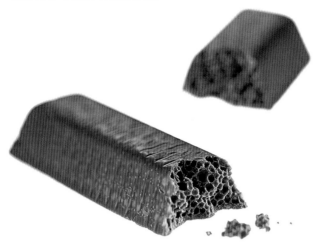

the usual indulgences	Calories	Fat (g)
Standard bar of dairy milk chocolate	255	14.8
Aero Chunky	194	11.3
Creme egg	175	5.9
Mince pie	250	9.0
Cream doughnut	180	11.5
Chocolate eclair	260	18.0
Average 100 g (3½ oz) slice of chocolate fudge cake	400	20.0
Salted peanuts, 50 g (1½ oz) pack	295	24.0

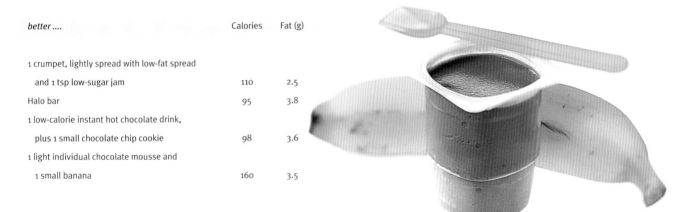

better	Calories	Fat (g)
1 crumpet, lightly spread with low-fat spread and 1 tsp low-sugar jam	110	2.5
Halo bar	95	3.8
1 low-calorie instant hot chocolate drink, plus 1 small chocolate chip cookie	98	3.6
1 light individual chocolate mousse and 1 small banana	160	3.5

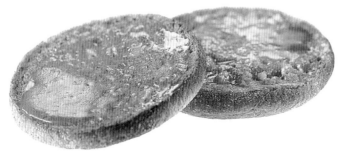

best ... ★★★★★	Calories	Fat (g)
One 125 ml (4 fl oz) tub of low-fat bio yoghurt and 1 medium piece of fresh fruit	140	2.0
1 wholemeal English muffin with a little spread and honey	180	4.0
50 g (1½ oz) ready-to-eat dried apricots, 1 banana	190	0.6
2 dark rye crispbreads spread with 25 g (¾ oz) home-made guacamole (spiced mashed avocado)	82	3.6
One 30 g (1 oz) slice of dark rye bread, spread with 1 portion Cannellini Bean and Basil Spread (page 213)	152	3.5

Ensuring a basic healthy diet

The sample seven-day diet plan opposite shows how an adult in normal health could put together all the preceding information into a delicious healthy everyday diet.

With the help of the recipe section later in the book plus the healthy eating tips you've learned in this section it won't be difficult to eat well indefinitely. Let's summarize those guidelines as follows:

1 Eat more complex carbohydrates — bread, potatoes, pasta, cereals, grains, pulses. Carbs low on the Glycaemic Index (page 195) may keep you feeling full for longer and regulate blood sugar levels.

2 Eat at least five portions of fruit and vegetables a day. Include plenty of leafy greens, and red and orange fruits and vegetables. Eat them raw, or cooked lightly and don't smother them in too much butter or commercial dressings.

3 Eat less fat, especially saturated and trans fats. Cook with less fat and go easy on bought foods high in fat, such as pastries, cakes, pies, cream and full-fat cheese and fatty cuts of meat.

4 Eat natural oily fats such as those found in pure vegetable, seed and grain oils, nuts, grains and seeds. These provide essential fatty acids. Use oils on salad and in cooking.

5 Eat less sugary and salty foods. For sweetness go for naturally sweet items like fruit. Use less salt in your cooking.

6 Eat more plant- and fish-based meals and less meat.

7 Get as wide a variety of foods as possible into your diet.

8 Eat the best quality foods that you can — fresh, wholesome, unadulterated food is best for your body.

9 Eat regularly throughout the day, having a breakfast, lunch, main meal and snacks.

10 Drink plenty of fluids and don't forget that water is one of the best drinks of all.

Most importantly — relax and enjoy your food. Make some time to plan your meal-times ahead and enjoy the pleasures of cooking.

The next section of the book contains special guidelines for diets to suit different lifestyles.

▧ The basic healthy diet

This diet is a guideline only, to help you plan your own eating. No precise portion sizes are given because this isn't a slimming diet — it is a healthy eating diet. If 'medium' portions are eaten, plus the milk and 'extras' allowance detailed below, you will be getting approximately the right amount for a maintenance diet.

Eat to suit your sex, size, activity levels and appetite. As a guide, if you are female, sedentary, and/or small you will eat smaller portions. If you are male, tall and/or active you will need to eat more. Try to get in touch with your appetite and be sensible about portion sizes. Eating more than you need will result in weight gain, even if your diet is healthy.

Unlimiteds
Unlimited are water, any leafy green vegetables and salad items, herbs and spices, herbal and 'no added sugar' fruit teas, lemon juice. Tea and instant or filtered coffee can be taken in reasonable amounts (using milk from the allowance below, if you wish). Fizzy calorie-free drinks and squashes should be limited to occasional use.

Milk
In addition to any milk mentioned in the plan opposite, you should have about 200 ml (7 fl oz) skimmed milk or calcium-enriched soya milk every day. If you don't want this, have a 125 ml (4 fl oz) natural low-fat yoghurt instead.

Extras
Allow yourself, in addition, 200 calories or so a day for a little indulgence. This could be 1-2 units of alcohol or something chocolatey. It could even be something like extra bread, or potato, or a milk drink at bedtime. It is up to you.

THE BASIC HEALTHY DIET

DAY ONE
Breakfast
2 Weetabix with skimmed milk, sprinkled
with chopped nuts and sesame seeds
1 slice of wholemeal bread with
sunflower spread and honey
glass of orange juice , 1 apple
Lunch
Spiced Lentil and Mixed Green Vegetable
Salad
200 g (7 oz), cooked weight, couscous
1 satsuma
Evening
Pasta with Milanese Sauce
large bowlful of mixed salad leaves with a
little olive oil and lemon dressing
portion of Greek-style yoghurt with
runny honey
Snack
1 Flapjack

DAY TWO
Breakfast
Mango and Peach Booster
multi-grain roll with sunflower spread and
low-sugar marmalade
handful of ready-to-eat dried apricots
Lunch
Anchoïade as a dip
wholemeal pitta crudités
Tomato and Bean Salsa
portion of vanilla ice-cream
Evening
Spanish-style Baked Trout
green beans , French bread , 1 banana
Snack
handful of dried fruit and nuts

DAY THREE
Breakfast
portion no-added-sugar muesli
skimmed milk , 1 orange
slice of wholemeal bread with sunflower
spread and honey
Lunch
Squash, Potato and Butter Bean Soup
large bread roll, 1 banana
Greek-style yoghurt
Evening
Spiced Chicken and Greens
portion of brown rice
Stir-fried Fruit Salad
Snack
1 Flapjack

DAY FOUR
Breakfast
Low-fat natural bio yoghurt
portion of blackberries
wholemeal English muffin with
sunflower spread and honey, peach juice
Lunch
large hunk of French or Italian country bread
with Feta and Pepper Spread
bowlful of mixed salad, red grapes
Evening
Winter Squash with Lentils and Ginger
portion of potato mashed with a little olive oil
portion of kale and portion of green beans
fresh figs
Snack
fromage frais with honey

DAY FIVE
Breakfast
Boiled egg
large slice of wholemeal bread with
sunflower spread, 1 satsuma
Apple and Apricot Shake
Lunch
Panzanella Salad, 1 banana
portion of low-fat bio yoghurt
Evening
Turkish Lamb Stew
large portion of bulgar wheat , broccoli
Mango Filo Tart
Snack
mixed dried fruit and nuts

DAY SIX
Breakfast
1 wholemeal English muffin with sunflower
spread and low-sugar marmalade
Greek-style yoghurt with chopped apple and
pistachio nuts
Lunch
Carrot and Orange Soup
Cannellini Bean and Basil Spread
French baguette, 2 tomatoes
Evening
Pasta with Olives and Sardines
large mixed salad
Snack
ready-to-eat dried apricots and prunes

DAY SEVEN
Breakfast
Banana and Strawberry Smoothie
large slice of wholemeal bread with
sunflower spread and honey
Lunch
Thai Salmon Salad, kiwi fruit
Evening
Chickpea and Vegetable Crumble
baked potato, spring greens
Snack
1 Flapjack

CHOOSING A DIET TO SUIT YOUR LIFESTYLE

So we've seen what the ideal diet is like — but how can you translate that into the way YOU live? In the next few pages we look at how healthy eating can fit into any lifestyle, from those of students on a budget to busy family cooks to executive dining.

Fast food for busy people

When your life is so busy that you can hardly find time to sleep, it is often 'proper' eating that suffers. Food is grabbed on the run, chocolate bars are a principal source of 'instant energy' and main meals always come carton-shaped. Here we look at what can be done to get your eating back into balance.

If you're busy, the chances are that you are busy earning money! If so, it is worth paying a small premium for time-saving food ideas from the supermarket.

For example: ready-peeled and -chopped vegetables; ready-prepared fruits, such as pineapple and oranges; ready-made chilled stocks, soups and sauces, and so on. All these can help you to eat healthily for only a little extra cost.

Much time can be saved if you freeze meals, sauces, soups, etc., that you have made yourself in batches on one of those rare less-busy days — it really is almost as quick to cook double or treble quantities.

If even the quickest and easiest cooking is out of the question most of the time, that doesn't matter. The trick is to swap fast fatty or low-nutrient food for fast healthy, high-nutrient food. Luckily, many foods you can eat with virtually no preparation are widely available. Fruits, salads, yoghurts, fromage frais, cheeses, milks, juices, bread, cereals — make these a sizeable part of your diet and who needs the take-away — a plate of wholemeal bread, goats' cheese and tomatoes is a fast food feast!

■ A head start in the morning

Breakfast is the meal most often missed by busy people; and yet, as we saw on page 42, breakfast is very important. A good breakfast can help your energy, your concentration, your memory and your alertness. So, for anyone pushed for time with a demanding lifestyle and decisions to be made all day, breakfast makes sense. It doesn't, though, necessarily have to be

FAST AND HEALTHY BREAKFASTS

* Muesli with milk and berry fruits
* Bread with spread, milk and nec-tarine or peach
* Bio yoghurt, shelled nuts, orange juice and banana
* Flapjack (see page 251), orange juice and banana

cooked, or large, or time-consuming. You simply need a fix of carbohydrate and protein, with a little fat and a good range of vitamins and minerals.

Try one or more of these strategies:

* Get ahead. Get your breakfast organized the night before. Put out cereals in their dish and cover them; pour out your juice into a glass and pop this in the fridge. Defrost a frozen bread roll. Do whatever you can so that in the morning rush you can still have some food.

* Pick a portable breakfast. Choose something you can eat on the way to work or as soon as you get there. Something based on bread or a pot of bio yoghurt and a banana is better than eating nothing. If you take a packed lunch to work, pack extra and eat earlier in the day.

* Choose a shake. There are several shakes based on milk or yoghurt in the recipe section. Any one will provide a quick breakfast, which you can make up the night before.

■ Time limits for lunch

The obvious answer for busy people is to persuade someone else to make you a healthy packed lunch — failing that, make it yourself. It will still save time on going to the deli or sandwich shop in between meetings, or whatever. The bonus of a packed lunch is that you know what is in it, you know when it was prepared, and you can tweak it to suit your own needs. You can also eat it at a desk, but it is best not to try to eat while working as that is a sure way to

digestive problems. You need to take a short relaxing break in which to enjoy your lunch, even if it is only 15 minutes.

■ Here is the blueprint for the contents of a healthy packed meal:

* Something high in complex carbohydrate. This can be bread for sandwiches, which is by far the quickest option. Cold cooked rice, bulgar, couscous or pasta are alternatives, which may be quick if you have some left over from, say, the previous evening's meal. Cooked new potatoes on their own make a tasty treat.

* Something with low- or moderate-fat protein. Fill bread, baguette or pitta with low-fat cheese or ham, vegetable pâté or tuna, or add to the rice, etc., for a salad.

* Add a dressing if you like. Keep a jar of ready-made vinaigrette handy. A little home-made mayonnaise also acts as a good spread, instead of butter.

* Add fresh veg. If you haven't time to chop, add items to your lunch-box whole — tomatoes, spring onions, peeled carrots. In cold weather, try a vacuum flask of vegetable soup.

* Choice of shelled nuts, fruit, dried fruit.

* A pot of yoghurt or fromage frais. This will be enough for many people, but men or very active people can also add:

* Malt loaf, flapjack, muffin or other semi-sweet bakery item.

■ If a packed lunch is impossible, here are some guidelines for other options:

Sandwich shop or deli: Order along the guidelines above. Pitfalls: lots of sandwich fillings are heavy on mayonnaise or French-type dressings. Go for dressings made with olive oil and, at least some days, ask for fillings and salad without dressing.

Fast-food outlet: Most burger bars can supply at least one or two items lower in fat — perhaps a fish or chicken patty on a wholemeal bun. Many fast-food bars provide little or nothing in the way of salads, vegetables or fruits, so pop your own fruit into your pocket.

■ Working from home

Many more people nowadays use the home as their workplace and find fitting in a healthy lunch just as much of a problem.

In summer, think 'everything basic', such as the breads, cheeses, yoghurts, fruits, tomatoes and so on, outlined above. In winter, think a bowl of soup, a hunk of bread and a piece of fruit. However busy you are, it is vital to stop for a break and something sustaining to eat. You will work better afterwards if you do.

■ Fast tracks to an evening meal

Don't always rely on a take-away or pizza delivery for your evening meal! The main secret to having yourself a delicious and healthy meal ready to eat within half an hour or so of coming home — and with not a great deal of effort on your part — is to have a well-stocked storecupboard. If you're busy, stocking it up is best planned as a once-a-month exercise which will save you time in the long run. Items you must have include:

* Dried pastas of various shapes and at least some wholewheat versions.
* Quick-cook wholewheat noodles.
* Couscous and quick cook rice.
* Brown and green lentils.
* Ready-to-eat dried fruits, shelled nuts and seeds.
* Cans of fish, such as tuna, mackerel and sardines.
* Jars of black olives, mixed peppers, artichoke hearts (all canned in water if possible or, if using those canned in oil, well drained).
* Cans of pulses, such as mixed beans, chickpeas, red kidney beans, cannellini beans and borlotti beans. Even baked beans in tomato sauce are fine.
* Lots of tomatoey-things, such as jars of passata, tubes of tomato purée, packs of sun-dried tomatoes, tubs of sun-dried tomato purée and cans of chopped and whole tomatoes.

QUICK DO-IT-YOURSELF SOUP

This soup will almost make itself while you do something else, and it can be varied according to what you have in the larder.

To make 4 servings, take 750 ml (1⅓ pints) ready-made vegetable or chicken stock. Take a pack of ready-prepared and chopped supermarket vegetables, e.g. carrot, onion, parsnip (even leftovers from your own fridge will work), about 450 g (1 lb) in all, add them to the stock in a pan with a 400 g (14 oz) can of chopped tomatoes. Simmer for 30 minutes. Drain a can of mixed pulses and tip them in. Heat through. If you have time, purée half the soup in a blender and return to the pan. If not, it doesn't matter. Stir in 1 tablespoon ready-made pesto and add sea salt and pepper to taste before serving. Leftover potatoes are also very nice in this soup.

* Packets of dried Italian and Chinese mushrooms.
* Herbs and spices, and a few bottles of seasonings and sauces, such as light soy sauce, Worcestershire sauce, chilli sauce, plum sauce, oyster sauce, and so on. These can be high in salt, but are used in small quantities.
* Low-sodium vegetable stock cubes, which are useful as standbys when you haven't got any fresh stock.

If your freezer also contains a selection of the following then you have the basis of a very healthy quick evening meal most nights of the week, especially if you have a microwave oven for quick defrosting:

* Frozen vegetables, a good selection, including peas, broccoli, sweetcorn.
* Ready-made tomato sauce.
* Ready-diced, -sliced or -minced chicken, turkey or lamb.
* Pizza bases.
* Ready-grated half-fat mozzarella cheese and some home-grated Parmesan.

In the fridge, the following will keep for weeks rather than days and will be welcome additions to your diet:

* Fresh chillies, ginger and garlic. Keep in the salad crisper.
* Yoghurt, fromage frais, eggs, cheeses.

Tomatoes, sweet peppers and Chinese leaves will all keep well in the fridge for a week or more, as will fresh carrots, courgettes and white cabbage. So will oranges, satsumas, kiwis and other fruits, depending on the condition they are in when you buy them. If you add these to your basic quick meals you will also be getting more vitamin C.

A large bag of potatoes will last a long time in cool dark conditions, so if you have a microwave you can add baked potatoes to your list of quickie dishes.

From all of this you can make dozens of different dishes. Here are just a few ideas (you will also find plenty of quick recipes in the recipe section):

* Pasta with tomato sauce, with added black olives, and Parmesan.
* Pasta with a sauce made from fromage frais, reconstituted Italian dried mushrooms and a little grated mozzarella cheese.
* Pasta with (frozen or jar) pesto.
* Noodles with a stir-fry of diced chicken, frozen stir-fried vegetables, ginger, garlic and soya sauce.
* Pizza topped with tomato sauce, grated cheese, sliced olives and reconstituted mushrooms.
* Rice or baked potato served with quick chilli, made from tomato sauce mixed with canned beans, fresh chopped chillies (lean thawed minced meat can be added if liked).
* Couscous reconstituted and topped with a jar of drained mixed peppers in oil, heated with drained canned chickpeas in 1 tablespoon of the pepper oil.

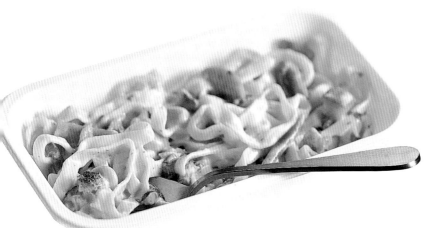

COTTAGE PIE: LOW IN FIBRE AND VEG, AND QUITE HIGH IN FAT — TRY TO ADD SOME HIGH-FIBRE VEGETABLES SUCH AS CABBAGE, WHICH WILL ALSO ADD VITAMIN C.

PASTA PRIMAVERA: HIGHER IN FIBRE, CARBOHYDRATE AND VEGETABLES, AND LOWER IN FAT. A MIXED SIDE SALAD MAKES THE DISH EVEN HEALTHIER.

CONVENIENCE MEALS

Many people rely on ready-cooked, chilled or frozen convenience meals for their supper — anything from a chicken curry to a Chinese meal for one or a roast dinner. But are they any good for you?

Of course, the answer is that they vary tremendously in nutritional content. For an average person (not trying to lose weight) many are too low in calories to satisfy the appetite. The main problem, however, is that many of them don't contain a reasonable balance of carbohydrate to protein and fat, although some manufacturers are making an effort in this respect.

If you need to rely on such meals more than occasionally, look for:

✱ The label. It should tell you how much fat the meal contains. and what proportion is saturated.

As a guide, under 10g fat in the whole meal is low, 10-20g is medium and over 20g is quite high. More than 25g for women or 30g for men per portion is probably too much, though this obviously depends on what else is eaten during the day. Look also for words on the pack like 'healthy eating' or 'low in fat', which will be another guide, though not infallible.

✱ Vegetables included in the meal.

✱ A good carbohydrate content (if appropriate), such as rice, pasta or noodles. (If you buy a ready meal which is just, say, meat or chicken in sauce, then you need to add some carbohydrate, even if it is just bread, and some fresh fruit or vegetables, (just a couple of tomatoes will do). If you choose wisely, you can fit ready meals into your diet — but try to fill the freezer with home-made soup and casseroles, so that you don't have to rely on them too often.

■ Take-aways

Nearly £3 billion is spent every year in the UK alone on just three kinds of take-away meals — burgers, pizza and fried chicken. This is equivalent to every single person in the country eating one of these types of take-away at least once a week. Add to that total the number of other kinds of take-away — fish and chips alone, for example, and you begin to see that the nutritional quality of the take-aways is a matter of importance.

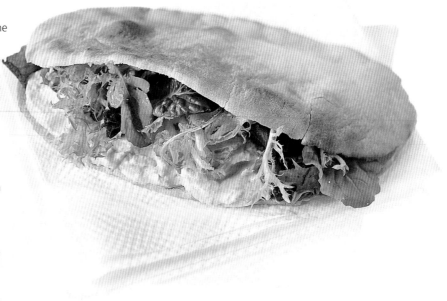

It is not possible to make many generalizations about take-away food as there are so many varieties, but one major UK survey found that up to 60% of the total calories in take-away meals comes from fat, with three-quarters of meals analysed over the recommended fat limits. Saturated fat is also likely to be high, and over half are high in salt. Considering that many take-away meals are high in calories, many also fall significantly short on a wide variety of nutrients, especially fibre, vitamin C, B group and E.

Here we look in more detail at some of the most popular types of take-out meal, examine their nutritional content and make some suggestions for the most balanced options to be found in each kind.

Burger in a bun with chips Meatburgers in a bap tend to be high in total fats, saturates and calories, and are low in fibre, vitamin C and some other vitamins, but are good sources of protein, iron, calcium and zinc. A medium portion of French fries is also high in fat, with a little fibre and vitamin C. The complete meal will also contain, on average, almost a whole day's recommended salt intake.

A typical quarter-pounder burger in a bun with medium fries would give you around 800 calories and 50g of total fat, of which approximately 25g will be saturated, depending upon the fat used.

Adding cheese to the burger increases the calorie, salt and fat content. Other types of burger available at fast-food outlets, such as chicken, fish and vegetable burgers, will be as high — or nearly as high — in fat as meat burgers. If you add a milkshake and a portion of apple pie to your meal, the fat content could reach a total of nearly 75g — an average whole day's maximum intake.

Wisest choices at a burger take-away are a plain small burger in a bun (about 250 calories, 10g fat), with orange juice, side salad and light vinaigrette, but salad and low calorie dressings are still not offered at many burger outlets. A beanburger is also a reasonable choice.

Pizza Pizzas can be a reasonably good bet for healthy eating, depending on which you choose and size of portion. An average whole take-away pizza can go up to 1,000 calories and would thus be hard to fit into a slimming diet, but would be fine for an average hungry man. Most pizzas are quite high in salt, especially those rich in cheese.

WATCH TAKE-AWAYS IF ...

* You are vegetarian. Many seemingly vegetarian take-aways contain animal fat (e.g. chips fried in lard).
* You suffer from allergic reactions. Some take-aways contain, for instance, dyes (pilau rice, perhaps fish batter, even chips), flavour enhancers such as monosodium glutamate (Chinese meals) and soya products (batters, burgers, pasties) and other additives.
* You should be following a low-fat diet.
* You are slimming. Only a few take-aways are suitable for a slimming diet if eaten regularly.
* You rely on them more than occasionally. A diet high in all but the most carefully chosen of take-aways is likely to be high in calories and fat and low in fibre, fresh fruits and vegetables and certain vitamins, such as C and E. Some fresh fruit or salad added to any take-away will increase its nutritional profile.

Pizzas contain plenty of carbohydrate in the base, the cheese provides protein and cheese and base provide calcium. The tomato sauce is a good source of carotenoids, including lycopene. An average single-portion pizza margherita will contain around 750 calories and 20-25g fat. Any pizza with a generous portion of vegetables on top — peppers, for instance — is a good bet, as are seafood pizzas. One of these pizzas, plus a side salad without added fat, would provide a reasonably balanced meal.

Fish and chips If you can find a fish-and-chip shop which serves generous portions of white fish encased in a light home-made batter fried in fresh vegetable oil to order, along with chips made out of good-quality potatoes and fried, again, to order — then a fish-and-chip meal can be quite nutritious, if high in calories and fat (though not saturated fat). The meal contains protein, carbohydrate, fibre, and a good range of vitamins and minerals, including some vitamin C in the chips. You could make it better balanced by adding peas or baked beans.

Sadly, however, much take-out fish and chips isn't carefully made. The fish and/or chips will often be twice fried, increasing fat and decreasing vitamin C. The proportion of fish to batter may be low, again increasing fat content. The fat used to fry may be lard, high in saturates, or it may be vegetable oil which has oxidized through over-use to a trans fat.

An average portion of fish and chips weighing 450 g (1 lb) may contain around 1,000 calories and 50 g fat.

Chinese/Japanese Many of the choices on Chinese take-away menus are high in fat, calories and salt. Some of the higher-fat dishes include sweet-and-sour pork in batter, duck dishes, and special fried rice. Dishes lower in fat and calories may include stir-fried vegetable dishes (with or without prawns or chicken), chop suey,

beef or chicken with green peppers, prawns in a chilli sauce, and barbecued spare ribs, plain boiled rice and noodles.

For a balanced meal go for plainly cooked rice or noodles with a vegetable dish containing some lower-fat protein, such as prawns, chicken or tofu.

Sushi is a good takeaway at 150–200 calories for an average individual box of mixed sushi and only 3–5g fat. Salmon nigiri or sushi is high in omega-3s.
■ Some average values per portion:
Beef chow mein: 600 calories, 25g fat
Chicken chop suey: 500 calories, 15g fat
Spare ribs in sauce: 800 calories, 50g fat
King prawns in ginger and chilli sauce: 250 calories, 10g fat
Large spring roll: 450 calories, 25g fat

Indian/Thai There are still many take-away 'curry' shops which will sell you a dish literally covered in oil. All the meat, onions, other vegetables and spices have been fried in oil, which later rises to the surface. Balti curries may be lower in fat because of the method of cooking; they are also a good source of iron.

Curries based on vegetables and pulses may be a good choice as they are high in fibre — for the regular take-away eater, this can be important as most take-aways are not. Prawn or chicken curries (chicken off the bone and without skin) can also be good — but with chicken, choose a tandoori (dry) curry or one with a stock-and-tomato-based sauce rather than the high-fat 'tikka masala' or any curry with coconut cream. Meat curries tend to be high in fat, as do many of the 'snack type' Indian take-away foods, such as bhajis and samosas. Naan bread is high in fat and calories — a better bet is chapati, which is cooked without fat.

Pilau rice is fried and contains about a third more calories than plain. A good side dish is a lentil dhal, providing fibre, protein and iron — in fact an ideal Indian take-away would be dhal with plain rice or chapati and a small vegetable curry.

■ Some average values per portion:
Tandoori chicken: 350 calories, 15g fat
Chicken tikka masala: 700 calories, 30g fat
Vegetable curry: 400 calories, 20g fat
Chapati: 150 calories, 1g fat
Naan: 300 calories, 16g fat
Lentil dhal: 200 calories, 8g fat

Baked potato A take-away baked potato is high in fibre and carbohydrate and low in fat, with moderate calories.Lower-fat toppings are tuna in low-fat dressing, cottage cheese, baked beans, chilli beans or fromage frais with chives. All also contain protein, helping to a better balance. An average 250g (9 oz) baked potato with a high-fat topping will be about 350 calories; with a lower-fat topping, about 250 calories. A bowl of salad balances the meal.

Doner kebab A kebab made from lean lamb and stuffed into pitta bread, with a generous portion of salad, can be a fairly well-balanced meal, containing carbs, protein and fat in reasonable proportions, as well as iron, fibre, calcium and other vitamins and minerals. However, it may be high in salt and, if the lamb is fatty and if a high-fat dressing is added, fat content may increase to 40g or more.

For those wishing to avoid meat, a pitta stuffed with salad and hummus would be a good idea — the hummus contains a lot of fat, but mostly unsaturated, and the chickpeas are nutritious.

Fried Chicken This is usually breaded (with fatty skin on) and then deep-fried, turning a low-fat source of protein into high-fat. An average small piece (90g with bone) contains around 200-250 calories and about 10-15g fat.

Side dishes may include coleslaw, high in fat at around 11g, and in calories, with 120 per small portion, or baked or barbecued beans, which are a better bet at around 100 calories and only 1-2g fat per portion, plus plenty of fibre and iron.

Vegetarian eating

A vegetarian diet is typically thought of as very healthy — and, certainly, that can be true. However, if you — or any of your family — are thinking of joining the estimated 3.5 million vegetarians in the UK, it is important to understand the possible pitfalls, as well as to enjoy the benefits that giving up meat may bring.

One-quarter of households now have a family member who is vegetarian; the meat-free meals market is growing at a rate of 90% a year, and at least 25% of all females aged between 16 and 24 are vegetarian. Statistically, if you choose to go vegetarian — eating no meat, poultry, fish or flesh of any kind — you are choosing an option that should boost your chances of living a long and healthy life. Large research studies conducted over the past decade agree that, compared to non-vegetarians, vegetarians have up to 30% less heart disease, up to 40% less cancer, 20% less premature mortality, less obesity, lower blood pressure and less occurrence of several other disorders.

However, statistics are not always as straightforward as they may seem — these results may also reflect the fact that most vegetarians have other lifestyle factors which may influence their health. For example, many are non-smokers and the level of alcoholism amongst them is low. Vegetarians may generally be more health-conscious; for example, taking more exercise.

The health-giving properties of a typical vegetarian diet may also not simply be due to it containing no flesh. The benefits may be, for example, from eating more plant foods, such as fresh fruits and vegetables, grains and pulses, thus bringing the diet more in line with the healthy blueprint outlined in the previous pages of this section — more carbohydrate, more fibre, more vitamin C, more phytochemicals. Vegetarians, on average, have a lower body weight than non-vegetarians, and lower calorie intake has also been linked with longer lifespan. The vegetarian diet will also probably be higher in unsaturated fats (though this isn't always the case) and higher in essential fatty acids than that of a meat eater.

Indeed, other statistics back up the theory that it isn't just giving up meat that procures the health benefits for the vegetarian. For example, health benefits similar to the vegetarian diet have been found in non-vegetarians who tend to eat high amounts of fruit and vegetables and little dairy produce. The population of the Greek island of Crete in the Mediterranean has extremely low rates of heart disease, cancer, obesity and early death, while eating meat in moderation and above average amounts of fish.

That is significant because there are certainly many vegetarians who, despite getting no saturated fat from meat, will be getting just as much saturated fat as meat eaters by replacing meat protein with an increased intake of dairy-based protein foods, such as cheese, milk and eggs. There are also unknown numbers of vegetarians who eat little fresh fruit and vegetables and exist on a vegetarian version of a junk diet. Teenage vegetarians seem particularly prone to eating an unbalanced and/or unvaried diet (see the Teenage Section, page 166).

The moral here appears to be that a healthy diet — whether vegetarian or non-vegetarian — is one high in natural plant foods (fresh fruits and vegetables, grains, nuts, seeds, pulses), low-fat and non-animal fat sources of protein, and natural oils. If a vegetarian diet fits in with this blueprint then it will be healthy. The things to watch out for when starting a vegetarian diet are:

✳ Don't just give up meat and not replace it with other sources of the important nutrients that meat contains, particularly protein, selenium, iron and B vitamins.

✳ Don't just use dairy produce as a meat replacement — if you do, you are likely to be eating too much saturated fat. However, low-fat dairy products, such as skimmed

---

VEGETARIAN SOURCES OF:

Iron - curry powder, cast-iron cooking utensils, ground ginger, seaweed, fortified breakfast cereals, lentils, cocoa powder, sesame seeds, pumpkin seeds, soya beans, soya mince, dried peaches, haricot beans, red kidney beans, cashew nuts, pot barley, couscous, bulgar wheat, dried apricots, dark green leafy vegetables, eggs, brown rice, baked beans in tomato sauce, broccoli.
Selenium - Brazil nuts, lentils, sunflower seeds, wholemeal bread, cashew nuts, walnuts.
Calcium - poppy seeds, Parmesan cheese, Gruyère cheese, Cheddar cheese, Edam, sesame seeds, mozzarella, Brie, tofu, Danish blue cheese, feta cheese, white chocolate, almonds, soya beans, figs, milk chocolate, yoghurt, haricot beans, spinach, brazil nuts, chickpeas, kale, white bread, milk, prawns, broccoli, spring greens, white cabbage.

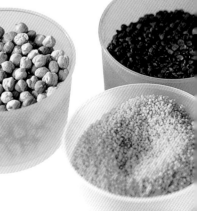

THE VEGETARIAN STORECUPBOARD

Here is a list of items you will find invaluable in your store if catering for a vegetarian or converting to vegetarianism yourself. Remember even store-cupboard items deteriorate with time, so don't buy large packs for one person, as they may not be eaten soon enough. When buying for the storecupboard, as much as when buying fresh foods, buy the best quality you can.

✳ Dried pulses of several kinds, including various lentils and an assortment of differently coloured and textured beans, plus chickpeas.

✳ Canned beans, chickpeas and lentils as above; especially good if you are busy. Chickpeas are an ideal standby for a quick snack — puréed with olive oil and garlic, they make a quick and tasty hummus.

✳ Grains which don't take long to prepare, such as quick-cook rice, couscous, bulgar.

✳ Other grains, such as barley and millet, which are useful for casseroles — or you can buy packs of mixed grains.

✳ Selection of pastas and noodles, at least some wholewheat, and some quick-cook polenta. Breakfast oats and muesli.

✳ Flours of various kinds, such as buckwheat and wholewheat (useful for pancakes, which can be made and frozen).

✳ Dried fruits, including peaches, apricots, prunes, figs, dates, sultanas.

✳ Cans of tomatoes and other vegetables which are good in cans, such as sweet peppers and artichoke hearts.

✳ Cans of ready-made hummus, pasta and pizza sauces.

✳ Dried spices and herbs, chilli sauce, soya sauce, black bean sauce.

✳ Jars or tubes of tomato paste, passata, black and green stoned olives, olive pâté, pesto.

✳ Vegetarian stock cubes and Worcestershire sauce.

✳ A good selection of oils and vinegars.

✳ Honey and good-quality unrefined sugar.

---

milk and low-fat natural yoghurt, are good — providing calcium as well as protein. Eggs are a good source of iron and vitamins, and also provide protein. Their saturated fat and cholesterol content mean that they shouldn't be relied on too heavily, especially for anyone who has been asked by their physician to follow a low-cholesterol, low-fat diet.

✳ Do eat plenty of plant sources of protein, such as pulses of all kinds and soya-based products, such as tofu, and, if you like it, textured vegetable protein (TVP). Quorn is a protein food made from a commercially manufactured mycoprotein similar to the protein to be found in mushrooms.

✳ Do take care to eat plenty of vegetarian sources of iron, selenium, and calcium (see box opposite). Red meat is rich is easily-absorbed iron (haem iron); the iron from plant sources (non-haem iron) is less well absorbed, but with care a vegetarian diet can provide enough. In a recent survey, selenium levels have been found to be low in vegetarians and vegans, but this varies from area to area. Vegetarians cutting down on dairy produce may have a problem, therefore, maintaining calcium intake and should eat plenty of seeds, tofu, pulses, nuts and leafy vegetables.

✳ Do be wary of eating too many sweet foods, such as pastries, biscuits, cakes and chocolate. These are all often high in fat, trans fats and calories, and eating

too many of them will almost certainly mean you are less likely to be filling up on more nutritious foods.

✳ Do get plenty of the foods rich in essential fatty acids, such as nuts, seeds and plant oils. If you don't eat fish you will be missing out on the omega-3 fatty acids EPA and DHA, but these can be converted in the body from alpha-linolenic acid, and linseeds (flaxseeds), linseed oil, hemp seeds and hemp seed oil, and walnuts are some of the best sources. The healthiest vegetarian diets are those that:

✳ Follow the general principles for healthy eating as outlined in this section.

✳ Contain a wide variety of fresh, natural and whole foods.

✳ Do not contain too much high-fat dairy produce to replace meat poultry and fish.

✳ Do not rely on too many sweet low-nutrient foods.

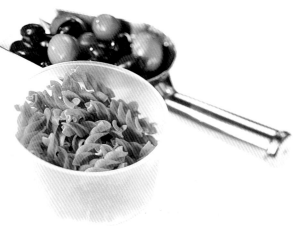

Plant protein versus animal protein

Until recently it was thought that, because most plant proteins (excluding soya beans) were 'incomplete' (i.e., not containing all eight of the essential amino acids), vegetarians should combine different protein sources at each meal to obtain all eight amino acids to provide 'complete' protein. The latest advice, though, says that a varied diet on a daily basis, containing a wide range of vegetarian protein foods, is sufficient, without worrying too much about providing 'complete' protein at every meal.

However, the Vegetarian Society makes an exception for pre-school children, whose parents are advised to use the combining method at every meal, to ensure adequate protein intake. This method means mixing pulses with grains (e.g. beans on toast, pitta and hummus, rice and bean salad), grains with a dairy product (e.g. cheese on toast, cereal and milk), or pulses plus starch (e.g. potato and lentil casserole.)

Studies of adult vegetarians show that they tend to consume lower levels of protein than non-vegetarians. However, as we have seen earlier in Section One, many of us tend to eat more (sometimes much more) protein than we need.

For more on protein see page 20. For more on children and teenagers and a vegetarian diet, see page 168.

The lone vegetarian in the family

Catering for a sole vegetarian may seem daunting, and can create extra work. Here are some ideas to make catering easier:

* Gradually introduce more non-meat meals into the whole family's menus — many of the recipes at the back of the book should inspire you. Meat lovers will appreciate the robust flavours and textures of brown or green lentils and several of the pulses, especially Egyptian brown beans, borlotti beans and black beans.
* Make full use of pasta — you can cook pasta with a vegetarian sauce based on tomatoes or pesto, for example, freezing the surplus sauce in batches, and serve a sauce with added meat for the rest of the family. Again, vegetarian pasta dishes make an excellent dish for meat eaters anyway.
* Some vegetarian dishes are easy to cook ahead and freeze. Things like bean casseroles, curries based on potatoes, aubergines, squash (freeze undercooked), nut and bean burgers and loaves all freeze successfully.
* Make main-course salads for the whole family and substitute non-vegetarian items for the lone veggie, e.g. salade Niçoise for the family, but use silken tofu instead of tuna for the vegetarian.
* For lunches or suppers, make chunky soups which are basically vegetarian and committed meat eaters can add chunks of chicken, ham, prawns, etc.
* Pizzas please everyone — and, again, you can add small amounts of shellfish or meat topping as required.
* Pulses are an important nutritional source for vegetarians — canned, pre-cooked beans are fine, and widely available, but if you do soak and boil your own pulses you can freeze leftovers in individual bags for another occasion.
* There is now a wide range of healthy non-meat and non-dairy burgers, rashers, sausages and patties available in the supermarkets, many of which also contain no trans fats.

It is important to find out just what a vegetarian will and will not eat before cooking anything for him or her.

See the box on the left for different types of vegetarian. See the second box on the right for a list of items which may also be on the 'banned' list if the vegetarian is strict.

DIFFERENT TYPES OF 'VEGETARIAN'

Demi-vegetarian: Will (usually) eat everything except red meat. Sometimes poultry is also excluded, but fish is included, though may be eaten only infrequently.

Lacto-ovo-vegetarian: Will eat all dairy produce and eggs, but no flesh of any kind.

Lacto-vegetarian: Will eat all dairy produce, but no eggs or flesh of any kind.

Vegan: Eats only plant foods — no dairy products, eggs or flesh. (See The Vegan Diet opposite.)

Fruitarian: Eats only fruits (at least 75% of diet), uncooked vegetables (mostly leafy vegetables), raw nuts, seeds and beansprouts.

Sproutarian: Eats mostly sprouted seeds, grains, pulses and rice.

Macrobiotic: Excludes all meat, poultry, dairy produce and eggs, but at initial levels may eat fish. Diet may progressively become more and more restricted, with the final level being a diet of brown rice only.

NOTE: These last three are not diets recommended by qualified nutritionists, as they will fall short of a variety of nutrients. The more restricted any diet is, the more chance that your full nutrient quota will not be met.

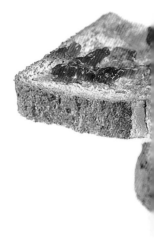

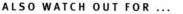

SAMPLE DIET

DAY ONE
Breakfast
muesli with skimmed milk
wholewheat bread with olive oil spread and
marmalade
1 orange
Lunch
Chunky Vegetable and Lentil Soup
pitta bread
slice of vegetarian cake
banana and yoghurt
Evening
Pasta with Basil and Ricotta
large mixed salad
Raspberry Gratin

DAY TWO
Breakfast
porridge with skimmed milk
wholemeal bread with olive oil margarine
and Marmite
fruit juice
Lunch
Chickpea Salad with Peppers and Tomatoes
pitta bread
Evening
Winter Squash with Lentils and Ginger
kale
1 orange

ALSO WATCH OUT FOR ...

Rennet: This enzyme from the stomach of animals is used in the production of many hard cheeses (as a curdling agent) and, therefore, these cheeses are unsuitable for most vegetarians. If a hard cheese isn't labelled 'vegetarian', it probably does contain rennet. Many hard cheeses are now being produced without rennet, using plant curdling agents, and these are widely available.

Gelatine: Derived from the bones of animals (often cows) and therefore obviously unacceptable to most vegetarians. Can be present in any commercial dessert or product requiring a setting agent — e.g. mousses, moulds, jellies, even fruit yoghurts. The vegetarian alternative is agar-agar, derived from seaweed and fairly easy to obtain.

Worcestershire sauce: Usually contains anchovies, but some brands don't, so read the label.

Stock cubes: Vegetable stock cubes are usually free of animal produce, but it is worth reading the label.

Margarine: May contain fish oils. Read the label.

Honey: Some vegetarians and most vegans won't eat honey; best to check.

When catering for any type of vegetarian it is best to talk to them to discover just exactly how strict they are. Some vegetarians also require the use of organic produce and/or whole foods.

The vegan diet

Vegans eat no dairy produce of any kind, or eggs, or anything from an animal, including honey. Nutritionally, a vegan diet is quite restricted. Calorie consumption is consistently lower in vegans than in non-vegetarians and in vegetarians, because the diet contains more high-bulk/low-calorie foods like fruits and vegetables, and protein intake is about 75% of average. The nutrients that may be in shortfall are calcium, selenium, iodine, vitamins B12 and vitamin D, and possibly riboflavin.

However, the average vegan diet provides MORE than the national average of vitamin C, magnesium, copper, folate, beta-carotene and essential fatty acids.

Total fat intake is about 25% lower than average and saturate intake is 50% lower than average, while average carbohydrate intake is nearly 55% — an optimum level, and fibre intake is also higher than the national average and higher, indeed, than in ordinary vegetarian diets.

Several recent studies have found that a vegan diet may hold back children's development physically and impair their mental agility – damage which can't be reversed by reverting to a non-vegan diet after 16. However, these findings are disputed by the pro-vegan lobby, and children on a vegan diet which is as comprehensive and varied as possible may not be at risk.

✱ Vegan sources of:
Calcium: Fortified soya milk, white bread, baked beans, dried figs, leafy green vegetables, tofu, nuts, muesli, pulses.
Selenium: Brazil nuts, lentils, sunflower seeds, wholemeal bread, cashew nuts.
Iodine: Seaweed, Vecon, kelp supplements.
Vitamin B12: fortified breakfast cereals, fortified soya milk, Vecon, fortified bread.
Vitamin D: Fortified vegetarian margarines, fortified breakfast cereals, fortified soya milk, sunlight.
Riboflavin: fortified breakfast cereal, soya milk, fortified soya milk, Marmite, Vecon.

Eating out and entertaining

As eating out and having friends round to dinner are such enjoyable things to do, it is a shame that special-occasion meals so often seem to incur guilt and result in several pounds of weight-gain. Here's how to pick the wisest choices from the menu or the cookery book — and still have fun.

The degree to which eating out or entertaining affect your nutritional status — and your size — is dependent upon two factors. First, how often you do it. If your eating out is restricted to a few times a year, then it really doesn't matter a great deal what you choose or how much you eat (with the proviso that, if you suddenly indulge in an over-rich large meal after a lengthy period of eating more healthily, your digestive system may well complain, see Heartburn and Indigestion, page 118).

However, many people find that if they add up business lunches and dinners, private invitations and restaurant meals, they are eating out almost as often as they eat at home. In such a case, it is very important to pick and choose from what is on offer to please your health as well as your taste-buds. This is the second factor — making sensible choices.

For those who experience 'special occasion' eating all too frequently, the next few pages of this section really are required reading.

Lunching

Eating out at lunch-time is much more likely to be a 'duty' lunch these days than a long, lingering pleasure lunch. If the latter, read the notes about restaurant meals below.

The average business lunch, luckily for our waistlines, no longer needs to be an over-indulgent, overlong affair. For most occasions, it is perfectly acceptable to restrict the meal to one — or, possibly, two — light course(s), usually avoiding a dessert. Alcohol figures less and less at lunch-time; if you are doing the entertaining, always offer alcohol but don't feel obliged to indulge too — iced water is fine.

If you are choosing the lunch-time venue and are lucky enough to have a wide choice nearby, suitably light menus can be found at fish restaurants, Japanese restaurants, modern English or French restaurants. Most top chefs, whose ideas are often multinational, are very aware of the demand for light and healthy meals.

When picking from any lunch-time menu, try to remember the guidelines for healthy eating at lunch-time (see page 46), remembering that a starchy high-carbohydrate meal, such as a large pasta dish, may leave you less than alert all afternoon. A salad or light fish dish would be ideal, with a fruit starter and some good bread.

Consider also what you will be eating later in the day, if you know, and choose a lunch to balance that out.

For further guidelines on specific healthy and less healthy choices, read the tips below.

Evening eating

It has been estimated that the average person who goes to a restaurant or to someone else's house for an evening meal, will eat in that one meal at least a whole day's normal calorie intake and probably more. Statistics also show that food eaten outside the home contains, on average, more fat and saturated fat than that eaten inside the home — an average of 50% of the calories in 'outside' food comes from fat. So anyone who eats out regularly will almost certainly be putting on weight and eating a diet unhealthily high in fat and saturated fat.

The two major considerations, then, may be to restrict the calories in your restaurant meals and to cut the fat. Protein needs are normally more than adequately met by the average restaurant meal but, as with take-aways, some thought may be needed to pick a meal which contains adequate fibre and fresh fruit and/or vegetables.

Here are some general tips which will help you to achieve this:
* Take some plain bread from the bread basket, but avoid the butter.
* Vow to pick only one rich course at any meal; make the others light.
* Unless unavoidable, have only two courses.
* Try to pick at least one course based on fruit and/or salad — e.g. a salad starter, a fruit dessert.
* Choose plenty of vegetables with your main course. Avoid restaurants where vegetable portions are minuscule.
* Watch out for added butter, fats, cream and cheese in each course. Anything fried, sautéed or sauced may be very high in fat.
* If enjoying a private informal occasion, many calories and much fat can be saved without lessening enjoyment if you share a dish. For example, there are six of you at a restaurant meal. None of you are hungry after your main course, but you want to taste dessert. You choose just two or three different desserts and pass them round. Most restaurants accept this solution with good grace.
* If the meal is the kind where you serve yourself, serve small portions of the high-fat items.

■ Now we look at some popular types of restaurant and pick out the best choices for health, and the less good.

French Traditional French cuisine has always been very heavy in calories and fat; everything cooked in butter, cream and buttery sauces. More modern French chefs are moving away from this and producing lighter healthier versions of old

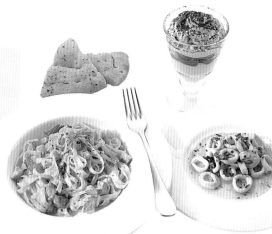

TYPICAL ITALIAN RESTAURANT MEAL

2,050 calories, 100g fat (approx).

Choose this meal — 45% of which is fat — and you will be eating all your day's calories (for most women) and more than a day's fat allowance for women OR men in one go. The meal is also low on fresh fruits and vegetables and fibre. Italian garlic flat bread, 75 g (approx. 350 calories, 12 g fat)

Starter: portion of calamari (fried squid), (approx 300 calories, 15 g fat).

Main course: portion of Pasta Carbonara (approx 900 calories, 45 g fat). This dish of pasta with a sauce made from eggs, cream and bacon is very high in fat and saturates.

Dessert: Portion of tiramisu (approx 500 calories, 30 g fat). Made from eggs and mascarpone cheese, this trifle is a typically rich Italian dessert.

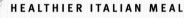

HEALTHIER ITALIAN MEAL ★★★★★

1,150 calories, 41 g fat (approx).

With almost half the calories and less than half the fat and plenty of fresh fruit/ salad. Plain bread, 75 g (approx. 240 calories, 5 g fat)

Starter: Melon and Parma ham (approx 150 calories, 5 g fat). Melon provides vitamin C and fibre, and average portion Parma ham weighs only 50 g or so, so fat content is relatively low.

Main course: Spaghetti Napoletana (approx 450 calories, 10 g fat). Large mixed side salad with olive oil dressing (120 calories, 10 g fat). Sauces based on tomato are ideal Italian food — seafood or a little grated cheese can be added for protein. The salad provides vitamin C, and fibre. The dressing provides healthy olive oil.

Dessert: Portion zabaglione (200 calories, 11 g fat). A fairly low-calorie treat.

favourites. In general, however, many French restaurants still seem reluctant to give decent amounts of vegetables and rely too heavily on the 'protein first, forget the carbohydrates' approach. The further south the influence, the healthier a French meal may be, becoming more Mediterranean in outlook.

* Go for: 'Provençal' cooking, e.g. dishes rich in tomatoes, peppers or onions, for instance. These may be high in olive oil and therefore calories, though, so choose a very light starter or dessert to balance the calories out. Grilled fish and mussels marinière are also good choices.

* Think twice: anything 'meunière'; in a rich butter sauce; cream sauces, creamy mousses; hearty French casseroles made with lardons or pork, for instance; profiteroles, gâteaux.

Italy Northern Italian food can also be very high in fat and calories — it is the southern Italian food which is healthier, although high in calorie-rich olive oil. Many of the Italian restaurants found in the UK mix the cuisine of both north and south Italy, but the good news is that in almost all Italian cafés there will be a good choice of healthy alternatives.

* Go for: vegetable and fruit starters, such as grilled vegetables or artichoke salad, figs and Parma ham or a healthy bean soup; pasta dishes without a creamy sauce, e.g. tomato-based sauces, seafood sauces, pesto; chicken cacciatore, tuna and white bean salad; grilled calves' liver and broccoli, squid (casseroled not deep-fried).

* Think twice: pasta dishes laden with cream and cheese, such as cannelloni or carbonara; pasta dishes with meat, such as Bolognese; deep-fried calamari; antipasto platters heavy with fatty deli meats. Most risottos in restaurants are very high in butter and/or oil and perhaps cheese too.

Pizzas are extremely variable — meat and cheese toppings are high in fat and calories, but tomato and seafood and vegetable toppings are better. Many Italian deserts are extremely high in calories and fat, so stick with granitas, fresh fruit or baked peaches most of the time.

Far East Chinese, Thai, Japanese and most Far-Eastern cooking will be able to provide you with a reasonable amount of healthy choices, but you need to be careful. You may find portion sizes quite large and fat content may be high, especially in Thai cooking, which uses a lot of coconut cream. However, many dishes are rich in vegetables, fibre and vitamin C, although many Eastern dishes are high in salt.

✱ Go for: chicken and sweetcorn or hot-and-sour soup; stir-fries of vegetables and prawns, pork, tofu or chicken, rice or noodles; casseroles of chicken, tofu or prawns and vegetables; spare ribs (dry), teriyaki, plain cooked rice, chilli prawns or crab; sushi; lychees.

✱ Think twice: spring rolls, deep-fried dumplings, deep-fried pork (etc.) in batter; tempura, special fried rice, spare ribs in wet sauce; coconut curries; caramel bananas.

Indian Much traditional Indian cuisine is well balanced nutritionally, with plenty of complex carbohydrate and vegetables and much protein coming from plant sources. However, many Westernised Indian restaurants cater to the Western taste and offer more dishes rich in animal proteins, fat and cream. Try to find Indian restaurants which base their cooking on traditional lines. Even so, if you are watching your weight, be aware that many Indian dishes may be very high in oil. Spices can be good for the digestion, stimulating and metabolism-boosting.

✱ Go for: vegetable-based curries, lentil dhal, rice, flat breads including chapati; tandooris, fresh fruit salads, mangoes.

✱ Think twice: masalas and korma curries containing cream; coconut curries, deep-fried samosas, bhajis.

Traditional English/Steak Bars/Carveries
If you often eat at traditional British restaurants and carveries you will, unless you are very careful, be getting an unbalanced diet, high in protein, high

MENU IDEAS FOR ENTERTAINING:

Marinated herbed shiitake mushrooms
Seared tuna with lemon grass
Blackberry Ice

Baked baby tomatoes and basil
Turkish Lamb Stew
Stir-fried Fruit Salad

Cucumber and Mint Soup
Parcels of Tilapia, Tomatoes and Olives
Mango Filo Tarts

Mushroom and Red Pepper Skewers
Thai Guinea Fowl with Cashews and Pineapple
Citrus Granita

in fat, low in carbohydrate, fruits and vegetables. A typical steak bar meal of prawn cocktail, steak and chips, gâteau or cheese and biscuits will probably contain at least a day's recommended maximum fat, saturated fat and protein.

✱ Go for: melon; grilled/roast chicken, turkey, salmon, trout; baked potatoes; large salad bowl; sorbet; strawberries, ice-cream.

✱ Think twice: pâté, prawn cocktail; large steaks, French fries; apple pie and cream.

■ Healthy eating at home

If you like to entertain, you have total control over what you serve and so choosing a healthy but delicious menu shouldn't be a problem. People no longer feel cheated if they aren't served a meal rich with butter, cream and thick sauces at every course. Tastes, colours and presentation are important, and a well-planned ethnic-style meal will always be appreciated.

Many of the recipes in this book are ideal for entertaining and some suggested three-course menus appear in the panel above. Here are some more tips

to help you plan a special, but balanced and nutritious meal.

✱ For pre-dinner nibbles, serve crudités, and perhaps Italian sesame breadsticks, with one of the dips that appear in the recipe section — such as anchoïade, skordalia, rouille or baba ganoush. These are much less salty than most crisps and salted nuts.

✱ Decide on your main course first and then plan a starter and dessert to balance it. For instance, a meat main course would require a vegetarian or light fish or shellfish starter. Whereas, if you are serving a high-carbohydrate main course, such as pasta, your starter could be a small portion of a high-protein food, such as crab or prawns. Try to include salad/vegetables or fruit with every course — e.g. a crab salad starter, a roast vegetable and grain main course and a fruit dessert.

✱ Quick, healthy and easy starters are grilled peppers in a vinaigrette on herb salad; asparagus spears with balsamic vinegar; artichoke hearts bottled in oil, drained and served with quails' eggs.

✱ If you are short of time, don't bother to make a dessert — a selection of fresh fruits with goats' cheese and oatcakes is ideal. Quick hardly-any-cooking desserts are fresh fruit compotes (e.g. lightly cooked summer fruits simmered in wine) or flambéed pineapples and bananas.

■ Before you think of drinking and driving

If you eat out in the evening, it is easy to notch up several alcoholic drinks. If you have to drive, however, be wary of how many units you take, however sober you may feel. As we saw on page 36, a unit of alcohol contains 8g of pure alcohol and safe limits for health are up to 3 units a day for women and 4 for men. To most people, though, this means little in terms of how much they can drink before their blood alcohol concentration rises to a level which means it is unwise to drive.

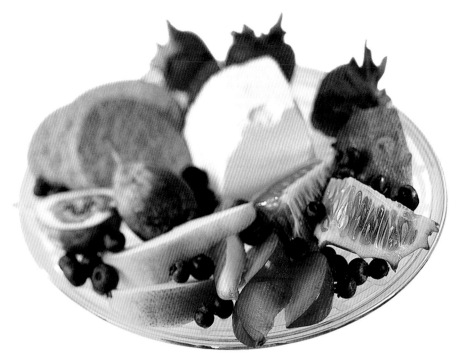

In the UK, you are 'over the limit' if your blood alcohol concentration is more than 80 mg alcohol per 100 ml blood (though this may soon be lowered by 50 mg in the UK). As a guide, a man can drink up to seven units of alcohol in an evening (four hours) with food, and a woman up to five units, before going over the limit. However, not everyone will have the same blood alcohol concentration after drinking the same amount. Generally, taller, heavier people can drink more than shorter, lighter people before reaching 80mg/100ml. Also, young people and people not used to drink will probably be more easily affected by the alcohol, and women are more quickly affected than men because they have a higher percentage of body fat and lower percentage of body fluid (for dilution of the alcohol) than men.

Moreover, if you drink quickly, your blood alcohol concentration will also go up more quickly. If a man takes five units, or a woman 3-4 units, in just one hour instead of in a whole evening, he or she will almost certainly be over the legal driving limit. It will then take a wait of 1 to 3 hours to get the levels below 80mg/100ml again.

The chart below gives a guide to what constitutes being 'at the limit' — but remember, it is only a guide, and different people may reach their limit on less alcohol. Even after just one or two units, judgement is impaired and, even though you may be below the legal limit for driving, it is safest not to drive after drinking any alcohol at all. The following tips may help you reduce your alcohol intake — and/or blood alcohol concentration — when eating socially:

✻ Remember that food slows down the absorption of alcohol. Try not to drink anything alcoholic before you start to eat; on an empty stomach it will rapidly cause a rise in your blood alcohol levels.

✻ Don't start the evening by quenching thirst with alcohol — quench it with water. You will find that you drink much more slowly then.

✻ Drink slowly. Alternate alcohol with water as much as possible.

✻ For your own guests, make sure there are plenty of low-alcohol or alcohol-free drink alternatives available — in winter, a low-alcohol punch, in summer a low-alcohol sangria (see page 254), plus juices, mineral water and alcohol-free beers and wine.

✻ Don't think that strong coffee will 'sober you up' or lower blood alcohol levels. Neither will running round the block or drinking water or vitamin C. Once the alcohol is in your body, nothing can do this except time. A healthy liver 'neutralizes' the alcohol at the rate of approximately one unit per hour (though this varies with individuals).

Alarmingly, this could mean that, if you have had a very heavy evening's drinking — say, two large gins, a bottle of 12% alcohol by volume wine and a large brandy (15 units altogether) — you would still be over the legal driving limit the following morning.

THAT'S THE LIMIT

You will probably reach your blood alcohol concentration limit if you drink:

Men			
10 stone	3 units in 1 hour	5 units in 3 hours	6 units in 4 hours
12 stone	4 units in l hour	6 units in 3 hours	7 units in 4 hours
Women			
8 stone	2 units in 1 hour	3 units in 3 hours	4 units in 4 hours
10 stone	2½ units in 1 hour	4 units in 3 hours	5 units in 4 hours

FOOD FROM FARM TO TABLE

The one healthy eating issue that seems to concern most people these days is that of food safety. In this section we analyse every area of this understandable concern — right from the beginning, down on the farm.

Modern 'factory farming' is the result of our international quest for cheap and plentiful foods, in the face of a growing population. However, such intensive farming has brought all kinds of problems and these do need to be faced.

We look at crop farming and the methods employed by the arable farmers in order to maximize their yields. Chemical farming is of increasing concern to many of us — so the facts and the alternatives are discussed. Similarly, especially since the BSE crisis, people are worried about intensive animal farming, so we look at just how good or bad factory-farmed produce IS for your health, and offer alternatives where possible and if necessary.

Food preservation is another area of possible concern. We are all so keen on being able to buy a wide variety of produce out of season, all year round, that we may not always realize just how some foods look so fresh ...

And the ones that DON'T look fresh inside those packets and cans, shrink-wraps and jars — are they OK, or should we give them a miss? Are our Governments protecting us enough from harmful additives — or is there still cause to worry?

The issue of food poisoning is discussed in detail and we look at ways to avoid the risks, again from farm to table. We also look at all the other food safety issues that each of us can help to prevent by buying, storing, preparing and cooking our food properly. From the shop to YOUR table — food safety really is in your hands.

In fact, in a way all food safety is in our hands. The choices we make about the things that we buy, where we buy them, and how much we are prepared to pay, are what will make the difference to the quality and the safety of the food that we eat in the long term.

When it comes to food, the choice IS yours. Let it be the right one.

Food production

The way in which we grow our crops, rear cattle and even fish the seas has changed dramatically in the last generation.

Crops

After the Second World War, the use of chemicals in the production of our food crops — everything from grains to vegetables, fruits and salads, from field to orchard to greenhouse — quickly became standard procedure. It seemed nothing but a good idea to use pesticides to kill insects and other creatures that were damaging crops, herbicides to kill weeds that were choking them and fungicides to cure diseases, as well as applying artificial fertilisers to help maintain the fertility of the new-style large-scale farms where, with the help of modern mechanization, food production could be vastly increased by growing just one type of crop on the same land, year after year.

Within a decade or two we had — almost miraculously — food that was plentiful, cheap and widely available. Most crops were also better to look at and more regular in shape, and as they appeared clean they no longer needed scrubbing before use... 'advantages' that most people now take for granted.

As the agri-industry took off, farms became vast and specialized; hedges, woods, ponds and wildlife disappeared and, by the '80s, hundreds of different chemicals were being used to bring us our food as a matter of course. Chemicals which often lingered on in the food that we ate but which were declared safe.

Nowadays, many crops are also sprayed after being harvested with preservatives and inhibitors to prolong their life for transportation, storage (sometimes for months) and shelf-life. Such sprays are even more likely to linger as residues on the food that we eat.

TIPS ON MINIMIZING RESIDUES

* Wash all fruits and vegetables thoroughly before eating
* Peel vegetables and fruits where appropriate
* Discard outer leaves of lettuce, cabbage, etc
* Never eat the green end of a carrot — remove at least 2.5 cm (1 inch) of the carrot below the stalk and peel a thick layer off carrots before use; residues of toxic organophosphates have, in past years, been found to be over safe limits.

By the '90s, the drawbacks of intensive farming were beginning to become apparent. Many people did not enjoy the idea of eating foods which might well be contaminated with chemical residues. They also began to worry about the effect of the agricultural industry on the environment, as it became clear that it has destroyed much of our wildlife by killing off the insects at the lower end of the food chain, by denuding the countryside and destroying natural habitats, and by polluting rivers. It has also interfered with traditional natural processes, such as pollination, because pesticides can't tell the difference between 'pests' and 'good' insects like bees. It has also helped to deplete the ozone layer.

Ironically, as the '90s progressed, it also became apparent that many common pesticides no longer actually work — the pests and diseases are becoming resistant to the chemicals the industry uses. Nowadays it can take only as little as two years for a pest to develop complete resistance to a new chemical. Fertilizers, too, often need to be used in larger and larger quantities to achieve the required results, and artificially fertilized soils may well be quite deficient in vital nutrients such as selenium.

■ What controls are there for our food safety?

Since 1977 there has been a working party on pesticide residues which spends about £2 million annually (a very small sum, in fact) on policing food production, and produces an annual report on levels of residues found in spot-checks throughout the UK. This working party is responsible to the Food Standards Agency, an independent organization launched in April 2000. The FSA is responsible for setting standards in UK food safety and nutrition, and reports to the Government. Acceptable and maximum residue levels are set by law, and any food producer found to exceed these levels may be prosecuted. In recent years, maximum safe levels have been exceeded in many chemicals on a variety of different crops, and in 2006 39% of sampled crops in our stores had residues present and 2% of these were above the MRLs. Over the years, the Government has been unable to bring down these residue levels. In a similar 2006 survey, 66% of school fruit was contaminated.

Another problem may be that, even if maximum levels are not being exceeded in isolation, if we take official advice and 'eat more fruit and vegetables' and more plant foods to prevent diseases such as cancer and CHD, we will inevitably be consuming more and more of these toxic chemicals — for that is what they are. The exact cumulative effect of a range of killer chemicals eaten over a person's lifetime, in doses individually declared officially safe, is yet to be assessed. Perhaps we should also remember that, from time to time, chemicals previously generally thought to be safe are withdrawn from use.

More and more crops are being imported into the UK, and these may be even more difficult to police. So, for those of us who believe that modern intensive agriculture has too many drawbacks, what are the alternatives?

Integrated crop management (ICM)

This is a kind of 'halfway house' between modern agrochemical and organic farming, and has been promoted and invested in heavily by all the major UK supermarkets in the past few years. ICM 'borrows' organic and traditional ideas, such as crop rotation and using natural predators to control pests. It also uses innovations (with the help of gene technology, see opposite), such as disease- and pest-resistant varieties of crops, but doesn't ban the use of chemicals in certain circumstances (e.g., 68 different pesticides are still permitted on potatoes), simply trying to ensure 'broad-spectrum' chemicals are avoided where possible and that preventative mass crop spraying is discouraged.

Organic farming

Sales of organic food in the UK are increasing at around 12% a year, and is worth £1.2 billion annually. Now, organic farmers can't keep pace with demand from people willing to pay extra for food they perceive to be unadulterated, healthy and environment-friendly.

It is estimated that only 4% of UK farmland is organic at the moment, and 70% of the organic food that we buy imported. The UK's organic farming movement receives less government subsidy than those in other EU countries, but even so the amount of organic food produced here is sure to rise slowly — organic farming can take up to 5 years to establish.

Only a handful of chemicals (as opposed to about 300 in standard farming), including derris and pyrethrum, are allowed in organic farming under rules laid down in the UK by the Register of Organic Food Standards (UKRoFS), which allows 7 bodies, such as the Soil Association, to inspect and certify farms. Methods used are based on the traditional ones of keeping crops healthy with good soil, rotation and natural fertilizers, wherever possible, and choosing suitable crops for the local environment. Pests and weeds are normally controlled by natural predators and methods.

ORGANICS – PROS & CONS

Pros:

* Generally much lower residues of potentially dangerous chemicals and antibiotics.
* International studies confirm frequently much higher level of nutrients; important as, in general, levels of many essential vitamins and minerals in food have declined by up to 75% over last 50 years.
* Trials confirm that the longer growing/maturing periods and lower water content generally result in better-tasting plant and animal produce.

Cons:

* Usually 50–70% more expensive.
* Some say that UKROFS organic standards are too low. E.g., organic chicken and fish may still be kept in cages, and organic chicken and eggs come from hens given 20% non-organic feed.
* Imported organic food has travelled many air miles, and some foreign organic standards are lower than ours.
* Some organics needs to be consumed quickly because of lack of preservatives.

Genetic engineering

Huge multinationals have spent several years developing bio-technological ways to improve plants, so the need for chemicals will be minimized... they say.

However, the entire area of genetic modification is causing much debate — its ethics, its safety and so on. We look at the subject in more detail later in this section.

Animal and dairy production

As with crops, intensive farming of meat and other animal and dairy produce has brought us relatively inexpensive and plentiful food. The idea of 'factory farming', with animals kept in conditions far removed from nature, is now taken for granted by most of us. Even food sources once considered 'wild', such as salmon, trout and novel meats like ostrich and crocodile, are being farmed intensively all over the world production all right for our health?

■ Meat and poultry

How cheap meat is produced

Low-cost meat, in general, means animals that grow quickly and take up as little space, food and labour as possible in so doing. In order for this to happen, intensive farming may take on board several practices with which many people find they are becoming disenchanted.

* *Keeping feeding costs low*: To put animals out to graze on foods that are natural to them, such as grass, is highly space-consuming, and is not a fast way of adding weight. Therefore it is expensive. A much cheaper method is to keep them indoors and feed them on manufactured foods, such as pellets made from the ground-up remains of other animals. It is thought that such an unnatural diet may be one of the causes of BSE in cattle, for instance.

* *Restricting space*: By feeding animals and poultry on man-made produce they no longer need to roam fields. They can be kept in small spaces, such as barns and pens, which obviously means much less land is needed. Unfortunately, the animals don't get enough exercise, so they become less healthy with weak muscles. They also become more prone to infections, which can quickly spread through a farm. This means antibiotics need to be used almost constantly. Antibiotic residues can last through the food chain until our meat and dairy food is on the plate.

Animals that do graze on 'natural' pasture may be eating food that has been sprayed with chemical weed-killers and fertilizers, which may show up later in the meat and milk (see below).

Industry, too, may increase toxic residues, for instance the highly poisonous chemical dioxin is a by-product of several industrial processes or waste clearance. Radiation discharges from nuclear sites around the country also show up in all of our food, albeit in levels which the Government has decreed safe.

* *Speeding growth*: Intensively reared animals and poultry are often 'force-fed' on a diet unnaturally high in calories, with added nutrients, given automatically and regularly so that weight is gained uniformly and quickly. Today this is often not seen as good enough, and hormones which speed growth-rate, such as clenbuterol, are apparently finding their way into a small amount of our meat, even though the practice is illegal in Europe.

Legal drugs, such as antibiotic growth-promoters, are widely used in certain areas of meat farming. Waste products from intensive farming are also increasingly polluting our rivers.

All this means that it is impossible to prevent traces of toxic chemicals and drugs from arriving in the food chain, at least in some foods, some of the time. Residue levels are officially monitored, but there is concern, for example, that because we may unwittingly ingest antibiotics in our food, we too will become resistant to them.

For example, in 1997 it was reported that, in humans, over 80% of infections with a salmonella bug were resistant to a wide range of common antibiotics; a result, a leading public health doctor was reported as saying, of farming practices rather than medical overuse. A range of new, hormone-related illnesses and problems are also being noted in humans and may be related to the food chain.

Food poisoning with bugs such as E. coli is another increasing problem — meat is frequently the culprit, sometimes because of unhygienic handling or storage anywhere from slaughterhouse to table. Much stricter rules are being enforced by Government to help beat this problem, but it will take some time. This subject is dealt with in detail on page 81.

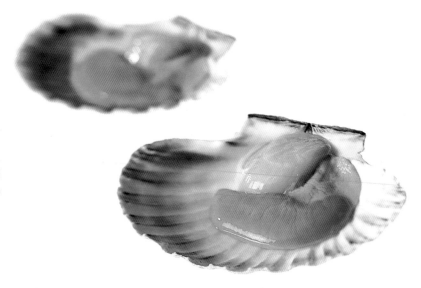

Making the meat you eat safer

✱ Organic outdoor-reared meat should be free from residues of artificial chemicals, antibiotics and hormones, though foreign imports may have been produced to lower standards than that of UK meat. Production is increasing and, although it is 30% more expensive than mass-produced meat, a little tends to go a long way — an idea that helps us eat a better-balanced diet anyway. Organic meat is produced using natural traditional rearing and living methods.

Many supermarkets, farm shops and websites now sell organic meat or, at least, offer a range produced using less intensive methods.

If you can't buy organic, aim to buy and eat lean meat. Residues tend to accumulate in fatty tissue. Think 'wild' – game meats are unlikely to be contaminated. And buy local, from a butcher you know and trust, and ask about the meat you're buying.

Beef and sheep

While the BSE scares of the late 20th century have largely died down, it is still present in the UK and other countries, and there is still a risk of variant CJD in humans exposed to BSE. The FSA says that the risk from BSE can't be completely removed, although strict safety measures make this risk very small.

You can reduce the risk further by following the tips here and:

✱ Buy only steaks and joints; avoid cheaper products like cheap sausages, pies and burgers.

✱ Buy organic beef – organic herds have very little incidence of BSE.

Meanwhile, a brain disease found in our sheep flocks – atypical scrapie – may be the 21st-century BSE. While the risk to humans is presently unknown, it is known that infected animals are entering the food chain but, by avoiding older meat and casings made from sheep's intestines (e.g. in traditional sausages), any risk of infection may be limited.

■ Fish and seafood

We are all being encouraged to eat more fish. It would therefore be nice to believe that at least the fish we eat is clean, with no residues of poisons, antibiotics, hormone-disturbing chemicals, etc.

Sadly, this is no longer the case. In Britain, the North Sea and river outlets are increasingly polluted by industrial waste, such as PCBs (polychlorinated biphenols) and dioxins. High concentrations of cadmium have been found in the livers of fish in the North Sea. Investigators have found that one-third of plaice had skin complaints, which were probably pollution-related.

Human waste in sewage can also cause some shellfish to harbour high levels of bacteria, and recent research found that industrial oestrogen-mimicking chemicals released into some of our river waters are causing up to 60% of male river fish to change sex!

Yet the alternative source of much of the fish that we eat — fish farming — also has its problems. Farmed salmon is reared in huge cages in lochs or coastal sea. These fish are often hosts to parasites, called sea lice, which are killed by means of antibiotics.

The farmed salmon usually also live in conditions not dissimilar to intensively reared animals, meaning diseases and other pests are becoming more common, and may be fed dyes to make them look pinker. Most worrying, though, is that they may be fed concentrated feed made from fish from polluted waters. Research has shown levels of PCB in one 100g portion of farmed salmon at over WHO limits.

FOR SAFER FISH

✱ Look for the MSC (Marine Stewardship Council) label on fish.
✱ Buy organic.
✱ White fish from the deeper waters, such as cod and haddock, is less likely to be affected by pollution.
✱ Scallops, crabs, lobsters and the prawn family are less likely to be affected by pollution/bacteria than shellfish that live on the shoreline, like mussels and oysters. The latter are cleaned before sale, or cultured, in which case they should be sold as such and be pollution-free naturally.
✱ Farmed organic fish, including cod, bass and other white sea fishes, is a good alternative to farmed salmon.
✱ Oily fish and fish livers are more likely to be affected as toxins such as cadmium and dioxins are stored in fat and liver. The FSA advises only one portion a week of farmed salmon.

Dairy produce and eggs

Nutritionally speaking, battery-raised eggs are not greatly different from free-range or organically-produced eggs. However, salmonella in eggs is still a big problem with intensively reared hens, and tests in 2000/1 showed traces of potentially harmful drug residues in 10% of eggs. Advice is still for the elderly, pregnant and ill not to eat raw eggs. More on how to avoid food poisoning appears on page 81.

Egg types and what they mean

* Battery eggs: These won't be labelled as such on the pack but nearly 90% of eggs sold in the UK are still from hens living in battery cages. These are the cheapest eggs to buy, and the hens are fed on a manufactured mixed diet that may include animal carcass by-products and medicines to keep diseases at bay.
* Barn eggs: Represent 4% of eggs sold; the hens live in barns and are free to move about, but may be overcrowded and their diet similar to that of caged hens.
* Free-range eggs: The conditions in which free-range hens are kept differ tremen-dously. Kept at the minimum standard required they may still only have cramped living conditions, with access to an out-doors area, but not necessarily to natural food. Their beaks may be clipped so they can't forage anyway. Perches and litter may or may not be provided; it isn't law. It is hard to tell from egg boxes just how free-range the hens who laid the eggs were.

Kept at a standard above the basics, free-range hens may lead a much more natural life, only going indoors at night and fed on fairly natural foodstuffs. The producers of this standard of egg will probably explain all this on the label as the eggs will be more expensive again.
* Four-grain eggs: The hens who lay these eggs have been fed only on foods natural to hens, and not on animal pro-tein. There is no medicine included in their food. They are still, however, likely to be barn hens rather than free-range.

MAKING DAIRY PRODUCE SAFER

* Low-fat milk will contain fewer residues than full-fat milk because fat tends to store toxins. The same applies to other low-fat dairy produce.
* Very fresh eggs, from whatever source, will contain fewer bacteria than older eggs, so try to find a source of eggs where the laying date can be established. Organic eggs and best-quality free-range eggs are also less likely to be contaminated, and 'Lion Quality' eggs are innoculated against salmonella, and guaranteed British.

* Freedom Food eggs: Sanctioned by the RSPCA, these may be free-range or barn eggs.
* Lion eggs: These have been produced to higher than minimum EU standards.
* Organic eggs: These are hard to find for most of us, but will be from hens whose beaks aren't clipped and who live in a flock of less than 500 (Soil Associa-tion standard) or 3,000 (Organic Farmers and Growers Standard). They lead natural lives, ranging over organic pasture, and all other food offered must be natural.

For more information on choosing healthy eggs, see page 77.

Milk — and products such as butter, cheese and yoghurt — is similar to meat in that any pollutants that the animal has eaten or been given or picked up elsewhere will show there, even if in minute amounts. Cows that graze on sprayed fields and who eat pelleted food containing contaminants will yield milk containing these items. One recent Government survey showed a high percentage of milk containing the toxic pesticide lindane. DDT has been found in butter, and a bacterium linked to Crohn's Disease has been found in 10% of milk samples. Like other foods, milk is regularly monitored and declared safe by the Government. However, more people are turning to milk from organic herds.

Pasteurization destroys much harmful bacteria and virtually all milk on sale now is pasteurized. The FSA is investigating claims that BSE can be passed to humans via cows' milk.

There has recently been much debate across the world about the use of BST, a man-made hormone which increases milk yield in cows. It is already in use in the USA but is banned for use elsewhere for the time being.

Food processing and preserving

■ Fresh food - but is it?

Once food is harvested or slaughtered, much of it is sold unprocessed via the shops. When you go to buy it, however, all is not necessarily as it seems. How fresh is 'fresh', for instance, and does it matter to your health? There are various ways the food industry can keep things looking fresh for weeks or even months.

✱ *Post-harvest spraying*: Many fruits, including apples, pears and grapes, and some vegetables, including potatoes, may be treated with preservative sprays (E 230-233) to prolong life. There is no way of telling which have been sprayed, but as these chemicals are toxic — indeed, one has been banned in the USA — a person eating a healthy diet rich in fruits and veg may be getting quite a dose. Organic food should not be sprayed.

✱ *Controlled-atmosphere storage* and packaging: The two biggest-selling fruits in the Western world, apples and bananas, are routinely harvested and then stored in a controlled atmosphere with reduced oxygen and increased nitrogen and carbon dioxide. This prevents ripening and ageing. When needed, they are artificially ripened with ethylene gas.

✱ *Modified-atmosphere packaging* is used for many foods, to improve shelf-life and keeping, e.g. bagged salads. The gases have been shown to deplete vitamin and antioxidant content of the food.

✱ *Waxing*: Citrus fruits, apples and various other fruits and vegetables are often wax-coated. This keeps natural moisture in, gives a shiny appearance and extends shelf-life. Vegans will not be pleased to hear that a substance often used in waxing, shellac, is derived from insects. There is no obligatory labelling, but 'unwaxed' fruits are usually labelled as such.

✱ *Genetic engineering*: For more on this see page 82, but basically food scientists can now inject 'long-life' genes into various foods, such as tomatoes, pineapples and bananas. These raw foods are currently not on sale in the UK.

✱ *Irradiation*: Due to huge public resistance against irradiated food, although the process (hitting fresh food with ionizing radiation to kill micro-organisms that make food age and rot) was made legal under licence in the UK in 1991, virtually no food is irradiated here, with the exception of some herbs and spices.

However, it is thought that much irradiated food may arrive, unlabelled, from the Continent, where the practice is much more prevalent. No blanket testing for irradiated imported food is in place, but 39% of samples of fish and shellfish sent for testing by trading standards offices in Suffolk had been irradiated. Another test found 18% of a variety of groceries and food supplements also contained irradiated items.

Irradiated foods permitted to be sold in the UK currently are: herbs, spices, seasonings and condiments; potatoes and yams; onions and garlic; vegetables and pulses; fruits; mushrooms; cereals;

FOOD PRESERVATION METHODS COMPARED

Canned: can store for several years.
pros: convenient, low cost, can be stored at room temperature.
cons: brine-canned foods high in salt; syrup-canned foods high in sugar. Vitamins B and C depleted. coated cans may leach chemicals into foods.

Bottled: over half of coated cans tested in 2001 leached the oestrogenic chemical, bisphenol-A.
pros: can store for several years.
cons: vitamin depletion.

UHT: can store for up to 6 months.
cons: vitamin loss and taste change.

Ambient: (processed food stored at room temperature, such as jellies) can store up to 3 months.
cons: generally high in chemical preservatives.

Chilled: can store up to a week
pros: fresh.
cons: cost, need to keep cool.

Frozen: can store 1-12 months.
pros: similar nutritionally and in appearance to fresh.
cons: not suitable for all food; energy-costly.

Vacuum-wrapped: can store up to one month.
pros: convenient.
cons: may have preservatives added.

Dried: can store up to a year.
pros: convenience.
cons: destroys vitamin C and B, taste loss, texture change.

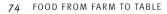

poultry; fish and shellfish. However, irradiated food must be labelled 'irradiated' or 'treated with ionizing radiation'. Much irradiated food on sale is not.

The main drawbacks of irradiated food, apart from 'factor X' (unknown long-term effect of a diet high in irradiated products), are that they deplete vitamins in food by up to 90%, and destroy 'good' bacteria along with the bad.

Processing

In general, the more a food is processed, the more it is likely to lose in terms of its natural nutrients, and the less 'natural' it will be. As a very simple example, strawberries are high in vitamin C and fibre, but add them to sugar and make 'economy' strawberry jam in a factory and you lose almost all of those two nutrients. Highly processed food, again in general, tends to lose its vitamins and fibre most frequently.

Where some things are taken away, however, others are added. Processed food is notoriously rich in high-calorie ingredients such as sugar, saturated fat and trans fats. Cream is skimmed off milk (we are now drinking more skimmed milk than ever before, for our health's sake) and put into our bodies via processed food. We replace sugar in our tea and squashes with artificial sweetener — only to eat even more of it in processed desserts, cakes and biscuits. And so on!

Processed food often contains fortifying ingredients to replace lost vitamins and minerals (as in many breakfast cereals, for example, or in the case of white bread which, by law, is

fortified with calcium), perhaps adding fibre and other 'healthy' things (see more about this in Functional Foods on page 83). Less welcome than these additions, though, are the ones that are put in the processing pot for other reasons.

■ E numbers and additives

Processed food labels may well contain a long list of E numbers, additives and items that you wouldn't consider necessary. Yet it is estimated that each of us eats about 2.25 kg (5 lb) of additives a year.

* *Colours E100-E180:* Used to make perhaps less-than-attractive foods look better or to restore a 'natural' colour to items where colour has been lost in processing.

* *Preservatives E200-E285, E1105:* Used to prolong product life and prevent bacteria build-up. Even 'healthy' foods, such as dried apricots, will probably contain preservative (in the case of dried fruit, usually sulphur dioxide, a known allergen).

* *Antioxidants E300-E321:* Used to stop the product going rancid.

* *Emulsifiers, stabilisers, thickeners E322-495:* Used in products such as fat-reduced desserts, soups and sauces to enhance texture and stop separation.

* *Processing aids E500-E578:* Used for a variety of reasons.

* *Flavour-enhancers E620-E640:* Used to improve flavour in processed foods.

* *Glazing agents E901-E914:* Used to add glaze and shine, and attractive appearance to foods.

* *Flour-improvers and bleaches e.g. E920-E926:* Used in baked goods and breads to improve texture, cooking quality and whiteness.

* *Sweeteners e.g. E420/421 and E953-959:* To add sweetness in place of sugars.

* *Miscellaneous E999-E1518*

In addition to these, your product may also contain one or more flavourings which don't have E numbers and needn't be declared on the label.

For people without known reactions, the additives are deemed safe (at normal levels of intake) by the Government. However, nobody really knows what long-term effects there might be on, say, a person who eats a diet high in additives (a typical 'junk food diet') from early life on, and research indicates that some additives can cause cancer in animals.

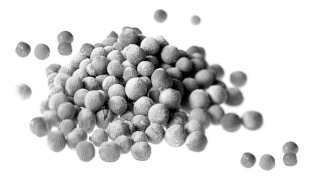

In Your Hands

Food and health from the shop to the table

Healthy eating is not just about knowing your nutrients. The health issues of concern from shop to table are that the food that we buy is the best quality we can find and/or afford; that it contains its full quota of nutrients and is safe to eat.

For instance, there is a world of difference in the nutritional content of a just-picked organically grown red pepper, displayed in cool conditions, taken home in a cool bag, stored and prepared correctly before being lightly cooked, and a red pepper of dubious origins which has been displayed too long on a sunlit counter, taken home in an overheated shopping bag and kept around on the veg rack for a week before being chopped too early and eaten too late. The first may contain its full quota of vitamin C (around 100mg) while the latter will probably have none at all.

Also, penny for penny, there is much more vitamin C content in a top-of-the-range 100%-fruit long-life juice than there is in a lower-cost 'juice drink', which — on reading the small print — contains only 10% juice and a lot of sugar and additives.

Finally, there is a far greater chance of contracting food poisoning from a piece of chicken purchased just on its sell-by date, bought at the start of a day's shopping, and left in a warm kitchen before cooking in an old microwave oven than there is from a long sell-by date piece which is only out of cool conditions for minutes and is cooked thoroughly.

This section is all about being a sensible food shopper and handler.

■ Where to shop
Corner shop? Specialist store? Supermarket? Health-food shop or farm shop? Where you buy your food is quite important. Here are a few checkpoints to help you decide:
* Pick shops with a high turnover of goods — produce will then be fresher.
* When it comes to fresh foods, avoid shops which keep produce on the roadside, in hot, light conditions (e.g. a display window for greens and fruit). Vitamin C and B content will be considerably diminished.
* With much food, you tend to get what you pay for, so consider how much you can pay for good food. If keeping costs low is vital, buying direct — e.g. from farm shops — is usually cheaper. Goods from small independent grocers will, sadly, usually be dearer.
* If you live in a 'food desert', with miles to the nearest store (a growing problem both for city dwellers and remote communities), contact your local council, more and more of whom are running free transport and/or free food-delivery services for such areas. The Soil Association runs a scheme in Devon (see the Appendix).
* Buy locally produced foods if possible.

When to shop
To buy and keep food at its best:
* Try to do your main regular shop soon after the major deliveries have taken place, if supermarket shopping. These will tend to be after the weekend rush on a Monday. If you shop Sunday afternoon or Monday morning you may find stocks —

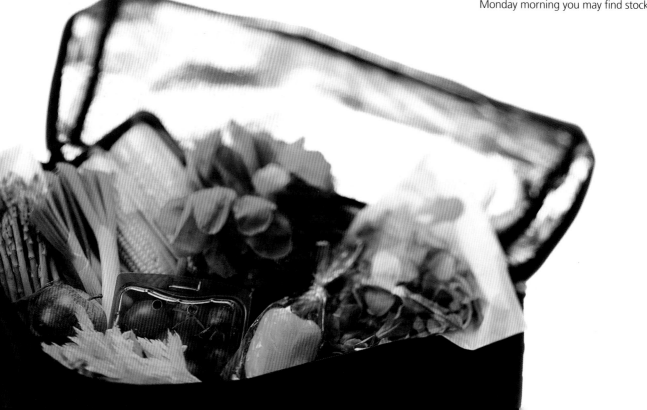

particularly of fresh fruits, vegetables, fish, and meats — are low and what is left is not what you would have ideally chosen.
* Don't shop for perishable items if you can't get them back into suitable cool conditions promptly — e.g., if you have to keep them by your side at work all day. This gives bacteria a chance to build up to unacceptable levels and also reduces vitamins B and C in your food.

Menus and lists

Before you do a major shop it is wise to plan out menus for the week ahead, balancing them for health and pleasure. Then write a list. It will help if the list runs in the order in which you will shop.

For safety it is best to purchase chilled and frozen foods last — carried round a warm shop in your trolley while you do other shopping, they may de-chill or begin to defrost, a possible safety hazard. It is also a good idea to purchase light-weight fruits, salads, etc. after heavy items like cans and bottles, as they may otherwise get crushed, which destroys vitamin C and spoils keeping qualities.

Getting quality in fresh foods

Here are some pointers for choosing the best available food:
* Use your eyes. Look for foods that look fresh and 'happy'. Use your nose, if food isn't in a sealed container. It should smell fresh and sweet.
* Meat need not look bright (often a sign is hasn't been hung long enough); it can look dark red (for beef) or pale pink (pork or lamb), but it shouldn't look grey. It shouldn't smell at all, except in the case of some game. In butcher's shops, watch that the butcher doesn't mix serving fresh and cooked meats without washing hands, and make sure he uses separate utensils and areas of the shop for both.
* Fish is often packed for sale atmo-sphere-controlled (see page 74) so it is hard to evaluate by smell — but fresh fish sold loose should not smell anything

other than sweet, fresh and perhaps vaguely of the sea. Any ammonia-type smell or anything 'fishy' means don't buy it. Shellfish MUST be really fresh both for taste and texture — and to avoid food poisoning. If wild, not farmed, salmon/trout etc. is on offer, buy it. Go for undyed smoked fish if available.
* Fruit and vegetables: buy organic when-ever you can. Pesticide residues are often highest in lettuces, strawberries, bananas, carrots and celery, so it is well worth buying organic in these instances. Look for fruit and vegetables in season, locally grown fruit and vegetables, and produce which isn't bruised or damaged (this will lose vitamin C and not keep well). A few blemishes are OK. Consider how long you need fruit to keep — ripe fruit will not keep long; unripe fruit can be ripened at home. (Controlled-atmosphere fruit, page 74, may follow its own rules!)
* Eggs should be perfect, not cracked or broken. They should be clean. Look for a recent packaging date. At present, a laying date isn't required. Free-range or organic eggs will be stated as such — 'farm fresh' or 'country fresh' are meaningless. All boxes must be stamped with the method of farming used.
* With all protein foods — meats, fish, eggs — look for quality assurance labels, which may not mean a great deal but are better than nothing. Look for descriptions of where or how the animal or fish was reared or in what circumstances hens were kept. With these protein foods, be prepared to pay a little more for quality or organic produce; if necessary, forgo the quantity — you only need small portions of protein for good health.

Getting quality in processed foods

As processed foods make up a fair-to-large proportion of most of our diets, it is vital that what we eat is the best we can get. With a little care it is possible to pick produce that isn't too high in satu-rated or trans fats, salt, sugar, etc. It is

possible to avoid the less pleasant aspects of processed food, such as mechanically recovered meat (MRM), indiscriminate use of additives, etc.

It is only by buying the quality, healthier options and leaving the rubbish on the shelves that we will eventually get the food we want. Here are some pointers for choosing good-quality cans, packets, jars, etc.

Reading the labels

* The name and description: If you glance at the photographs on some packs, you may find that all is not as it seems. For instance, a UHT carton with a tempting photo of citrus fruits on the front, calling itself 'citrus juice drink' may contain as little as 10% real juice, the remainder being made up of water, sugar, colourings and flavourings. NOT quite so good for you. And this is legal. Strawberry flavour yoghurt may never have been near a real strawberry or even real strawberry juice or extract; it will simply use artificial flavouring. This, too, is legal. Meat in cheap 'pork' sausages and other meat products, such as burg-ers, can include mechanically recovered meat, a kind of slurry removed by machine from a carcass after all the other meat has been removed. 'Meat' can also include rind, skin, sinew and gristle. Another problem is that the percentage content of what you would consider to be the main ingredients in a product may, in fact, be quite small. For instance, you may be getting only a small percentage of meat in a 'steak pie'. Yet another problem arises for those avoiding certain ingredi-ents for health or other reasons. Say you're trying to avoid all beef products. You may be surprised to find, on reading the ingredients list, that a chicken stock cube contains beef extract. Or, you're trying to go vegetarian — only to find that many yoghurts contain gelatine, which is made from beef bone. Read the small print carefully to find out what you're

Fat:

free: ←---0.15g/100g
low: ←---5g/100g
reduced: 25% less
less: x% less

Saturates:

free: ←---0.1g/100g
low: ←---3g/100g
reduced: 25% less
less: x% less

Sugars:

free: ←---0.2g/100g
low: ←---5g/100g
reduced: 25% less
less: x% less
no added: no sugars, or foods composed mainly of sugars, added to the food or its ingredients

Fibre:

increased: 25% more and ---}3g/100g serving
more: x% more
source of: ---}3g/100g or per serving
high in/rich source of: ---}6g/100g or source of per serving

Sodium:

free: ←---5mg/100g
low: ←---40mg/100g or per serving
reduced: 25% less
less: x% less
no added: no salt or sodium have been added to the food or its ingredients

really buying; even then it may not tell you the whole story. However, the EU is currently reviewing labelling laws and new guidelines from the FSA's Food Advisory Committee recommend a crackdown on the use of misleading words and phrases on packaging.

✱ *Special health or product claims*: Words like 'natural', 'traditional', 'farm-fresh' have very little meaning when applied to processed foods. For instance, farm-fresh eggs are usually battery eggs. Pictures of country scenes mean nothing. Some manufacturers banner claims such as 'free from artificial colourings and preservatives' in their products to distract from the fact that they do contain, say, artificial sweeteners and flavourings. As another example, there is no legal definition of the term 'low-sugar', though maximum 5% by weight is a guideline. 'No added sugar' banners may also be misleading as many such products contain high amounts of other, similar, sweeteners, such as syrup, honey or concentrated fruit juices. Even the term 'organic' can mislead, as processed foods, containing a number of ingredients, may contain up to 5% non-organic ingredients.

As 70% of the salt that we eat is in processed foods, it is worth seeking out 'low in salt' and 'reduced-salt' products if you eat them a lot. However, these may be harder to find than 'low-fat' or 'low-sugar' products — the UK food industry has, apparently, spent the last few years being somewhat reluctant to reduce the amount of salt it uses in manufacture, thus keeping our taste for salty foods high. If the manufacturers won't cut down — perhaps we should cut down on the amount of high-salt processed foods that we put in our basket (a list of high-salt foods appears on page 33). It is called voting with your purse. It is currently hard, however, to find out exactly how much salt is in foods. There is no law to say the amount has to be declared, either in the ingredients list or in a nutrition panel (see opposite).

The fat content of food is a strong selling point — not only do we have various 'low-fat', '90%-fat-free', etc. claims, but now also such things as 'high in monounsaturates'. The table on the left lists various claims for the major nutrients and what that should mean, according to DEFRA (formerly MAFF) guidelines set in 1993. However, one omission is that there are none on what constitutes 'lean' or 'extra-lean'.

Another anomaly regarding fat claims is that the percentage of fat content often quoted (e.g. chips — only 5% fat) is misleading to say the least. By this, the manufacturer means that the chips contain 5% of their total weight as fat - i.e., 5g fat per 100g food. This does not mean that the chips only contain 5% of the total calories in the food as fat. All food — including chips, meat, cheese, and so on, contains a high or fairly high percentage of water (e.g. lean meat is 74% water, oven chips are about 60% water, hard cheese is about 36% water) which is calorie-free. So 5% of fat by weight turns out to be a much higher percentage of the total calories. Five grams of fat equals 45 calories, as there are 9 calories per gram of fat. There are about 160 calories in 100g of oven chips. So the real amount of fat in the chips is 28%!

A reduced-fat cheese may say something like 'only 15% fat' (i.e. 15g fat per 100g cheese). Working out the fat content on the only sensible basis — as a percentage of total calories — in fact it contains nearly 52% of its calories as fat. This is the kind of information you really need in order to balance your diet, and yet currently the only way to work out fat content as a percentage of nutrients is to take a calculator with you when you shop! For more on nutrition labelling, see below.

Fibre content can also be a good selling point. To be claimed high in fibre, a food needs to contain at least 6g of fibre in an average portion. However, sometimes a food is high-fibre because of added bran. High bran intake can inhibit absorption of some minerals such as iron and it is better to get fibre from natural sources such as pulses, whole grains, fruits and vegetables.

Vitamins and minerals can be good promotional value — by law, to be a 'rich source' of any of these, a product has to contain at least 50% of a day's recommended intake per serving.

QUICK GUIDE TO NUTRITION LEVELS ON FOOD LABELS

per serving	A lot	A little
Fat	20g or more	2g or less
Saturates	5g or more	1g or less
Sugars	10g or more	2g or less
Fibre	3g or more	0.5g or less
Sodium	0.5g or more	0.1g or less

GUIDELINES ON DAILY NUTRIENT INTAKES (MAFF)

	Women	Men
Total fat maximum	70g	95g
Saturated fat maximum	20g	30g
Sugar maximum	50g	70g
Fibre minimum	16g	20g
Sodium maximum	2g	2.5g

Lastly, reduced- or low-calorie content may be a selling point for weight-watchers. A reduced-calorie (energy, joules) product must have 75% or less energy than a similar product for which no energy claim is made, and a low-calorie product must have a maximum of 40 calories per 100g product.

List of ingredients

So if you can't tell exactly what you are buying from the banner descriptions and illustrations, you must check the ingredients list. You should now find percentage quantities of at least the main ingredients listed (in accordance with the EC Quantitative Ingredient Declarations directive).

Ingredients are listed in descending order of content by weight, i.e., the ingredient contained in the greatest amount is listed first, and so on, so that the last ingredient listed is the least. E numbers must be included in this list, but may be expressed by name alone, making it hard to detect which you are eating unless you have their names handy, but additives used in an ingredient (e.g. dried fruits in a fruit cake may have been preserved using sulphur dioxide) needn't be mentioned and neither need flavourings. Sugars, as explained above, come in a variety of guises, including glucose, dextrose, fructose, glucose syrup, lactose, maltose and treacle. Concentrated fruit juices used as sweeteners, honey and brown sugar are all similar to basic sucrose and no better for the teeth.

Trans fats (see page 17) will usually appear on the ingredients list as 'hydrogenated fats or oils' or 'hardened fats'. Look out for them in margarines, cakes, biscuits, pies and pastries, though they will be in many more products too. Some ingredients need not be listed and some foods and alcohol are exempt from having to declare their ingredients.

The nutrition panel

Currently there is no legal obligation on manufacturers to provide nutrition information (fat, sugar, salt, fibre content, etc.) on their packs unless specific nutrition claims are made (e.g. 'low-fat'). However, many do, although it is not always easy to interpret the figures, which are usually given in g or mg per 100 g / ml of product and sometimes also in g or mg per serving. Knowing how much, say, fat there is in 100g of product when you are not sure of the weight you will be eating is not ideal. Trans fats are not listed (though they will be included in the total fat column). Sodium content is not the same as salt content — for the total salt content you need to multiply sodium content by 2.5.

Some supermarkets and manu-facturers are adopting the 'traffic light' scheme, which shows boldly on the front of the pack how much fat, saturated fat, sugar and salt the product contains by banding each as Red (high), Amber (medium) or Green (low) in that item.

The criteria for these colours are per 100g food: fat – high, more than 20g; medium, 3–20g; low, under 3g; saturates – high, more than 5g; medium, 1.5–5g; low, under 1.5g; salt – high, more than 1.5g; medium 0.3 – 1.5g; low, under 0.3g; sugar – high more than 22.5g; medium 5–22.5g; low, under 5g.

But not all companies are using the traffic light scheme. The chart (above left) approved by the Government offers a simple guide to what is a high content and what is a low content of fat, sugar, fibre and sodium per serving. The second chart, also approved by the old MAFF, gives total amounts of all the major nutrients that you should be eating a day. Take it with you shopping and it is quite easy to see whether or not a product can fit in with a broadly healthy diet. For example, if a single-serving can of soup contains 2g sodium you can see that it provides a maximum day's sodium intake for women.

Several pressure groups and health professionals, as well as the FSA, are lobbying for a complete rethink on food labelling laws — it is certainly long overdue – but the UK cannot make changes to labelling laws independently of the EU.

* *Use-by dates:* You should always check the 'use-by' dates which are provided on most packaged foods. A 'use-by' date means that the food should be eaten by that date at the latest. Sometimes you will find different use-by dates within the same group of foods on the shelf — pick the pack with the furthest date. 'Best before' dates are for foods with a longer life. They may be fine after that date, which is a guide only.

Foods at home

■ Storing foods

✱ Fruits, most vegetables and salad items: These should ideally be kept in the fridge until needed, unless room temperature is needed for ripening. These should be stored in crisper compartments, in ventilated boxes or plastic bags with holes pierced in them. Mushrooms should be stored in brown paper bags. Bananas are best kept in cool conditions outside the fridge. Potatoes should be kept in cool (but not frosted) dark conditions. If fruit and veg are stored in warmth and light, they lose their vitamin C quite rapidly. Even in a fridge, fruits and vegetables will gradually deteriorate, so use up items on a rota basis and discard any that are wrinkled, browned, dry, yellowing, woody or mouldy.

✱ Frozen foods: These should be transferred immediately to the freezer. Keep different types of frozen food together — e.g. raw meat in one place, frozen desserts and cakes in another. Place raw meats at the bottom of the freezer.

✱ Food to be frozen: These should be blanched (in the case of vegetables) or otherwise prepared, cooled if necessary, and frozen in containers or heavy-duty plastic bags as soon as possible after purchase (in the case of fruits and vegetables, to retain maximum vitamin C). Fresh foods should be frozen using 'fast freeze'.

✱ Fresh meats, dairy produce and all chilled food: These should be stored in the fridge. Store raw meat, ideally in a covered leak-proof container, in the bottom of the fridge, well away from cooked meats, to avoid cross-contamination and possible food poisoning.

✱ Opened jars: These should be kept covered and stored in the fridge.

✱ Opened cans: These should be decanted into glass or china containers, or at least heavy-duty plastic ones, and the contents used within 24 hours, as chemicals from the insides of the cans may leach into the food.

✱ High-fat items, such as cheese, butter, pâté and fatty meats shouldn't be wrapped in cling-film, as this may contain chemicals which can migrate into these foods.

✱ Cheese: This should be stored in its own container, which should have air-holes. Individual cheeses may be wrapped in greaseproof paper. If bought wrapped in cling-film, remove it.

✱ Once a bottle, can, jar, pack, etc., is opened, it will NOT keep indefinitely.

■ Preparing food

Careful food preparation can retain water-soluble vitamins B group and C and minimize risk of food poisoning.

✱ *Avoid* chopping, peeling or tearing fresh fruits, vegetables and salads until the last possible minute before cooking or eating, as cut and exposed surfaces lose vitamin C and begin to oxidize.

✱ *Don't* leave vegetables soaking in water (hot or cold) as this too leaches vitamin C.

✱ *Cook* vegetables for the minimum amount of time to retain nutrients.

✱ *Defrost* meats, fish and meat products thoroughly before cooking, unless the label advises otherwise. Poultry MUST be thoroughly defrosted — feel the cavity to check before cooking and check portions with a sharp knife. Meat that comes out of the fridge very cold should also be brought to room temperature before cooking (but don't leave meat for longer than necessary to achieve this). The problem with cooking chicken (etc.) which isn't thoroughly defrosted is that the centre may remain pink even if the meat looks cooked, meaning bacteria won't have been killed. Don't stuff poultry as the stuffing may also prevent the inside of the bird from thoroughly cooking.

✱ *Microwave defrosting.* Always make sure that frozen foods defrosted in a microwave are turned from time to time for even defrosting.

✱ *When handling raw meat* in the kitchen, use a clean chopping board reserved just for raw meat. A marble board may harbour fewer bacteria than those made from wood or plastic, though some plastic boards now come impregnated with an anti-bacterial compound. Chop and put on a plate, and cover if not putting directly into a cooking pan.

Wash hands and utensils plus chopping board thoroughly after use. Steep utensils in boiling water if practical. Dry hands well before handling other foods. Anti-bacterial cleansers may help prevent bacteria build-up. Clean tap handles which may have been touched with infected hands.

✱ *Keep* all work surfaces, fridge, cupboards, food containers and eating utensils and dishes thoroughly clean.

✱ *Cook* all meat thoroughly to prevent food poisoning. Minced meat, chicken, sausages and burgers should have no pink left in their centres at all. All microwaved food should be piping hot in the centre.

Reheating and leftovers

* If food has to be kept after cooking, allow it to cool and transfer it to a fridge (or freezer) as quickly as possible. If hot food is to be kept for, say, less than an hour, cover it and keep at room temperature then reheat to piping hot, or keep in a low oven just simmering. Vitamins B group and C will diminish in food kept warm for long periods. In general, it is better to allow a meal to cool and then reheat it than keep it hot for long periods. Meals shouldn't be kept at room temperature for any longer than an hour.

* All reheated food should be reheated until piping hot.

* Leftover food, if still in good condition, should be wrapped or put in containers (preferably glass or china), covered and kept in a fridge. Use or throw away within 24-48 hours.

* Discard any leftover food that has discoloured, has an unusual smell, mould or white patches appearing on it, if it has a film on top or has dried out, or in any other way doesn't appear fresh and appetizing.

How to avoid food poisoning

Reported cases of food poisoning and deaths from food poisoning are on the increase. In the UK in 1982 there were only 14,243 reported cases; in 2001, the FSA estimated that there are now up to 4.5 million cases of food poisoning in the UK a year,

No one knows the exact reason for this increase, although as the highest percentage of cases are caused by food 'eaten out', the rise in restaurant, café and take-away eating is an obvious cause. Food eaten in the home accounts for one in six cases and it is thought that demand for a reduction in the amount of preservatives, including sugar, in processed foods, is causing this rise. Another factor is the increased 'food miles' produce travels, and increased number of handlers.

The most common sources of food poisoning are bacteria, although fungi and viruses can also cause it. Worryingly, many cases are caused by bugs virtually unheard of 20 or so years ago. To compound the problem, many food-borne bacteria are resistant to antibiotics, so food poisoning may be hard to treat. Risks can be reduced by following the tips on the right.

* Campylobacter: responsible for about half of all reported cases of food poisoning. A recent official survey found bacteria in 51% of intensively reared supermarket chickens and 68% of free-range. It is also found in meat, unpasteurized milk and doorstep milk pecked by infected sparrows. It can cause gastroenteritis, paralysis and death. Chicken and meat should be thoroughly cooked.

* Salmonella enteriditis: the second most common cause, accounting for around 40% of cases. There has been some improvement in recent years in the amount of salmonella in eggs, according to the DoH, and research suggests that now only 6% of chickens in the UK are infected. It is also found in meat and other sources. It can cause severe gastric upsets, and even death, especially in the young, ill, pregnant or elderly. Eggs and poultry should be as fresh as possible when eaten, as bacteria quickly multiply, and they should be thoroughly cooked. Poultry should be carefully defrosted and stored correctly. Eggs should not be eaten raw. Free-range and organic eggs and poultry have a lower incidence. New forms of salmonella are now infecting foods like salads, fruits and veg. Produce to be eaten raw should be washed thoroughly.

* Salmonella typhimurium: a newer salmonella strain very resistant to antibiotics and more likely in intensively reared animals. Follow advice for salmonella enteriditis.

* E.Coli 0157: is causing an increasing amount of poisoning. It has a very low infective dose and a common source of infection is meat, possibly contaminated during slaughter and processing. Under-cooked meat may then cause poisoning. Minced meat and under-cooked burgers

have been cited as particular risks because mincing may spread it through the meat. Dairy products can also be contaminated. The bacteria cause severe stomach upsets, even death, especially in vulnerable people. E. coli has even been found in apples.

* Listeria monocytogenes: bacteria found in soft cheeses, such as Brie and Camembert, in pâtés, and chilled ready-meals and deli foods, like pre-packed salads, pasta salads and hams. The bacteria can thrive at temperatures as low as 5°C (many domestic fridges function at around this temperature). It is dangerous for pregnant women, young children and people with weak immune systems.

Genetically Modified Food

Tomatoes that remain ripe without rotting, crops that resist weed-killer, cows that produce human-style milk, and animals without foot-and-mouth or BSE. Whatever you want in your food — it seems that the bio-technologists can do it, or will be able to do it soon. They are already promising us cancer- and heart disease-preventing vegetables and red meat low in saturates.

Over thousands of years, crop- and animal-breeders have tried to improve things like yield, disease-resistance, size, etc, through selective breeding, but this is a very slow process. Now, there is a much quicker way to alter the characteristics of anything from an apple to a bean to a cow. That way is broadly called genetic engineering or modification, a technology that has as many detractors as enthusiasts.

■ What is genetic engineering?

Every living organism has a 'blueprint' or pattern of genes, containing all the hereditary information needed to give it all its special characteristics. Until recently, genes have been passed on through each species via normal reproduction. Now, however, scientists know how to remove genetic material from one living thing and insert it into another, thus giving the second species a new characteristic and bypassing natural evolution.

This 'genetic modification' (GM) can not only be done from, say, fruit to fruit, but can also cross species — for instance, tomatoes have recently been given a gene from fish that helps them 'stay in shape' when frozen, and GM has produced a cow with 'human' breast milk, which could be used for healthier formula milk.

So far, GM has mainly been applied commercially in major world crops, such as soya, maize, oilseed rape, cotton, potatoes and tomatoes. There are, though, test sites all over the world, including the UK, for a wide variety of other GM foods.

■ How much genetically modified food are we currently eating?

Although no UK farmers currently grow GM foods for sale, the first GM food to arrive for sale in the UK, ten years ago, was tomato paste using GM tomatoes from the USA. Cheese made using a genetically produced enzyme (instead of rennet) has been widely on sale since the early '90s. However, 60% or more of the processed food we eat may contain significant amounts of GM soya because GM soya beans (engineered to be herbicide-resistant) now comprise half of the world's soya crop — these GM soya beans are mixed with traditional soya beans before distribution — and soya is now contained in about two-thirds of all processed foods. GM maize is also being used in processed foods. GM potatoes, apples, wheat and other GM foods are being tested in trial grounds throughout the UK and the world. The truth is that, due to cross-contamination, very small quantities of GM foods may be in virtually everything we eat. Also, GM soya and maize go into animal feedstuff – 30% of their diet can be GM food.

■ What are the advantages of GM for food consumers?

Companies promoting GM food say that the new technology can have many benefits for the consumer by making food keep fresh for longer, taste better and have a healthier profile. For instance, scientists in the UK have isolated the gene material in broccoli which contains sulphorophane (see page 96), the anti-cancer agent, and are working on implanting it into other vegetables. They also say that if, as a result of genetic engineering, there will be increased yield and less waste — for instance, through production of pest- and weedkiller-resistant strains or faster-growing animals and fish — then there will be more food available, and this should be reflected in price control.

■ What are GM foods' drawbacks?

Aside from the ethical arguments relating to 'tampering' with nature, one of the main problems is that no one knows what the long-term effects of eating genetically modified food may be, nor of their effect on the environment. For instance, much genetic engineering involves using antibiotic 'marker' genes, which, some experts worry, will make antibiotic resistance in humans even more widespread and affect our ability to fight disease. It is also thought that genetic engineering may produce new toxins and allergens, and may decrease nutrient content — for example, weedkiller-tolerant soya beans have been shown to contain significantly lower levels of beneficial phyto-oestrogens.

Other experts say that, in engineering pesticide-resistant crops, 'superweeds' will develop (indeed, mutant weeds have been found growing near GM rape crops in Cambridgeshire), leading to the need for even stronger herbicides to kill the new weeds. Risk of cross-contamination is high, as pollen can travel miles, but separation between GM and non-GM crops can be as little as 200 metres, particularly worrying for organic producers, who lose their licence if contaminated.

There is also growing concern about weedkiller residues on weedkiller-resistant crops sprayed with glyphosate (in Roundup from Monsanto, one of the largest multinationals involved), linked with negative effects in humans, animals and plants. Despite this, permitted residue levels have just been increased.

■ How easy is it to avoid GM foods?

Unfortunately, it is quite hard. The EC's consumer affairs department has said ALL processed food will have genetically modified food in it, even if only in tiny amounts, because of cross-contamination and the inability of manufacturers to be 100% sure crops they buy are GM-free.

But at least in 2004 the labelling laws concerning GM foods in the EU were revised. Now, if a food contains or consists of genetically modified organisms (GMOs), or contains ingredients produced from GMOs, this must be indicated on the label. For GM products sold 'loose', information must be displayed immediately next to the food to indicate that it is GM.

Products such as maize and soya flour, oils and glucose syrups have to be labelled as GM if they are from a GM source. But products produced with GM technology (cheese produced with GM enzymes, for example) do not have to be labelled.

Products such as meat, milk and eggs from animals fed on GM animal feed also don't need labelling.

Any intentional use of GM ingredients at any level must be labelled. But there is no need to label small amounts of GM ingredients (below 0.9% for approved GM varieties and 0.5% for some other varieties) that are accidentally present in a food.

If you wish to avoid GM foods, the only alternatives currently are to read labels and avoid all produce containing soya and maize and their derivatives, or choose organically grown soya, maize and products, as the Soil Association, which monitors organic standards, has strict rules to minimize cross-contamination, and genetic modification is not allowed in organic standards.

Soya is found in a wide variety of processed foods, including confectionery, margarines and spreads, mayonnaise, cakes, breads, biscuits, gravy, soups, stock cubes, meat dishes and many more.

■ What official safeguards are there?

Currently the FSA has to ensure full safety evaluation before any 'novel' food is allowed on sale. Some GM foods are considered 'novel' enough to qualify for a full safety evaluation before being

allowed on sale; others may come under a category described as 'Substantial Equivalence' which, briefly, means that they are indistinguishable from the conventional product and therefore have a 'fast track' route to approval and need not be labelled. There are also several independent lobbyists, such as the Food Commission, Sustain and Friends of the Earth, working hard to ensure that our food is, and remains, safe to eat.

Other food innovations

Progress is being made in other areas of food research, without the application of genetic engineering, which may be of benefit to our health.

For example, after several years of development we now have access to dairy produce and eggs high in omega-3 oils. Plant breeders in Wales are also using a variety of rye grass very high in the essential fatty acid linolenic acid to feed to cows and thus help promote milk that is lower in saturated fat than normal. Cows at another English research station are being fed a diet high in heat-treated soya and rape seeds, which also results in milk high in unsaturated fat.

In the USA, a device has been patented which will kill virtually all food poisoning bugs in a millisecond without harming the food itself, and scientists at the UK's Institute of Food Research have pinpointed fruits and vegetables which can protect against E. coli.

■ Functional foods

Functional foods are those that claim enhanced health properties or nutritional We've seen bread that is said to reduce hot flushes in menopausal women; and a fermented milk drink which claims to increase the 'friendly' gut bacteria, i.e. it is pro-biotic (see page 152). Several foods now have added 'omega-3 oils' and claim to help reduce heart disease; as do the

margarine spreads containing sterol esters to reduce blood cholesterol. Hundreds more similar products appear annually.

Nutritionists are often sceptical about these products. They may work, but it is believed that, as with some vitamin and mineral supplements, the 'active ingredients' would be better eaten as part of the food in which they naturally occur. For example, omega-3 fish oils in fish, lignans in natural linseeds, and so on. In other words, the benefits of food are best enjoyed in as natural a way as possible.

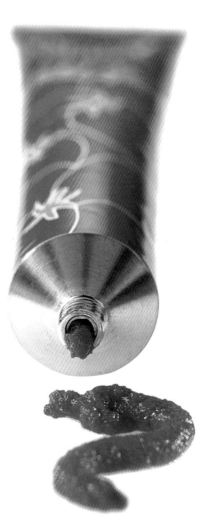

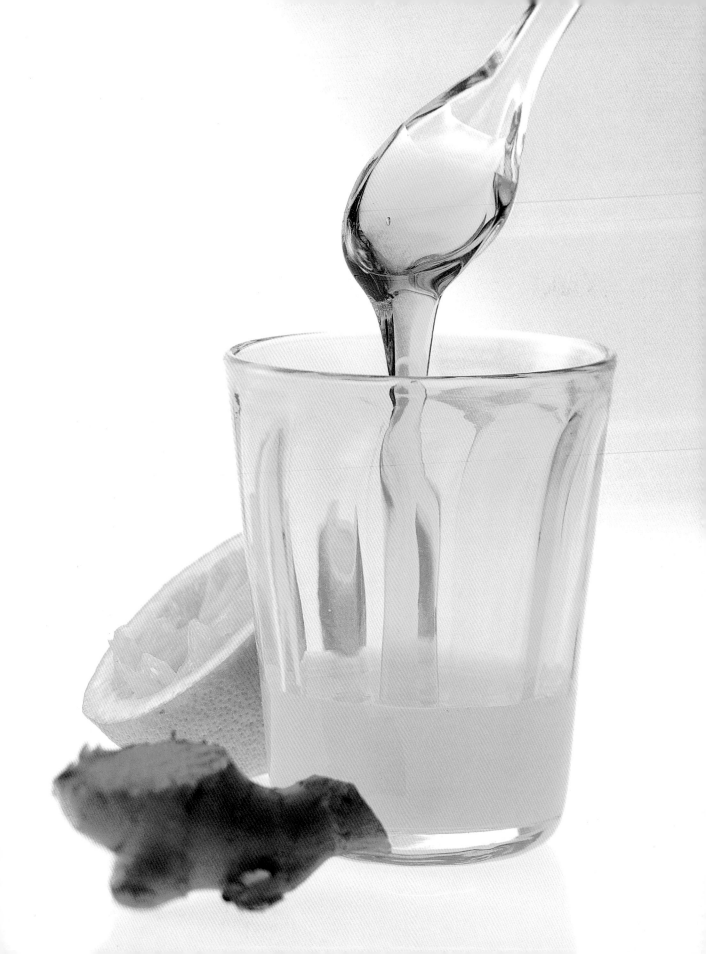

Food as medicine

Twenty years ago, who would have believed that we would be being urged to drink up our red wine for a healthy heart, or would be told to eat up our tomato ketchup to help prevent cancer? The last few years have seen a massive increase in interest in the idea of food as medicine — and yet it is nothing new. For thousands of years the medicinal value of plants and food has been appreciated throughout the world. Garlic was first used as a medicine at least four thousand years ago. Five hundred years ago it was known that fresh fruits and vegetables could cure scurvy. Two hundred years ago a powerful effect of the foxglove flower (*Digitalis*) in helping heart problems was discovered, and 150 years ago salicylic acid (the natural forerunner of today's aspirin) was first isolated from the bark of the willow.

Even as recently as the turn of the century, the largest proportion of medicines were herbal-based. It is only in the mid-to-late century that Western medicine has become so sceptical of the power of plants — and so reliant upon man-made chemical drugs to effect cures. Now people in their hundreds of thousands — including the medical profession and scientific world themselves — are realizing the major drawbacks of a society dependent upon drugs for their health. Drug resistance, drug dependence and unwanted side effects are three main reasons why alternative, more natural methods of cure and prevention are regaining popularity. Diet is a first choice in this change. We all need to eat — so if what we eat can act like medicine, too, then isn't that a marvellous solution?

Now, with the advantage of modern scientific techniques we know so much more about food, what is in it and how it works, that we can fine-tune our diets to suit almost any illness or condition. We are no longer reliant upon the local witch-doctor to provide cures without question. We have the greatest minds in the most well-funded laboratories in the world, seeking the answers to food as medicine.

ACNE AND SPOTS

ACNE IS CAUSED by over-production of sebum — oil — which sits in the pores of the skin, particularly on the face and back. The pores become clogged and are then easily infected. This over-production of sebum usually occurs in the teenage years, because of increased production of the sex hormones, and is more common in boys than girls. Acne can carry on into the 20s and can also occur in women before menstruation, and a mild version may also occur at menopause. Some experts believe that acne is exacerbated by stress, in which case the Anti-stress Diet tips on page 138 may be used in conjunction with these.

SOLUTIONS

All teens should eat a basic healthy diet and follow the particular instructions for them given in Section Three, The Teenage Years (page 167). It is also useful to increase quantities of foods rich in beta-carotene, such as carrots, apricots, sweet potatoes and broccoli (best sources list on page 23). In the body, beta-carotene converts into vitamin A, which is known to be important in maintaining a healthy skin. Sufferers should eat plenty of zinc-rich foods, such as shellfish, lean meat and nuts (best sources list on page 31), as acne may be linked with a zinc deficiency. They should also eat vitamin E-rich foods, such as vegetable oils, nuts and seeds, to aid skin healing (best sources list on page 24), and most experts also agree that a diet high in vitamin C (fresh fruits and vegetables) to fight infection is also important. If an acne sufferer refuses to eat a healthy diet such as this, it may be worth considering supplements of vitamins E, C and zinc.

A diet high in chocolate and saturated fats has often been cited as the cause of acne and spots, but this is still unproven and most experts now believe that there is no link, except that if people eat too many sweet, fatty and 'junk' foods then they will not be getting enough of the nutrients they do need. There is some evidence, though, that a high-salt diet may be a contributing factor, so it is worth avoiding salty snacks and foods.

Doctors often prescribe antibiotics for acne, which can help the condition, but if antibiotics are taken for long periods they can upset the gut microflora which, ironically, may make acne worse! Eat lots of live bio yoghurt or take acidopholus supplements to help avoid this. Live yoghurt may also help acne if applied to the skin at night rather like a face cream. The herb agnus castus, available as a supplement, may help to balance the hormones.

AIDS AND HIV

HIV AND AIDS ARE IMMUNE system deficiency diseases in which the body's natural defences break down and leave the sufferer at much greater risk of infections, such as bronchitis and pneumonia, viruses like herpes and cold sores and cancer.

SOLUTIONS

There is as yet no cure, but help can be obtained through the right diet which will help to keep the immune system functioning well. The Immune-strengthening Diet — rich in vitamins beta-carotene and A, B group, C, E and zinc, — which appears on page 143 is a good basic diet for sufferers who should, however, show the diet to their physician for approval.

The antioxidant mineral selenium, found in Brazil nuts, lean pork and fish (best sources list on page 31), for example, may also be lacking in the diet and research has shown that low selenium levels may be linked with some cancers.

It is important to try to eat enough, as weight loss and malnutrition are common side effects of AIDS. Sufferers should consult a dietician approved by their physician for help with their own personal eating plan, depending upon the course their own illness is taking.

ALCOHOL ABUSE

IN OTHER PARTS OF THIS BOOK the benefits of light to moderate drinking are well documented — for example in connection with a protective effect against heart disease and Alzheimer's. Safe drinking limits for men and women are outlined on page 36 and sensible social drinking and drink/drive limits are discussed on page 66. However, alcohol abuse remains one of the most important causes of ill health throughout the world.

Alcohol is a drug and an intoxicant, and alcohol addiction and dependence is widespread. Experts believe that 33,000 premature deaths a year in England and Wales alone are related to excessive alcohol consumption. Alcohol consumption is linked to 80% of suicides and 40% of road traffic accidents and up to 30% of all hospital admissions. Up to 15 million working days are lost each year because of alcohol abuse. The safe drinking limits outlined by the DoH (see page 36) are exceeded by approximately 27% of men and 15% of women. The higher above these limits your alcohol intake, the more likely it is that you will become dependent and incur a variety of side effects and illnesses.

ALCOHOLISM

A PERSON IS USUALLY described as an 'alcoholic' when problem drinking has turned into dependence and full addiction, with bouts of — or chronic — intoxication, cravings for alcohol that can't be controlled, increased tolerance so that more and more alcohol is needed to achieve intoxication, psychological and physical dependence (withdrawal symptoms such as headache, sweating and tremor), and marked social problems (such as aggression, inability to work, and depression) and a lack of concern over their appearance.

PROBLEM DRINKING

But how to tell if your enjoyment of alcohol is turning into abuse? If you find you can tick several of these statements you are probably becoming a problem drinker, or are in danger of becoming one:

* I drink for comfort or confidence.
* I drink when alone.
* I drink every day — or nearly every day — above safe limits.
* I feel agitated if I can't have a drink when I usually do.

Alcohol dependence — the CAGE questions

Doctors often use the 'CAGE' questionnaire when trying to ascertain if a person has become dependent upon alcohol. If the person can answer 'yes' to two or more of the four questions, then it is likely that he or she has become dependent upon alcohol:

1 Have you ever felt you should CUT down on your drinking?
2 Have people ANNOYED you by criticizing your drinking?
3 Have you ever felt bad or GUILTY about your drinking?
4 (EYE-OPENER) Have you ever had a drink first thing in the morning to steady your nerves or get rid of hangover?

■ Alcohol-related problems

People who regularly drink over the safe limits, whether or not they are described as alcoholic, will almost inevitably find themselves facing health problems, illnesses and symptoms associated with alcohol abuse sooner or later, unless they change their drinking habits. (And, even then, for people over 40, some alcohol-induced symptoms may not be reversible.) Here are the main problems the long-term heavy drinker may have to face:

* *Nutritional deficiencies* — alcohol affects the absorption and metabolism of many nutrients, including the vitamin B group and vitamins A and D, the minerals zinc, calcium and phosphorus, and the essential fatty acids, and may deplete the body of magnesium.

* *Heart and circulatory problems* — heavy drinking — binge drinking or regular intake of nine or more units of alcohol a day — is associated with abnormal heart rhythms, increased risk of heart attack, high blood pressure and strokes.

* *Increased risk of some cancers,* particularly of the breast, mouth, larynx, pancreas, oesophagus, colon and liver.

* *Increased risk of digestive tract problems,* including gastritis and duodenal ulcer.

* *Increased risk of gout and diabetes,* and damage to the immune system.

* *Impotence and infertility*

* *Possibly brain and nerve damage* — although a recent large long-term study found no link between cognitive function and heavy drinking, other studies link alcohol abuse with blackouts, fits, confusion, memory loss, hallucinations, etc.

* *Liver damage* — enlarged liver, fatty liver, jaundice, liver cancer and cirrhosis, which may be more likely if drinks are mixed, e.g. beer and scotch.

* *Foetal alcohol syndrome* — causing mental retardation/abnormal growth.

* *Early death*

■ Prevention or cure?

In the light of all this evidence, surely the most sensible solution is to stay within the safe drinking limits and enjoy the benefits this will bring. It is much easier to do this than to try to beat dependence later in life. For many people, however, it is too late to do this. Proven methods of cutting down alcohol intake or, perhaps, cutting it out altogether, are by enlisting your doctor's help, attending a 'drying out' clinic, joining Alcoholics Anonymous, and, particularly, by also getting help in sorting out any contributory social, emotional or lifestyle problems.

It also helps to have a strong motivation if you are to succeed in cutting down alcohol — for example, parents may realize that their drinking is affecting their children's emotional and everyday life; someone else may realize that he will lose his hard-earned career if he doesn't cut his alcohol intake.

ALLERGIES

AN ALLERGY IS an over-aggressive response by the body's immune system to a substance — for example, an airborne pollutant, a chemical, a plant, an animal's fur or feathers — or a food or food additive (though many, many things can be allergens). An allergic reaction can produce a wide variety of symptoms, the most common being skin reactions (eczema, urticaria, for example), digestive reactions (such as vomiting, stomach-ache, bloating or diarrhoea) or respiratory tract reactions (like wheezing, runny nose, rhinitis and other asthma-like symptoms). Other reactions can include headache, flatulence, fatigue, fluid retention and palpitations.

When an allergic reaction is so severe that it can be life-threatening, this is called anaphylactic shock. The immune system releases a 'hit' of histamine within seconds after the allergic individual has come into contact (even slightly) with the allergen; the throat may swell and make breathing difficult, so the sufferer will wheeze, the face may swell, rashes, stomach cramp and vomiting may occur, and unless adrenaline treatment is given quickly the sufferer may die.

Diagnosed anaphylactics – numbers of whom have doubled in the past few years – carry their own emergency kit for treatment. Anaphylaxis usually starts in childhood and is not outgrown. The most common foods to cause this type of reaction are peanuts, other nuts and seeds, fish and shellfish, and eggs.

The tendency to be allergic (or 'atopic') may run in families and may only involve a reaction to one food. However, where there is an adverse reaction to a food but the traditional allergy tests are negative, the term 'food intolerance' may be used, although it is still possible that immune reactions may be involved in some way. There may be a nutritional connection – recent research published in *The Lancet* found that adults who consumed the most vitamin E-rich foods had fewer allergy-related antibodies in their blood. The increase in numbers of people with food intolerances may also be related to our obsession with cleanliness and avoiding exposure to germs, which, some experts feel, may leave us more susceptible to allergens.

Intolerance may frequently involve more than one food item and larger quantities may be needed to produce a reaction. However, this term may also be used to describe a specific condition e.g. lactose intolerance. Normally the digestive enzyme lactase breaks down lactose, the sugar found in milk and dairy products. If this enzyme is deficient, lactose passes into the intestines resulting in bloating and diarrhoea.

Some experts say that up to one in six people in the UK suffer from allergic reaction to some degree; however, there is evidence that many more people think they are allergic to certain foods, etc., than actually are and other trials put the figure as low as less than 2% of the population.

There is little doubt, though, that instances of food allergies and intolerances are on the increase and have been implicated in a number of other conditions such as arthritis, migraine, IBS, PMS, ME, Crohn's disease and hyperactivity in children.

There is now a scientific test for true allergic reaction, the RAST test, which measures the amount of immunoglobulin E antibodies (IgE) a person has to a specific substance. There are also 'skin prick' tests, in which a tiny amount of the suspected allergen is placed on the arm and a scratch made in the skin, then any reaction (swelling, redness) noted, but this method is more suitable for non-food allergens, such as dust mites, feathers, pollen, etc., and is useless for most food intolerances.

Other tests, such as hair tests by post or unspecific blood tests offered by alternative practitioners, are probably of little real use in most cases. According to research, some private allergy clinics are notorious for giving out long lists of 'problem' foods to people with no known complaints while failing to spot true allergies.

The most reliable test for food sensitivity is the exclusion diet, which should be discussed with your doctor and supervised by a dietician. This involves a diet usually consisting of a few foods which almost never cause allergic reaction (lamb, bottled water and rice are prime examples), which is followed for a number of days and then, if symptoms have improved, one by one other foods are introduced, at intervals, starting with foods less likely to produce a reaction. If there is no reaction, they can stay in the diet. Once any newly added food triggers a reaction, it should be removed from the diet (possibly for good, although see Living with a Food Allergy or Intolerance overleaf).

A simpler form of exclusion diet involves removing one or two suspect foods from the diet for about 2 weeks and if the condition clears the food is then reintroduced. If the symptoms return it is assumed that the reintroduced food is to blame. This type of exclusion diet is best attempted with professional advice.

■ Foods most likely to cause allergy

Almost any food, additive or drink can cause allergic reactions, though some, like rice and lamb, do so less often. Here are the most common food:

* Cows' milk and dairy produce: see lactose intolerance on page 88. Some people who can't tolerate cows' milk may be able to have goats' milk. Others find that they can drink skimmed milk and low-fat milk products but not full-fat varieties. Common in babyhood and may be outgrown.

* Eggs: often egg whites rather than the yolks are the problem. Eggs are an ingredient in many products, so label-reading is crucial. This allergy is most common in toddlers and again may be outgrown.

* Grains: wheat intolerance is common; gluten is not always the 'culprit', though it may often be. Any grain can cause allergic reaction, but rice and corn are less likely to do so. Again, grains, particularly wheat and gluten, appear in many products and so vigilance is needed. See Coeliac Disease.

* Fish and shellfish: allergic reaction to these is increasing, possibly because of increasingly polluted waters. Most common allergens seem to be prawns, oysters, crabs and white fish.

* Nuts and seeds: peanut allergy is the most common, and it is now thought that around one in 200 people are sensitive to peanuts. Sufferers may be advised to avoid groundnut (peanut) oil, although a recent study showed that only 10% of peanut-sensitive adults tested were allergic to unrefined peanut oil and none to refined oil. Unrefined oil is more likely to be found in ethnic foods and refined oil can be contaminated if peanuts have been cooked and the oil is re-used. Many other food products may be cross-contaminated with peanut traces. Cosmetics sometimes even contain peanut oil.

Other common nut allergens are walnuts, brazils and cashews. There is a growing allergy to sesame seeds — found not only in hummus, tahini, sesame seed bread and sesame oil, but also often in vegetable burgers, Oriental meals and cakes.

* Fruit: strawberries and oranges are often cited as allergens, as well as other members of the citrus family, kiwi fruits, apples and cherries.

* **Soya beans:** soya beans and soya bean products, such as tofu and soya flour, can cause a reaction, particularly digestive upsets. Soya is found in a multitude of commercial products and avid label reading is necessary for those with a soya intolerance.

* **Sugar:** sugary drinks, sweets and juices, and other high-sugar products, including chocolate, may be badly tolerated and can contribute to candida or gut dysbioses, food cravings, and many other problems that may have an allergy link.

* **Additives:** artificial food additives, such as preservatives and colourings, have long been suspected of causing allergic reactions and are especially linked with hyperactivity in children. Likely 'culprits' are the azo dyes, such as tartrazine (E102), caramel (E150), benzoates (E210-219), sulphates (E220-229), nitrates (E249-252), glutamates (621-623), and artificial sweeteners such as aspartame. For more information on additives and health, see page 75.

■ Living with a food allergy or intolerance

Exciting new work has shown that a technique called enzyme-potentiated desensitization (EPD) may be helpful in treating a range of conditions where food allergy or intolerance may play a part, e.g. eczema, arthritis, irritable bowel syndrome, etc. The technique involves injection of tiny doses of the allergens together with a naturally occurring enzyme, producing the desensitizing effect. Doses are given at three-month intervals at the start, and then frequency is gradually reduced.

At the moment, however, this treatment is not really widely available and the most obvious course of action for most intolerance sufferers is for them to stick to a diet that excludes the food(s) to which they are allergic or intolerant. As self-diagnosis is often difficult, as has been proven by research, it is unwise to start any limited diet unless the allergy has been confirmed through your physician by using one of the techniques described above.

A suitable diet may then be a simple matter to follow (if, for instance, you are allergic to oysters only, it won't be too hard for you to follow a diet that doesn't include oysters). If a wider range of foods is involved, however, or if you have an allergy to one of our major foods, such as dairy produce or grains or even soya, the diet becomes much more restricted and advice from a dietician is needed so that you can safely avoid possible nutrient deficiencies.

The long-term outlook for an allergy sufferer isn't always bleak — sometimes your body will change and tolerate a food that you have had to avoid for a long time. In severe cases, however, returning to a food, particularly for anaphylactics, is a risky business and needs professional supervision if undertaken at all.

For addresses of several organizations that may help, see the Appendix at the back of the book.

ALZHEIMER'S DISEASE

ALZHEIMER'S IS THOUGHT of as a disease of the elderly, but it can begin at the age of 50 or even earlier, often with barely noticeable small problems, such as poorer short-term memory, progressing at an unpredictable rate into severe memory loss and confusion. In those with Alzheimer's, plaques and deposits are formed within the brain, but the exact causes of this damaging process are still being unravelled.

The first theory in the 1980s was that aluminium intake was a factor, as a core of aluminium was found in these plaques, but now many experts believe that ingestion of aluminium is not a significant factor.

Tobacco smoking is now known to increase the risk of Alzheimer's. High blood pressure, diabetes, stroke, high cholesterol and having a fat stomach are all also known risk factors for the disease. There is also a genetic link.

SOLUTIONS

The starting point for everyone should be a basic healthy diet which can help to prevent or minimize all the conditions above.

A large 4-year New York study published in 2006 found that people who ate a Mediterranean-style diet high in fruit, veg, wholegrains, fish and a little red wine were up to 40% less likely to develop Alzheimers. The people who scored highest in reducing their risk ate mainly vegetables, beans, cereals, fruit and nuts, moderate amounts of fish and just small quantities of meat and dairy products. They ate virtually no saturated fats and chose olive oil, and had 1–2 glasses of red wine a day. The Healthy Heart diet on page 142 is a Mediterranean-stye diet.

Various other scientific trials have shown elements of the Mediterranean diet as having a protective effect against

---

WHO GETS ALLERGIES?

People who produce too much of the IgE antibody (see page 88) are 'atopic' individuals, who are more likely to suffer allergic reactions, and the tendency to this is probably inherited. It may also be that babies are 'sensitized' to allergens even before birth by what the mother eats, but this is still the subject of much research. Food allergies do, however, seem more common in childhood. The simple truth is that the experts don't yet have any concrete answer to who will get what allergy, or even when, which means that as yet there is no means of prevention.

Alzheimer's – including vitamin E, monoun-saturated fats, fruit juices and red wine.

Most scientists also believe that a brain 'well-used' throughout life is also an important factor in avoiding or post-poning Alzheimer's, as people who keep fairly mentally active seem to suffer less. In view of this, it may well be worth taking the supplement ginkgo biloba, which is said to improve the circulation of blood to the brain. There are other as-yet-unproven claims for the benefits of the minerals zinc and selenium in pre-venting Alzheimer's, as well as the com-pound co-enzyme Q10.

Some experts still stand by the aluminium theory and so it may be worth avoiding cooking foods, especially acidic foods, in aluminium saucepans, and avoiding the additive aluminium phos-phate, to be found in some baked goods, and aluminium hydroxide, used in several proprietary indigestion remedies, until further evidence for or against this theory emerges.

Once somebody has Alzheimer's dis-ease the above dietary measures should still be followed as far as possible, but emphasis should also be placed on pro-viding the sufferer with tempting food that is easy to eat and serve.

ANAEMIA

ANAEMIA IS A CONDITION in which there is a reduction in haemoglobin, the material in the blood's red blood cells that carries oxygen to the tissues in the body. The symp-toms of this lack of oxygen can be mild or more severe, including vary-ing degrees of tiredness up to total fatigue, weakness, pallor, breath-lessness, dizziness, lack of stamina and poor concentration.

The most common cause of anaemia is iron deficiency, and this can occur for several reasons. Women during their menstruating years are particularly sus-ceptible, especially if periods are heavy, as once iron is lost with the blood it takes a long time to to be replenished in the body. Any other form of major blood loss, such as haemorrhage, childbirth or accident, can also result in anaemia.

Pregnant women are also prone to anaemia, especially if iron stores are at a low at the start of pregnancy, as there is much more blood circulating in the body than normal and so more iron is needed to go round. To prevent anaemia in preg-nancy, women may be given supplements of iron with folate, a deficiency of which can also be a factor. Some illnesses can also produce anaemia — cancer and leukaemia, AIDS and stomach ulcers, for example. Lastly, a nutritionally poor diet may be to blame.

SOLUTIONS

With iron-deficiency anaemia, the solu-tion is to eat a diet containing plenty of iron-rich foods. For a best sources list, see page 30. Your physician will probably also prescribe a course of iron pills. Animal sources of iron, such as lean red meat, are absorbed more easily than veg-etable sources, but absorption of iron in the diet is helped by vitamin C, so eat a C-rich food at the same time as your iron-rich food. Tea, coffee and cola all hinder absorption, so avoid consuming these drinks within one hour of a meal. Phytates found in bran also affect absorp-tion, but this is not thought to be a sig-nificant factor as the body may adjust to this. Not all anaemia is caused by iron deficiency, however, so it is therefore important that you see your physician for a correct diagnosis.

Pernicious anaemia is anaemia caused by a lack of vitamin B12, or the body's inability to absorb it. Vegans, in particu-lar, may have a B12 deficiency, as it is only found in animal foods or in fortified vegetarian products. B12 supplements suitable for vegans and vegetarians can be obtained from health food stores or your physician.

Angina, see Heart Disease and Stroke

Anorexia, see Eating Disorders

■ ANXIETY STATES ARE OFTEN a response to an overload of stress in people's lives. When people are under stress, the body's 'fight or flight' system pumps adrenaline out in preparation for dealing with a crisis situation, but in modern life the crisis doesn't manifest itself physically — e.g. in a fist-fight or a long run away from danger, and the adrenaline simply stays around, making the person tense, nervous or anxious. This can be a short-term thing or, in some stressed-out people, an almost permanent state of affairs. Short-term anxiety can also be a perfectly natural response to worrying situations, such as a job interview or an exam.

Anxiety can trigger several other complaints, such as digestive problems, insomnia, muscular pain, skin complaints, palpitations, nausea and diarrhoea. See separate entries for all of these. Acute anxiety can take the form of a panic attack, a severe state of panic which may include palpitations, faintness, dizziness and fear. Sufferers should see their physician for professional help.

SOLUTIONS

Long term, try to seek out causes of anxiety and think about what changes you can make to your lifestyle to minimize these. Tackle anxiety by mimicking the 'fight or flight' response — take some exercise and do some deep breathing. This will help adrenaline to disperse and help you relax. The Bach Flower Rescue Remedy, may also help. Other causes of anxious feelings are alcohol abuse or an overload of caffeine drinks and products such as strong coffee, tea, cola and chocolate. If you are prone to anxiety it would be wise to limit these items

severely. Alcohol and, to a lesser extent, caffeine, can also disrupt sleep patterns, which may make anxiety worse.

Chronic stress depletes the body of B vitamins, so eating plenty of B-rich foods (see best sources list on page 26) and perhaps taking a B-group supplement is a good idea. Eat a good basic healthy diet including lettuce, which is a soporific, and plenty of calcium- and magnesium-rich foods. Herbal remedies for anxiety include valerian, camomile, passionflower and lemon balm, all of which can be taken as an infusion or in supplement form. Cloves, rosemary and lavender are all also said to be calming, and their essential oils are ideal in aromatherapy. Yoga and other forms of massage are also worth trying to alleviate symptoms.

■ SEVERAL CONDITIONS CAN BRING about a loss of appetite — anxiety, stress, depression and shock are four typical situations. Illnesses of many kinds can cause loss of appetite, particularly digestive disorders such as irritable bowel syndrome or peptic ulcer, viral and bacterial illnesses and food intolerance. Colds, catarrh and allergic rhinitis can lessen appetite, partly by reducing the sense of smell and taste, as can cigarette smoking. Drugs prescribed for various ailments can cause appetite loss — for example, those the side-effects of which may be nausea, or loss of taste or sense of smell. Hormonal changes through the monthly menstrual cycle mean that women's appetite may vary, usually being greater in the week preceding a period and lower in the few days afterwards.

Eating disorders such as anorexia nervosa may present themselves as poor appetite, though the sufferer may, in fact, have a normal appetite. Diminished appetite is fairly common in the elderly (see Section Three, Sixties Plus, page 182)

and this may be partly due to lessened needs as well as lowered physical activity and a general slowing down of hormone-based responses, of which appetite is but one example.

Poor appetite can also be brought about by a deficiency in certain nutrients — zinc deficiency may contribute to loss of taste and smell and therefore appetite; potassium and magnesium deficiency may also be to blame — likely if the person with a poor appetite has been taking diuretic drugs for fluid retention, as some varieties cause these minerals to be excreted in the urine. Alcohol can reduce the appetite if taken in excess regularly — one drink can, however, be an appetite stimulant. In fact, any kind of drink, including water, squashes and fizzy drinks, can depress hunger signals if taken before meal times. Children with a poor appetite should, in particular, be discouraged from drinking too much before a meal — in one study, 15% of pre-school-age children took just under 50% of their daily calorie needs in the form of drinks, especially squashes.

A short spell of poor appetite in an otherwise healthy person, when the reason is clear, is nothing serious to worry about and the appetite should return (often with a vengeance!) when the cause is gone. Any chronic loss of appetite should be discussed with your physician.

To tempt a poor appetite, small amounts of tasty and attractive food should be offered frequently. If possible low-nutrient 'junk' foods should be avoided, unless the main consideration is weight gain; meals and snacks should contain plenty of foods rich in vitamins B and C (which are water-soluble and the body can't store them for long), zinc, potassium and magnesium.

Arrhythmia, see Heart Disease and Stroke

ARTHRITIS

THERE ARE TWO MAIN TYPES of arthritis — osteoarthritis and rheumatoid arthritis. Osteoarthritis is a degenerative condition of the joints with a strong genetic component more common in older people. A normal healthy joint, such as the knee or hip (two very common sites of osteoarthritis), is covered by a smooth layer of shiny cartilage, which normally allows free gliding movement. In osteoarthritis, the cartilage becomes roughened, resulting in the underlying bone being worn. This is the commonest form of arthritis and is more common in women. Symptoms are pain, stiffness and loss of mobility in the affected joint(s).

Rheumatoid arthritis is determined by blood tests and history and is most common in adult women. It is a chronic inflammatory condition involving multiple joints and is thought of as having an auto-immune disease component. The immune system, which normally defends us against infection, appears instead to react against some part of the body. Rheumatoid arthritis often starts with pain and weakness in the hands and wrists. Joints may swell and may eventually become deformed. Inflammation may flare up and then disappear again, making it difficult to known exactly what 'works' to help. The causes of rheumatoid arthritis aren't fully understood, but there may be an environmental trigger such as a virus or bacterium. Even stress has been linked to rheumatoid arthritis.

SOLUTIONS

Diet doesn't really appear to play a big part in the prevention or management of osteoarthritis in most people, with the main exception that the symptoms of the condition — and the amount of trouble it causes — will be worse in someone who is very overweight or obese. The 'load-bearing' joints, such as the knees and hips, are put under much greater strain if the sufferer is too heavy. So, if you have osteoarthritis and are overweight, it is very important to lose the weight (see Section Four).

However, one recent trial in the USA has found that the progress of osteoarthritis can be minimized with high intakes of the antioxidant vitamins C and E, and with vitamin D. (Note: vitamin D can be toxic in excess but is fine in multinutrient supplements for regular intake up to 10 µg.) The essential omega-3 oils in cod liver oil and oily fish may also help. Glucosamine sulphate supplements have also met with success in minimizing pain in some trials and may even help restore joints to health (see page 151).

The role of diet and dietary factors in rheumatoid arthritis still remains quite controversial, but results of a number of trials suggest that diet does have a part to play in managing symptoms. A variety of diets have been reported to be helpful, but unfortunately, in rheumatoid arthritis what works for one sufferer may well not work for another. Moreover, as explained above, because symptoms often disappear for weeks or longer of their own accord, it is hard to know, when the sufferer suddenly feels better, whether it is diet or a period of remission. However, certain general guidelines seem to achieve the best results.

A good starting point is to follow all the healthy eating guidelines (e.g. the Basic Healthy Diet on page 53). Omega 3 fish oils and olive oil can subdue the enzymes that cause inflammation. One 2006 trial found that patients given daily fish oil plus 10ml olive oil showed significant alleviation of joint pain, morning stiffness and fatigue over a six-month period. A diet low in saturated fat will help these fats do their work. A diet high in fruit and vegetables provides antioxidants, which may be important. One US trial showed that people who ate higher levels of vitamin C were three times less likely to have progression of the disease than those eating the lowest; another US trial found that low levels of vitamin A and E were linked to the disease's development. Blood tests on people with arthritis have also shown low selenium levels. There is also research showing that the spice turmeric can help relieve inflammation and evidence that a healthy vegetarian or vegan diet can help minimize symptoms in some people.

An analysis published in the *British Journal of Nutrition* during 2000 showed a link between the eating of meat and offal and rheumatoid arthritis. It may also be helpful to try eliminating from your diet the plants of the nightshade family — potatoes, tomatoes, aubergines and peppers, which may exacerbate the inflammation of rheumatoid arthritis. Eliminate them for a period of eight weeks; if, by then the symptoms are improved, you may want to avoid those foods in future. Tobacco is also a member of the nightshade family and so smoking should be avoided if you do seem to have rheumatoid arthritis which is triggered by the other members of the nightshade family.

Many other foods are reported as 'triggers' for attacks of rheumatoid arthritis. Dairy foods and grains, especially wheat and corn, are the most common triggers mentioned. Coffee, nuts and fruits with pips have also been cited, as well as red wine and citrus fruits. However, because these vary so much and because some, such as dairy foods and grains, form such an important part of many people's diets, and eliminating them without proper dietary advice could cause nutrient and energy deficiency, it is important to be medically supervised if you want to attempt to pinpoint a particular trigger.

Recent trials using supplements of evening primrose oil and fish oil in cases of rheumatoid arthritis have shown encouraging results, but response takes time (up to three months). Linseed oil —

like fish oils, rich in omega-3 fatty acids — may have a similar effect. Some experts believe that supplements of vitamin E, C, and zinc and selenium may help, but this is still hotly debated. Various other supplements — including nettle tea, bromelain, collagen, green-lipped mussel extract and cider vinegar — are said to help some people, but the evidence is mainly anecdotal.

People who are on anti-inflammatory drugs for their arthritis may well become anaemic and should therefore be sure to eat plenty of iron-rich foods regularly. People who are on steroids should be sure to take plenty of calcium-rich foods. See also Gout.

ASTHMA

THE SYMPTOMS OF ASTHMA are wheezing, cough, tight chest and difficulty in breathing, due to air passages in the lungs narrowing. Asthma now affects one in seven UK schoolchildren, and research indicates rates among under-fives have almost doubled in less than a decade, while 5% of adults are thought to suffer. Asthma is the most common long-term disease in the West.

This may be due to a number of factors, including air, chemical and food pollution, but asthma may be triggered by many things, including house mites, cigarette smoke, household sprays, cold air, exercise, pollen, animals, and less commonly by some foods (often dairy produce) and food additives. If foods are involved, they may sensitize air passages and result in some other trigger causing an attack.

It is hard to find the food link in such cases, but certain items are known to be more sensitizing than others. Food additives containing sulphites (E220-E227) are common triggers and are mostly found in squashes, wines, beers, cider, vinegar, dried fruits, quick-frozen shellfish and some ready-prepared salads (read the labels to check) as are the azo dyes such as tar-

trazine (E102) found in drinks, sweets and other commercial products. Some asthmatics are allergic to the salicylates in aspirin.

An asthmatic reaction is possible in anyone with a food allergy or intolerance, but asthmatics should only carry out food avoidance or elimination under medical supervision, as serious reactions may result.

For more information, see page 88.

SOLUTIONS

Asthmatics can follow some dietary precautions to help minimize attacks even if a food intolerance isn't the problem. New research shows that omega-3 fatty acids in oily fish (and linseeds) can protect against asthma, while high intake of omega-6 fats, such as sunflower oil, may increase susceptibility in children. A low-salt diet is a good idea as salt can increase the reactivity of the airways. A diet high in magnesium may help as magnesium reduces the reactivity of the muscles in the airways and of certain allergy cells (MAST cells) — for best sources, see page 32. A diet rich in antioxidants — selenium and vitamins C, E and the carotenoids (for best sources, see pages 22-33) — can help boost the body's defence mechanisms against attack. Apples, rich in beneficial plant chemicals, are linked with improved lung function.

Asthma can begin at any age, so it is important to try to protect yourself against it. Research shows that people who eat a poor diet, low in fruits and veg, and therefore antioxidants, are more likely to get asthma. Several recent studies have found that lung function and asthma symptoms improve in both adults and children who eat plenty of fruit and veg. Apples, tomatoes, carrots, leafy vegetables and citrus fruits appear to have the greatest effect.

A new system called enzyme-potentiated desensitization (EPD) is showing promise in helping control asthma, where minute doses of allergens are injected up to four times a year; see the Appendix for addresses.

See also Allergies, Hay Fever.

Atherosclerosis, see Heart Disease and Stroke

Bad Breath, see Halitosis

BLOOD PRESSURE

■ HYPERTENSION (HIGH BLOOD PRESSURE) is an extremely common disorder, affecting approximately one-fifth of adults in Western countries. If left untreated, it can cause strokes, heart attacks and kidney disease, and yet symptoms are not easy to spot.

Some people have a hereditary predisposition to it, short people in particular are susceptible, and the middle-aged and elderly are more prone to it than young people, men more often affected than women (although incidence rises in women during pregnancy). People who smoke are also more likely to have high blood pressure, as are women on the Pill and people under stress.

SOLUTIONS

Medication can help to reduce hypertension, but there are also various nutritional methods of helping to prevent or control high blood pressure. One of the major factors is body weight — overweight and obese people are much more likely to have raised blood pressure; so, if you have hypertension — or any of the risk factors as described above — and are overweight, follow a sensible slimming plan such as that in Section Four and get down to a reasonable weight slowly. Yo-yo dieting is very negative and may actually make hypertension worse.

Alcohol is another factor — high intake may result in raised blood pressure, so if you drink more than the safe limits (see pages 86 and 66) you should cut down. Even 2 pints of beer or half a bottle of wine a day increases blood pressure, one large trial has found.

A study in the *New England Journal of Medicine* proved that reducing salt (sodium) intake does lower blood pressure – and combining a low-salt diet with increased fruit and vegetables has an additional beneficial effect. Try to limit salt intake to no more than 4g a day, equivalent to 1.6g of sodium, which is the RNI for adults in the UK, or take advice for your own case from your physician.

A list of the major sources of salt in the diet appears on page 33, and other tips for cutting salt intake are to stop adding salt to the cooking of vegetables and to food at the table, and to eat a diet as high in natural produce as possible, because it is highly processed foods which tend to contain most salt.

There are several salt substitutes available which you may find helpful, and nowadays there are many commercial foods which are 'reduced-salt'. It is also quite easy to wean yourself away from a taste for salty foods by cutting down on them gradually.

While cutting salt, increase your intake of foods rich in potassium (see page 32), such as dried apricots, pulses and nuts, because research shows that high potassium intake can help lower blood pressure. NOTE: do not eat a high-potassium diet if you have any sort of kidney disorder.

Two other minerals, calcium and magnesium, have also been shown to lower blood pressure (see their respective best source lists on pages 29 and 32), as have omega-3 essential fatty acids in the form of oily fish and linseed, garlic, dark chocolate, fruits high in soluble fibre (see the Food Charts) and moderate alcohol consumption (one or two drinks a day).

Data from the Vegetarian Society shows that vegetarians have less incidence of hypertension than meat-eaters. This could be for a variety of reasons, however; many vegetables are good sources of potassium, calcium, magnesium and vitamin C (500g a day has been shown to lower blood pressure). Ginger and the herb rosemary are also traditional herbal remedies for raised blood pressure.

BRONCHITIS AND COUGHS

■ BRONCHITIS is an acute or chronic inflammation of the bronchial tubes — the airways which lead to the lungs. There will often be an underlying infection. Bronchitis is accompanied by a mucus-producing cough and often a raised temperature. The most common cause of bronchitis is smoking, but it can also be caused by infection or viruses, pollution or an allergic reaction to, say, dust or airborne fumes.

SOLUTIONS

Avoidance of tobacco and known allergens is the obvious starting point in avoiding bronchitis. People who are prone to chest infections should also build up their immune system with a diet rich in antioxidants, zinc and other immune builders (see Immune-strengthening Diet, page 143). Some nutritionists advocate avoidance of 'mucus-forming' foods, such as dairy products, saturated fats and white bread, although this has never been proved.

Once bronchitis has taken hold it is important to take action quickly to minimize its duration and severity. Take plenty of fresh garlic; one of its active compounds, allicin, is a powerful antibiotic. To a lesser extent, onions and leeks are effective too. Increase your intake of vitamin C, with plenty of fresh fruits and salads. Manuka honey helps fight the streptococcus bacteria that cause sore throats – take twice daily with fresh lemon juice and a little warm water or use on bread.

The herbs hyssop and thyme are antiseptic and can be taken as an infusion daily (see Herbs for Health, page 154). It is also useful to inhale their oils in recently boiled water. Bronchial and other coughs and sore throat can be soothed with liquorice and with the honey drink mentioned left. A honey and cider vinegar gargle and zinc lozenges can also be effective in some cases.

Bulimia, see Eating Disorders

CANCER

■ A QUARTER OF all deaths in the industrialized world are due to cancers. One in three Britons is at risk of contracting cancer and about 153,000 a year die of the disease. There are over 100 different types of cancer and it is now believed that the causes and triggers may be almost as diverse. However, the consensus of opinion is now that 60-70% of all cancers could be prevented by doing just two things — eating the suggested healthy diet and giving up smoking.

The consensus report from the World Cancer Research Fund estimates that up to 40% of cancers — four million cases throughout the world — could be avoided by means of correct diet and body weight. Let's look at these consensus recommendations one by one:

Increase intake of a wide variety of fruits and vegetables

It seems that in the fight against cancers, fruit and veg may hold the key. Increased intake of them is linked with, for instance, decreased incidence of cancers of the stomach, lung, breast, prostate, mouth, pancreas and bladder. In one study, cancer deaths in vegetarians were found to be 39% lower than in others.

Not only do fruits and vegetables contain fibre, vitamins and minerals needed for health but we are now discovering the wealth of 'hidden' compounds they contain. These are the biologically active non-nutrients in food called phytochemicals.

Under that umbrella term there are many different groups of phytochemicals, such as flavonoids, indoles, sterols and phenols, and within each group are yet more specific compounds, each with its own function(s). It seems that many of these are marvellous at helping prevent, or block, or suppress, carcinogens or tumours. Here are some examples:

* *Tomatoes* contain the carotenoid lycopene, one of the phenol group, which protects against cancer-causing pollutants. One trial found that men eating ten servings of tomato a week were 45% less likely to get prostate cancer, but other trials have been less conclusive.

* *Broccoli* and other members of the brassica family contain indoles, a group of cancer-fighting agents. Broccoli contains glucosinolates, which break down in the body to form sulphorophanes which fight cancers of the lung and colon.

* *Brussels sprouts* contain another glucosinolate, sinigrin, a compound which helps to suppress pre-cancerous activity.

* *Watercress* is rich in phenethyl isothiocyanate, which is particularly good at helping to prevent lung cancer.

* *Carrots, broccoli* and all dark green, red, orange and yellow vegetables contain carotenoids, which help to protect the immune system and may help fight lung cancer.

* *Yams* are high in phyto-oestrogens, which may help to protect against breast cancer and other similar hormone-driven cancers.

* *Oriental mushrooms* such as shiitake contain lentinan, which strengthens the immune system and helps the body fight cancer.

* *Grape skins* and many other fruit skins are rich in resveratrol, a compound which inhibits cancer development and is also found in red burgundy wines. Grapes also contain ellagic acid, also

NUTRITION AGAINST CANCER

* Increase intake of a wide variety of fruits and vegetables (total weight per day 450g minimum). Choose organic produce, eat skins and choose less sweet varieties for much higher levels of cancer-fighting antioxidants.
* Increase intake of starchy plant foods in general, including whole grain cereals and pulses, again 450g / 1 lb a day minimum.
* Increase intake of dietary fibre (NSP) from a variety of sources (the first two points would achieve this). Intakes of up to 24g /³/₄ oz a day from natural sources (not added bran) are recommended by COMA.
* Reduce intake of saturated fats and meat. WCRF recommends reducing meat intake to less than 80g / 2 ³/₄ oz a day. It may be wise for people eating more than 90g / 3 ¼ oz a day to consider a reduction.
* Reduce total fat intake to approximately 30% of total calorie intake, but eat adequate omega-3 and monounsaturated oils.
* Avoid obesity — keep to a reasonable body weight throughout adult life.
* Limit consumption of alcohol to safe drinking guidelines (see page 36).
* Limit consumption of salt-cured, pickled, char-grilled and smoked foods.

found in cherries and strawberries, another cancer blocker.

* **Citrus fruits** such as oranges are high in antioxidant flavonoids, the phenol lutein and linolene to fight breast, colon and skin cancer.

* **Nuts and seeds** contain phytosterols, which help block colon, breast and prostate cancers, and gamma tocopherol, which may inhibit prostate and lung cancers.

And so on! For more information on the phytochemicals and their amazing powers, see pages 34-5. Many fruits and vegetables also contain rich levels of the important antioxidants, vitamins C, E and beta-carotene, which also offer considerable protection against some cancers.

Increase intake of starchy plant foods

Starchy, 'complex carbohydrate' foods, such as whole-grain cereals, rice, pasta, oats, pulses and potatoes, are high in fibre (NSP) and high intakes are linked to low levels of prostate, pancreas and breast cancer. Research also suggests that a substance called butyrate, produced by fermentation of complex carbohydrate in the bowel, is essential for colon mucosal health, helps prevent conditions which

promote cancer and increases rate of death of cancer cells.

Regular intake of soya may help prevent colon cancer.

Reduce intake of saturated fats and meat

High-fat diets, and particularly those high in saturated fat, have long been linked with increased incidence of cancers of the colon (more marked in males). A high-fat diet also seems to increase the risk of cancer of the prostate, ovaries and breasts. Intake of high-fat foods, such as full-fat dairy produce, fatty cuts of meat and high-fat convenience foods, should be limited to reduce saturated fat intake.

In 2005, a major European (EPIC) study found that high intake of red meat increases the risk of bowel cancer. The risk was one-third higher when eating more than two 80g portions a week. Eating a portion of fish every other day, conversely, reduced the risk by a third. One reason that meat-eating may be linked with cancer could be that meat increases levels of nitrosamines in the body. These are chemicals known to be cancer-inducing. Other chemicals in processed meats and hormones in fresh meat may also increase cancer risk. Organic meat may contain

OTHER NOTES ON CANCER AND DIET

* Garlic contains anti-cancer compounds, such as diallyl sulphide and s-allylcysteine, which help to prevent and suppress tumours by up to 60%. Fresh garlic is the best medicine — its compounds appear to be more effective than supplements.
* Green tea contains five times as much cancer-fighting antioxidants (EGCG) as black tea.
* The mineral selenium is an antioxidant and is powerful in fighting the free radicals which are thought to increase risk of cancer. Brazil nuts and tuna fish are two good sources of the mineral. For best sources list, see page 31.
* Aspirin appears to be anti-cancer. 300mg a day may reduce the risk of cancer of the colon and rectum.
* Nitrate fertilizers, used by commercial growers to fertilize

vegetables such as lettuce and greens, are no longer thought to be cancer-causing. In fact there is evidence that they turn into nitric oxide in the body and offer health benefits.
* Supplements of beta-carotene appear to be ineffectual in cancer protection. One trial found that smokers who took supplements of the antioxidant actually had more incidence of lung cancer. Neither do supplements of vitamin C or E appear to offer protection.
* Polyunsaturated cooking oils can oxidize if heated too many times or kept too long and may be carcinogenic. Oils should be stored in a cool dark place, and discarded after use.
* Smoked and cured foods, such as smoked salmon and bacon, are carcinogenic and should be eaten in moderate amounts.

---

fewer chemicals and will be hormone-free. Overcooked meats, barbecued, burnt and chargrilled meats have also been linked with increased incidence of cancer, probably because the high cooking temperature creates carcinogenic compounds.

Increase intake of omega-3 fatty acids
By following all the above guidelines our total fat intake should automatically reduce to within recommended levels (most cancer research agencies agree that this is a maximum of 30% of total calories). A high-fat diet is linked to several types of cancer (see above) and is a major cause of obesity and overweight (see next paragraph). However, some types of fat are necessary in the diet and probably have a role to play in cancer prevention. Adequate amounts of omega-3 fatty acids appear to protect against cancer of the prostate, lung, breast and bowel, probably by having a 'calming' effect against the inflammatory prostaglandins in the system. Omega-3s are found in oily fish and linseed (flax) oil. It is therefore a good idea to replace some of the meat meals in the diet with oily fish meals as well as plant-based meals. According to latest research, there is also a link between high monounsaturated (e.g.

olive) oil intake and lower risk of colon and breast cancers.

Avoid obesity and overweight
Overweight is linked to breast cancer, which is one and a half times more likely in overweight post-menopausal women. There is a less obvious link between cervical cancer and overweight, and cancer of the gall bladder in women and prostate in men. By following the advice above, a weight within the body mass index guidelines (see page 188) should be fairly easy to maintain for everyone.

Limit consumption of alcohol
Excessive alcohol intake increases the risk of several cancers, including those of the mouth, pharynx, larynx, oesophagus, breast and liver. It may also increase risk of rectal cancers. Beer can be a major source of nitrosamines, which are carcinogenic, and heavy beer drinkers appear to be more at risk from pancreatic cancer. Alcohol drinking should therefore be kept within safe guidelines (see page 36). A protective effect for bowel cancer has been shown in red wine, which contains resveratrol, also found in grape skins, but safe limits should still be observed.

See the Anti-cancer Diet on page 140. Helpful addresses appear in the Appendix.

Diet and breast cancer
The latest studies on breast cancer and diet show that the evidence linking a high-soya diet with reduced breast cancer risk is inconclusive and that clinical trials need to be done. Indeed, in 2006 the National Cancer Institute in the USA found that, for women with oestrogen-dependent breast disease, a diet high in oestrogen-rich foods or supplements (such as soya) could actually be risky.

Other work on diet and breast cancer indicates that a low-fat diet can help prevent recurrence; that a low Glycaemic Index diet reduces the risk of breast cancer after the menopause; and that a diet high in acrylamide (in foods such as crisps and chips) doesn't increase the risk.

CANDIDA

THERE ARE SUGGESTIONS THAT a yeast — Candida albicans — may be involved in causing a range of symptoms which are attributed to food sensitivity. However, this is highly controversial as there is no scientific proof that this is the organism causing such problems which may lead to such a 'Candida' diagnosis. It may be that the balance of micro-organisms in the gut is disturbed, with the beneficial bacteria being reduced, allowing other bacteria — or possibly yeasts — to establish themselves. This may particularly be the case where courses of antibiotics are taken, which kill off the 'friendly' gut flora, or after severe stomach infections. It has also been suggested that this perhaps should be called Gut Dysbiosis.

The most frequently seen symptoms are irritable bowel, wind and bloating, constant fatigue, mild depression, muscle or joint pains, headaches, vaginal thrush, a craving for sweet foods and an intolerance of alcohol. Other problems may include a sensitivity to foods containing yeasts and moulds and even sensitivity to musty or mouldy atmospheres and damp weather. Foods containing sugar, in particular those high in sugar, are commonly reported as causing symptoms. This could be due to the troublesome bacteria and yeasts that feed on sugar.

Candida-type infections can also occur in people whose immune systems are not functioning well, perhaps after a long illness or long period of stress. Long-term use of steroids, for conditions such as asthma, can make people more susceptible and deficiencies of vitamins and minerals can affect the immune system.

SOLUTIONS

The nutritional treatment of dysfunctional gut is three-sided:

1: Follow a special diet which may discourage the growth of the offending organisms. This can be achieved by avoiding foods containing sugars, and also yeasts and moulds (to which there appears to be some form of sensitivity). There is also some evidence that a diet high in garlic may help.

2: Take a course of prescribed anti-fungal medication from a qualified practitioner.

3: Re-colonize the gut with friendly bacteria, which can be achieved by taking a pre-biotic supplement known as fructo-oligosaccharides (FOS), which feeds the beneficial bacteria, together with a pro-biotic supplement containing lactobacillus acidophilus and bifidobacteria. These are also present in reasonable quantities in some live yoghurts.

There are many different 'anti-candida' diets being offered by private nutritional therapists and doctors. Some are unnecessarily strict — for instance, forbidding all grains or dairy products. Some patients respond to these diets because, in fact, their symptoms were not of candida-type infections at all but, say, a grain or dairy allergy. Other 'therapists' recommend avoidance of all fruit — a tactic which is neither necessary nor wise. The avoidance list which appears on page 141 (with the Anti-candida Diet) is the one that the top experts now agree achieves results, without being too strict.

Long-term, people who have had candida-like infections may, after treatment, be able to tolerate some or all of the 'forbidden' foods again. However, a healthy lifestyle and a good immune system (see the Immune-strengthening Diet on page 143) are the best bets to fight the condition. Turn to page 141 for the Anti-candida Diet and food avoidance list.

Cataracts, see Eye Problems

Catarrh, see Colds and Flu

Chickenpox, see Herpes Simplex 1

CHILBLAINS

■ CHILBLAINS, WHICH USUALLY APPEAR on the hands or feet, are painful swellings that may itch and burst like blisters. They are an extreme reaction to cold, caused by poor circulation to the extremities, and are therefore more common in cold weather.

SOLUTIONS

Smoking is a contraindication and should be avoided if you suffer from chilblains.

Aerobic exercise, which helps maintain good circulation, is the main prevention — chilblains are more common in people who take little exercise, and in the elderly, although young children also seem to be prone to them. For other advice on improving circulation, see Circulation, Poor.

Food methods of increasing blood-flow to hands and feet include regular consumption of ginger, chillies and mustard. One good idea is to drink a glass of ginger wine most evenings. External remedies include potato poultices, mustard baths and bathing in carrot juice, all of which are unproven but won't do you any harm so may well be worth a try. Lastly, keep hands and feet warm in winter, with good socks, gloves, etc., and have a warm foot bath every day.

Chronic Fatigue Syndrome, see ME

CIRCULATION, POOR

■ PEOPLE WITH POOR CIRCULATION often feel cold when others don't and may look a little pale, with pale hands and feet. Their metabolism may be slower and they may suffer from related problems, such as chilblains, sluggish digestive system, including constipation, problems waking up in the morning and a general feeling of lethargy. When blood is circulated, the heart pumps it through the arteries to all parts of the body. The blood is then returned with the help of muscular activity through the veins. Poor circulation can then be caused either by a weak heart muscle, or by the hardening of the arteries (atherosclerosis), when the blood is not easily able to move through the arteries because build-up of deposits such as cholesterol on the arterial walls have narrowed them. For more details of both these problems, see Heart Disease.

SOLUTIONS

A major factor in good circulation is regular aerobic exercise, such as walking, jogging or cycling, during which blood is naturally pumped faster. Also, exercise encourages the muscles to remain fit and strong and in 'good working order' — in other words, more efficient in helping the circulatory system.

Garlic, ginger, buckwheat and the supplement ginkgo biloba are all aids to circulation, and may be used as part of a healthy diet. Vitamin E and omega-3 fatty acids, such as fish oils and linseed oil, also help to 'thin' the blood and aid its flow through the circulatory system.

Cirrhosis, see Alcoholism

COELIAC DISEASE

■ AN INFLAMMATORY CONDITION of the gastrointestinal tract, coeliac disease is caused by intolerance of the protein gluten, which is found in wheat and rye, and similar proteins in barley and oats. The gluten damages the intestinal lining, thus reducing the sufferer's ability to absorb nutrients. This can then result in conditions such as malnutrition, anaemia, osteoporosis and other problems.

First symptoms may appear when gluten is introduced into the diet of susceptible children after weaning, but the disease can also present symptoms at any age. Adults may have only mild symptoms or, in some cases, none at all. One in 1,500 of the UK population suffers from coeliac disease and the average is higher in insulin-dependent diabetics and those who suffer from some other auto-immune conditions.

Symptoms can vary enormously but in children they commonly include poor weight- and height-gain, crying and general miserableness, diarrhoea, bloating and vomiting. In adults, there may be weight loss, diarrhoea or constipation, anaemia, tiredness, lethargy, flatulence, mouth ulcers and sore tongue, painful joints, depression, amenorrhoea or infertility.

SOLUTIONS

If you suspect coeliac disease see your physician, who will make arrangements for diagnosis to be made.

Once coeliac disease is diagnosed, management involves avoiding all foods containing gluten, wheat, rye, barley or oats. These include ordinary breads, biscuits, pasta, cakes, many breakfast cereals, pastry, puddings and pies. A recent study produced evidence that oats may not be harmful in adults; however, until there is further evidence, oats should still be avoided.

The avoidance list may sound daunting at first, but specially produced gluten-free foods are available, e.g. breads, biscuits and pasta, where the gluten is removed from the wheat, leaving gluten-free wheat starch; or some are made from grains, such as corn and rice, which are naturally gluten-free.

A small proportion of coeliacs may also need to avoid wheat starch if they do not improve and a smaller proportion still may be helped by a diet that is also milk-free.

Some special products are available on prescription. Specific dietary advice for coeliac sufferers should be obtained from a dietician and, once diagnosed, the diet needs to be life-long. In proven cases of nutritional deficiency, e.g. anaemia, appropriate supplements will be needed. A general multivitamin/mineral may be helpful for the first few months after diagnosis, but this should be discussed with your physician first.

The Coeliac Society (see address in the Appendix) produces an annual list of manufactured foods that are guaranteed to be gluten-free and this list is regularly updated.

COLDS AND FLU

◼ A COLD — symptomized by sneezing, blocked-up nose, perhaps cough and body temperature changes — is a viral infection, as is flu. Although colds and flu are 'caught' from an infected person, in the air or by touch, you are more likely to get a cold or the flu if you have a weak immune system — perhaps through long periods of stress or other chronic illness, or through poor diet.

SOLUTIONS

The Immune-strengthening Diet on page 143 will help to prevent colds and flu. This includes plenty of foods rich in vitamin C and zinc. It has been suggested that mega-doses of vitamin C — up to 5 g a day — help prevent colds, but this has never been proved in scientifically conducted tests. High doses of vitamin C

taken for more than just a few days can cause stomach upsets, diarrhoea, kidney stones and other problems. If you feel a cold coming on, however, its severity and duration may be lessened by immediately increasing your daily intake of vitamin C to 500 mg a day, and continuing at that level for as long as the cold lasts. It is quite hard to get 500 mg of vitamin C a day in your normal diet, so taking a supplement will be necessary — try a chewable one with added bioflavonoids and zinc.

Cold Sores, see Herpes Simplex 1

COLITIS

◼ THIS IS A GENERALIZED TERM for inflammation of the colon. Several conditions can be grouped under the name, including ulcerative colitis, Crohn's disease and irritable bowel syndrome (dealt with in a separate entry).

Ulcerative colitis is ulceration of the colon lining; symptoms include watery stools, which may contain mucus and/or pus, abdominal pain, tenderness, colic, and intermittent or irregular fevers. It is unclear how the condition is actually caused, although there may be an irregularity in circulating antioxidants, i.e. vitamins A, C and E and the minerals selenium and zinc.

Crohn's disease is inflammation that can attack any section of the gut from mouth to anus. Symptoms may be diarrhoea, abdominal pain which can be mistaken for appendicitis, fever, appetite loss, weight loss and a bloated feeling. It is not clear why the disease starts, but some trials have shown that there could be a food intolerance link and that avoiding the problem foods significantly extends the time before recurrence. Foods primarily found to be a problem include grains, dairy produce and yeast. However, a bacterium in milk – MAP – is particularly implicated. The UK's leading

SOME OTHER IDEAS FOR MINIMIZING YOUR COLD

* Garlic — a proven antibacterial and decongestant: include plenty of the fresh product in your diet and take garlic oil supplement.
* Oils of thyme and eucalyptus may help to clear congestion: use a few drops in boiling water as an inhalant and use thyme in your cooking.
* Ginger and chillies are stimulating spices which are said to help fight off the viruses and are decongestant: use plenty fresh in your cooking.
* Echinacea stimulates the immune system, and veg, nuts and seeds, contain sterols that regulate it.
* Drink plenty of fluids throughout your cold, preferably citrus-based.
* It may also help to avoid dairy products, chocolate and all foods high in saturated fat throughout your cold. These are said to be mucus-forming and might encourage your cold to develop into sinusitis or catarrh.

Crohn's expert believes that without MAP there would be almost no incidence of the disease. Normal pasteurization doesn't kill the bug, but heating milk at home to a minimum of 80°C does.

SOLUTIONS

Constipation may bring on an attack of ulcerative colitis, in which case a high-fibre diet will help such as that outlined on page 14, avoiding too many refined and low-nutrient foods. A basic healthy diet, including plenty of vitamin C-rich foods, will help to minimize symptoms. Research shows that, during an attack, 20% of patients have benefited from a milk-free diet.

Antioxidant supplements may be useful and fish oil supplements may help to speed up recovery and reduce the number of attacks — probably because the omega-3 oils from oily fish have anti-inflammatory properties.

Crohn's sufferers should first try heating milk to 80°C or avoiding it. They can also try a low-fibre diet, avoiding certain fruit and veg, such as citrus, pineapple, bananas and grains; although, in others, a high-fibre diet may reduce the recurrence of the disease. Again, supplements of antioxidants and fish oils may help in either case. If food intolerance is suspected it is important not to self-treat but to seek professional help from a dietician (via your physician).

See the Appendix for addresses of useful organizations.

Compulsive Eating, see Eating Disorders

Conjunctivitis, see Eye Problems

CONSTIPATION

■ CONSTIPATION — the infrequent passing of stools — is one of the most common physical complaints in the Western world. More than just an uncomfortable problem, if left untreated it can cause or contribute towards diverticular disease and haemorrhoids. Largely, it is our modern Western diet that is to blame, although lack of physical activity undoubtedly makes the problem much worse, and sometimes other factors can cause sudden constipation, especially stress or a change in daily routine.

To function correctly and regularly (which may be less or more than the 'once a day' people usually regard as normal), our bowels need high-fibre foods as well as plenty of fluids to help bulk up the stools and make them easy to pass — about 3-4 pints of water a day is ideal.

The total amount of fibre we need in our diets has been set by the DoH at 12-18 g a day, but some people may need much more than this in order to maintain a regular bowel, particularly if constipation is or has been a major problem in the past and if their general levels of physical activity are low.

SOLUTIONS

To get this amount of fibre you need to make a real effort to include some high-fibre foods at every meal. Prunes and rhubarb are also known to contain fur-

ther special compounds which produce a laxative effect, but they should not be relied on to the exclusion of a varied high-fibre diet. The food charts on pages 260-317 list the fibre content of over 300 foods and the best sources of fibre are listed on page 14.

Fibre is found in all fruits and vegetables, grains, nuts, seeds and pulses, but not in animal products, and so the best diet to prevent constipation is one that contains lots of natural unrefined plant foods. Refined produce such as sugar, white breads, white rice and manufactured cakes and biscuits, refined breakfast cereals and white pasta contain much less fibre than their natural, unrefined counterparts.

Some people add a spoonful or two of bran to their daily diet to help keep them 'regular' — true bran is a very good source of insoluble fibre, but many experts believe it is better to get fibre as a natural part of your foods, as bran in this form can hinder absorption of some minerals.

If stress rather than a low-fibre diet is causing your constipation, then a mild herbal relaxant taken for a few days should help the problem — try camomile tea twice a day or the supplement kava kava — and see what lifestyle changes you can make (See also Stress, page 134). Exercise not only helps regulate bowel movement but also helps you relax.

Millions of people currently rely on daily doses of branded laxative pills to try to help cure their constipation. However, these are best avoided except for really very occasional use as long-term they can make the problem much worse because your colon comes to rely on them instead of trying to work for itself. So when you stop taking them your constipation is likely actually to become much worse than it was before. It is much better to cure constipation slowly, by means of the appropriate diet, exercise and lifestyle modifications.

NATURAL REMEDIES FOR CONSTIPATION

Various other foods and herbal remedies are recommended for constipation. Some of the herbs, such as senna, are strong purgatives and the same applies to them as to over-the-counter laxatives (see below). More gentle remedies include rose hip syrup, olive oil, honey, liquorice, blackstrap molasses, and psyllium seeds infused in water. Strong spices, such as curry powder, ginger and chilli, have a laxative effect.

CHD (Coronary heart disease), see Heart Disease and Stroke

Coughs, see Bronchitis and Coughs

CRAMP

■ EVERYONE HAS A MUSCLE CRAMP now and again and it is unmistakable — an extremely painful, and sometimes prolonged, powerful contraction of a muscle, often in the leg, usually sudden. Cramp may be due to over-exercise, perhaps without sufficient prior warming-up of the muscles involved, and may be exacerbated by insufficient fluids and minerals before or during prolonged exercise.

SOLUTIONS

A range of minerals are involved in muscle contraction and relaxation. It makes sense to have adequate amounts of salt in the diet if you exercise a lot, particularly in hot conditions when you will lose salt in the sweat. However, salt intake should still not exceed healthy eating guidelines (see page 33). Adequate calcium intake is important, too, as is magnesium, which works with calcium in the body (best sources lists, page 29 and 32).

Drink plenty of fluids when exercising and see Circulation, Poor, for further information about nutritional deficiencies which may result in poor circulation. Cramp may also occur at other times — for example, in bed at night — and this is likely to be a circulatory problem.

Once a cramp has begun, the best way to relieve it is to massage the affected area and if possible, stretch it out. Try to relax and breathe calmly.

Crohn's disease, see Colitis

Cuts and Grazes, see Wounds, Cuts and Grazes

CYSTITIS

■ CYSTITIS is a bladder infection, the main symptoms of which are a need to urinate very frequently, but then finding that you can only pass a few drops, a burning sensation when you do pass urine, and, if the attack is left untreated, pain in the kidneys (felt in the centre of the back). Urine may be cloudy, or even red, through traces of blood, and you may feel generally unwell.

SOLUTIONS

Research shows that drinking 50ml of cranberry juice cocktail daily can halve the risk of getting cystitis, and may lessen the severity of an attack. At the onset of an attack it is essential to cut out tea, coffee and alcohol, and to drink plenty of water, which helps to dilute the urine and so makes it less painful to pass as well as reducing infecting bacteria. Sufferers should also obtain sachets of potassium citrate, available from the chemist, which neutralizes the urine, and should see their physician. A basic healthy diet, low in refined sugar and low-nutrient foods, will help to prevent infection.

DEPRESSION

■ DEPRESSION is usually treated medically with a variety of drugs that enhance mood but, unfortunately, few are free from side effects. However, with dietary alterations and other natural methods, many cases of depression can be helped or even cured. Symptoms of depression can be severe or mild, short-term or long-term. Cause is often difficult to pinpoint, but symptoms may often include a general 'slowing down' both physically and mentally; inability to concentrate; loss of self-esteem, loss of libido, insomnia, deep feelings of unhappiness and or worthlessness, fear of life in general and withdrawal from social life and feeling at odds with the world at large.

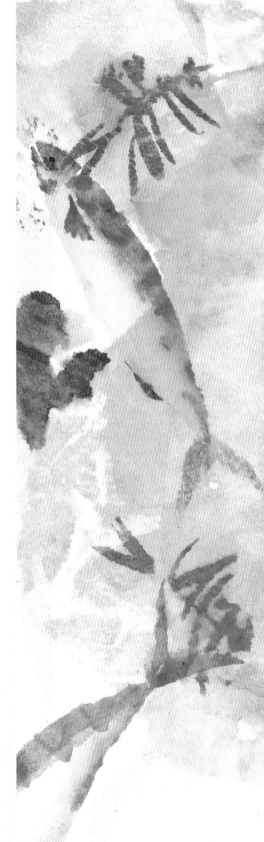

SEASONAL AFFECTIVE DISORDER

One common form of depression is SAD (Seasonal Affective Disorder) which is the term used to describe the depression that many people in northern Europe feel throughout the long dark winter months and thought to be the result of the lack of light, which in turn results in low levels of serotonin in the brain. This can be alleviated using all the methods outlined below and it has been found that regular light therapy works well in the winter months.

See also: Menopause (page 178); Menstrual Problems (126); ME (page 125); Fatigue (page 111) and Anxiety (page 92).

Depressives sometimes lose their appetite, possibly because of a knock-on effect from the 'slowing down' syndrome that is so symptomatic of depression, and possibly because the will to 'look after yourself' goes. Poor or meagre eating habits will result in nutrient deficiencies, which can also contribute to depression.

Other depressed people frequently turn to food for comfort, perhaps binge-ing on lots of high-carbohydrate foods, such as cakes, sweets and biscuits. This is a downward spiral, because comfort eating inevitably results in weight gain and even lower self-esteem.

SOLUTIONS

Interestingly, there is probably a genuine reason why so many people crave sweet foods when they are feeling miserable. There is evidence that high-carbohydrate, low-protein meals help in the metabolism of tryptophan. Due to the action of insulin, after such a meal, tryptophan is free to enter the brain for conversion to serotonin, a compound which enhances mood. (Incidentally, many of the new wave of anti-depressant drugs, including Prozac, also work by increasing available serotonin.) However, healthier carbohy-drate foods such as bread, fruits and dried fruits may help mild depression.

It is vital for any depressed person to be encouraged to eat a basic healthy diet. This will include regular portions of the protein foods such as lean meat, low-fat milk, cheese and eggs which are rich in the amino acid tryptophan, which con-verts to the mood-enhancing compound serotonin in the brain. Recent research in the UK showed that women deprived of tryptophan showed symptoms of depres-sion within hours.

Several studies have found a link between a low intake of omega-3 fatty acids, such as those found in oily fish, and high levels of depression and mental illness. As omega-3s are healthy anyway, it is worth including plenty of oily fish or a 1–2g daily supplement in the diet. The basic healthy diet should also include plenty of foods rich in the vitamin B-group (for best sources, see page 26), which keeps the nervous system healthy. Research has shown that people who follow a diet low in B vitamins suffer from more mood swings and are less happy. Vitamin C is depleted more easily in the body when it is under stress (which includes depression), so plenty of C-rich foods should be included. Vitamin C can also help in the production of serotonin. If the depressed person isn't eating prop-erly, then daily supplements of B group and C are indicated.

Alcohol should be avoided — in small doses it has a stimulant effect but after the first drink or so it is a depressant and likely to have an adverse effect on those prone to depression. Alcohol also robs the body of the B group vitamins and C. Caffeine can also make worsen depres-sion, so tea, coffee, cola and chocolate are best kept to a minimum.

It is important to try to take as much regular aerobic exercise as possible when depressed — there is much research to show that mood is enhanced by exercise because it releases endorphins into the body. A daily brisk walk would be good, as fresh air also has a stimulating effect and can banish that 'what's the point' feeling so consistent with depression. Taking that first step is all that is needed.

Herbalists will recommend the herb hypericum (St John's Wort) for depres-sion. Most research to date shows that it is effective as a mild anti-depressant, with few, if any, side effects and can be taken for periods of several weeks (in dosage as specified). Hypericum can be bought as dried leaf from some specialist shops and health food shops or as tablets called Kira.

DIABETES

THERE ARE approximately 1.4 million diagnosed diabetics — and perhaps half a million undiagnosed diabetics — in the UK alone and the figure is increasing. Diabetes mellitus is caused by lack of the hormone insulin, which is responsible for regulating levels of sugar in the blood and its utilization by tissues. Without insulin, the level of sugar in the blood rises.

The first signs of diabetes are increased thirst, frequent urination, weight loss, excessive tiredness, and perhaps skin and fungal infections and blurred vision. If diabetes is not treated it can damage the heart, kidneys, eyes and other organs. Urine and blood tests can diagnose diabetes, which can be either as Type 1, insulin-dependent diabetes (IDDM), or Type 2, non-insulin-dependent diabetes (NIDDM). Diabetics of both types are at greater risk than normal of cardiovascular disease, kidney disease, eyesight problems and infections.

NOTE: Anyone with diabetes should be regularly monitored and counselled by their physician and dietician. The notes below are for general guidance only. Any diabetic who wishes to follow any of the diets or diet tips recommended should get professional approval.

■ Insulin-dependent diabetes

People with this type of diabetes don't produce any insulin themselves and need to have regular daily injections of insulin coupled with correct diet (see below) in order to control the diabetes.

Who gets it?

About 25% of diabetics are insulin-dependent. This type of diabetes is more common in children and young adults and it is thought that about 10% of cases are found in people with one or other parent also IDD. There is some evidence of a link between a virus that attacks the pancreas, where insulin is normally produced, and the onset of diabetes. Sudden shock also seems to precipitate the start of diabetes. At the moment, however, there is no proven cause and no cure.

■ Non-insulin-dependent diabetes

People with this type of diabetes either produce a little — but not enough — insulin, or there is a defect in its use. However, the diabetes can be controlled either simply by modifications in diet (and weight) or in addition with the help of tablets.

Who gets it?

This is the most common form of diabetes, about 75% of all cases. It is most common in people aged 40 upwards, which is why it was often called 'mid-life onset diabetes'. More women suffer than men. Insulin production doesn't appear to decrease with age, but increased age may produce a resistance to insulin's action, probably because of weight gain and lack of physical activity.

Many people with Type-2 diabetes are overweight. People with a BMI (body mass index) over 30 are ten times more likely to develop diabetes than people of average weight, according to Diabetes

UK. People with a BMI over 35 are 80 times more likely. Even being slightly overweight (with a BMI over 26) increases the risk threefold. Losing surplus weight means less insulin is needed.

Type-2 diabetes may also be triggered by steroid medication or other factors which are less likely, and up to a third of Type-2 diabetics have other family members who are also diabetic. Diabetes occurs more frequently in people of Asian, Jewish or Afro-Caribbean races.

Prevention and management

The USDA Diabetic Prevention Program has found that keeping a sensible weight, eating a healthy low-fat diet and taking regular exercise offers the most effective protection against Type-2 diabetes. If you already have diabetes, following similar guidelines can offer control of the disease.

Type-2 diabetes can often be controlled by losing weight alone. If the diabetic is overweight, he or she should follow a sensible diet plan such as that in Section Four until the body mass index is down to the ideal range of 20-25. (For middle-aged people who have been severely overweight, a target of no less than 22 is probably realistic and sensible.) The British Diabetic Association says that it doesn't provide a 'special' diet just for diabetics, because the right diet for diabetics is similar to healthy eating recommendations for everyone.

This diet should be low in saturated fat and low in simple sugars, such as sugar itself and sweets, which cause sharp rises in blood sugar levels, and low-nutrient, highly processed 'junk' foods. It should include plenty of complex carbohydrates, fibre, fruit and veg, and adequate protein and essential fatty acids.

To help keep blood sugar levels from fluctuating too much, for many diabetics it helps to have regular small to medium-sized meals and snacks, including plenty of low-to-moderate glycaemic index foods (see page 195) especially pulses, oats and fruits, which are high in soluble fibre and also have the benefit of lowering blood cholesterol levels, which are often high in diabetics. (However, individual needs vary and a dietician's advice is needed.)

The nutritional requirements of a diabetic can be met by following the basic healthy diet in Section One, or the Healthy Heart Diet on page 142.

Plenty of water and fluids should be taken to help keep the kidneys working well, and a diet high in antioxidants, zinc and garlic will help to protect against infections. If you would like the odd sweet treat, chocolate or dessert, eat it with a main meal to help keep blood sugar levels constant.

New research also indicates that a diet high in fruit and vegetables, vitamin E and fish oils (which can be taken by eating more oily fish or as a supplement) is particularly beneficial for diabetics and can help prevent insulin resistance, the 'pre-diabetic' state. It also offers protection against cardiovascular disease, which is diabetics' leading cause of ill health and death, because of their increased levels of cholesterol and fat in the blood.

In people who are diabetic, supplements of 200μ chromium sulphate daily may help control blood sugars, and ginseng, cinnamon and high-cocoa-solids chocolate may also help.

Exercise

Some regular moderate exercise, such as walking, will help to get or keep surplus weight off and strengthen the circulatory and immune systems, as well as lower blood pressure and blood cholesterol. However, exercise 'uses up' blood sugars for energy and the insulin-dependent diabetic should take care to eat sufficient carbohydrate before exercise to avoid hypoglycaemia (a 'hypo'), when too much insulin is present and blood sugar levels crash. If this should happen, blood sugar needs to be raised quickly with glucose tablets or similar. After exercising, it is a good idea to have a healthy snack containing carbohydrate and a little protein, such as a banana and a yoghurt.

■ **DIARRHOEA** can be a symptom of several different illnesses or disorders. An acute (short-term) attack of diarrhoea is often related to food poisoning, when bacteria such as salmonella or E. coli are present in foods and have not been killed by appropriate cooking, and is also frequently experienced by travellers abroad who may drink contaminated local water or eat new foods. When abroad on long-distance travel it is sensible to drink only bottled water and stick with foods that have been well cooked.

Food allergy or intolerance is another common cause; for example diarrhoea is a symptom of lactose (milk sugars) intolerance and coeliac disease, which is caused by intolerance to the gluten in wheat and other products. Diarrhoea can also be the result of eating too much food which has a laxative effect — for instance, rhubarb or oranges. Many infections and illnesses may result in diarrhoea, particularly in small children. Zinc supplements can prevent diarrhoea in children.

SOLUTIONS

Sufferers from an acute attack should drink plenty of bottled water to which is added a little salt and sugar for rehydration, and eat no solids for 24 hours. When able to eat a little again, eat bland, easily digested, energy-rich low-fat foods, such as potatoes, rice, white bread and bananas. Also get plenty of potassium-rich foods, such as bananas, potatoes, seeds, lentils and nuts, into your diet as soon as possible as diarrhoea depletes the body's potassium levels and potassium is particularly important in stabilizing your body's fluid levels after a bout of diarrhoea.

Get back to a basic healthy diet when you can, paying particular attention to foods rich in zinc and B-group and C vitamins — water-soluble vitamins which will also have been depleted by the condition. Live bio yoghurt will also help to get the digestive system back to normal functioning by restoring its normal levels of healthy bacteria.

Diarrhoea that lasts longer than 48 hours or recurring bouts, for which you can find no simple explanation, need investigating by a physician. The cause could be irritable bowel syndrome, colitis

DIARRHOEA

'DIABETIC' FOODS — WORTH THE EXPENSE?

There is a huge range of commercial foods available, produced especially for diabetics and often sold in chemists or health food stores. These are items, such as diabetic jams, confectionery, biscuits and so on, and they are usually more expensive than ordinary products. Although they are often as high in fat and nearly as high in calories as their ordinary counterparts, they usually contain fructose (fruit sugar) or another sweetener, sorbitol, instead of sucrose. The BDA feels that these products are unnecessary.

These days, supermarkets carry a very good range of products low in fat and sugar which are equally suitable for diabetics. There is not really any such thing as a 'diabetic food' and, in any case, high intake of fructose and sorbitol can cause problems — such as diarrhoea or other digestive upsets. A diabetic should discuss the whole topic of how sweet foods can be included in the diet with their own dietician.

or several other more serious problems.

See also the entries on Allergies, Coeliac Disease, Colitis and Irritable Bowel Syndrome, and the section on Safe Food on page 81.

Digestive Disorders, see Heartburn and Indigestion

DIVERTICULAR DISEASE

DIVERTICULAR DISEASE is a common problem in older people, when small pockets or sacs form in weakened areas of the wall of the colon. Half or more of the population over 60 may have diverticular disease, but only 25 per cent or less will have the symptoms — abdominal pain, particularly in the lower left-hand side above the groin, and a change in bowel habits, e.g. alternating diarrhoea and constipation. If the pockets (diverticuli) become clogged with waste matter and infected, symptoms may also include fever and bleeding, and hospital treatment will be needed. The cause of diverticular disease is probably our highly refined Western diet, with inadequate amounts of fibre, particularly soluble fibre. This can easily lead to constipation and the diverticuli may form when straining to pass hard stools.

SOLUTIONS

To prevent diverticulitis follow the Basic Healthy Diet (page 53) or, if prone to constipation, a high-fibre diet. Follow all the tips in the separate entry for Constipation, paying particular attention to getting enough cereal fibre and soluble fibre in the diet, found in excellent quantities in pulses, fruits and oats. The Food Charts on pages 260-317 list the soluble fibre content of all common foods. On average we need 18 g of fibre a day, of which at least 6-8 g should be soluble.

Also make sure to get enough fluid in your diet — insoluble fibre needs fluid to form stools that are easy to pass. If upping your fibre intake, you should drink plenty of water — at least 1.75 litres / 3 pints a day. Fibre is best obtained through a natural high-fibre diet — avoid sprinkling raw bran on foods, as it may irritate the colon.

Duodenal Ulcer, see Peptic Ulcer

EATING DISORDERS

ANOREXIA NERVOSA, BULIMIA NERVOSA AND COMPULSIVE EATING are the three main categories of eating disorder, which most experts agree are an outward expression of psychological conflict rather than simply a problem with food and body image. In practice, it is sometimes not simple to categorize a sufferer as being precisely one or another of the three. For example, anorexics may later become bulimic; compulsive eaters may from time to time be bulimic, and so on. However, there are distinct differences between the disorders and their effects, described here in more detail.

■ Anorexia nervosa
The term means 'loss of appetite due to nervous reasons' but, in fact — at least in the early stages of the disease, most anorexics do feel hungry and do want to eat, but they don't allow themselves to do so. Later, appetite may indeed disappear and, even though the anorexic may want to be cured, she or he may find that that decision is no longer within her or his grasp (ironically, because anorexics frequently fear being out of control).

Neither is anorexia simply an obsession with becoming slim (although thinness is outwardly one of the anorexic's main goals), or a disease brought about by modern society's accent on good looks — anorexia was recognized as long ago

ZINC AND ANOREXIA

There has been some evidence that supplements of the mineral zinc can help anorexics to regain their appetite and taste-buds and may help the depression from which many anorexics suffer. It has also been suggested that a zinc deficiency may also be one of the factors in the development of anorexia, although this is yet to be proved.

as the Middle Ages and given its name nearly 130 years ago. Some cases, certainly, may be triggered by a need to have a particular body image (which is why the incidence of anorexia, and bulimia, is high amongst people like dancers, models and actors, many of whom have the 'anorexic personality type' as described below).

Anorexia nervosa is thought not to have just one cause, but several, although many sufferers do tend to have certain things in common. The disease is ten times more prevalent in females than males, and is thought to affect up to one in two hundred women, and up to one in a hundred girls in their late teens, although it can also effect older people (including menopausal women).

Many experts believe that there can be a genetic tendency towards anorexia, with extra factors acting as triggers. Sufferers tend to be high achievers and often from families where academic achievement is important. Many anorexics appear to be confident and efficient and perfectionist, wanting to be good at all they do (though some may be introverted and shy), but underneath may have a constant feeling of not being good enough, and of literally, being 'anxious' to please, particularly peers (including parents), and may feel that the parents don't care about the person so much as what is achieved.

Experts say that the two most common traits in the anorexic personality are perfectionism and obsessionality. It is thought that giving up food may be a way of exercising control over life, over others, and over oneself. Anorexia may be a solution to this personality type,

whereas others may turn to alcohol, drugs or crime, for example.

The symptoms of anorexia are a preoccupation with weight and weight loss, and perhaps with eating only foods perceived to be low in calories, such as lettuce or celery. Orthoroxia – a name coined for an obsession with eating only pure, natural, healthy foods – may disguise anorexic tendencies. Anorexics may go to great lengths to avoid eating food and become adept at making excuses for missing meals. Often, though, they will enjoy preparing and serving delicious meals for the rest of the family.

Weight loss is the obvious first physical sign, although many anorexics disguise this well with big and baggy clothes. Anorexics are often restless and hyperactive and may be obsessional about exercise and orderliness. In women, periods will cease. As the anorexia progresses, the sufferer will face severe constipation, malnutrition, will feel very cold all the time and may grow hair on the body while hair on the head may be thin. As time goes on, anorexics will tend to eat less and less, until eventually their diet may consist of a lettuce leaf and some water every day. Unless the anorexic is treated, death through starvation or related causes, such as heart failure, will occur.

The sooner the anorexic can be persuaded to accept treatment the more chance of recovery. Treatment often consists of a stay in hospital, where the patient is fed until sufficient weight is gained, coupled with psychological and practical counselling. It has been found that unless the underlying causes of the

original anorexia are addressed, the anorexic will often quickly lose weight again. Recovery often takes several years. About half of diagnosed and treated anorexics recover completely, others remain ill long-term, and about 5% die.

It is very hard for an anorexic to make a recovery without the support and help of other people, as many refuse to admit that they have a problem. Various private clinics and residential homes now exist where the anorexic can be helped to work through problems and be taught to eat again. The Eating Disorders Association has a network of support and self-help groups, which also have a high degree of success.

Some nutritionists who specialize in eating disorders have a programme which helps sufferers to eat normally again through a process of teaching them the real value of food and why the nutrients it contains are important for a healthy body; by suggesting several small meals a day, beginning with foods the anorexic feels she or he can manage to eat and learning to accept that the taste and texture of food is something to enjoy not fear, and then gradually reintroducing other healthy foods.

■ Bulimia nervosa

It is thought that bulimia nervosa — when the sufferer binges on, sometimes huge, amounts of food and then purges through vomiting, diuretics or laxatives — is much, much more common in the Western world than is anorexia, but because most bulimics feel shame at what they do and follow the binge/purge cycle in secret, many cases go undetected. Bulimia also affects predominately young women, though more and more young men and older people seem to be becoming sufferers.

The causes of bulimia may often be very similar to those of anorexia but, whereas the anorexic uses not eating as the 'answer' to her or his problems, the bulimic uses secret binges as a way to help them alleviate stress, loneliness, anxiety, or depression, feelings that she or he doesn't feel able to share with anyone else as it is very important for her or him to appear successful and self-contained.

This desire to binge is usually overwhelming in the bulimic, who seems to have no control over the binge sessions. Once a binge is over the sufferer regains control by purging, vowing never to binge again — but sooner or later is compelled to do so. Some bulimics begin purging themselves after fairly normal-sized meals, as a way to control their weight without conventional dieting, and then find it difficult to stop.

Typical binge foods are refined carbohydrates, such as cakes, biscuits, bread, chocolate and pastry. Cheese, butter, ice-cream and other fatty foods are also common binge components. However, some bulimics gorge on meat, and even fruits and vegetables.

Symptoms of bulimia in others are often hard to spot, particularly if the bulimic is of normal weight (as is often the case), appears to eat normal meals and may seem perfectly happy. Drastic fluctuations in weight may be an indication, however, and many bulimics do have long or short periods of semi-starvation before a binge. Also, in order to buy the quantities of food needed for a binge, some bulimics may resort to stealing money, or shoplifting.

Physical signs of bulimia will not, however, take long to appear. If vomiting is the main way of purging, the bulimic's teeth will quickly be affected. The acid in the vomit erodes tooth enamel and severe tooth decay follows. The bulimic may also face digestive disorders, including severe irritation of the lining of the intestines, severe chronic sore throat, gum disease, hair loss, general fatigue and depression, as well as malnutrition,

imbalance in tissue salts in the body and finally, possible kidney failure, even heart failure and death.

Sufferers of bulimia can be helped with the aid of counselling and advice on diet. The compulsive binges that bulimia sufferers experience are, at least in part, brought on by the periods of starvation and the imbalance in blood sugar levels these cause. The binge is the body's way of telling the sufferer that food is needed.

It is now known that female bulimics tend to binge more in the week preceding a period (when hormonal changes mean that most women do need to eat more at this time) than at any other time, and explanation of this and help with a suitable pre-menstrual diet and any other medical treatment as necessary is important.

One leading expert in bulimia advocates the 'little and often' theory for bulimics — several small meals a day, avoiding refined carbohydrates but including protein and fresh fruit. Most of all, bulimics need to be shown how to be around food in a normal manner again, to re-learn eating for the right reasons and eating a healthy diet without guilt and, if slimness was their main goal, to be shown what constitutes a sensible body weight for them, achievable without starvation or purging. As with anorexia, they also need to be helped to deal with any underlying psychological problems.

■ **Compulsive eating**

The third, and possibly largest, group of people with an eating disorder are the compulsive eaters — people who regularly eat very much more food than is necessary, often in the form of bingeing as bulimics do, but without purging. The result is that, inevitably, they gain weight and many compulsive eaters become chronically or morbidly (life-threateningly) obese. This over-eating and bingeing often begins when the sufferer faces particular problems in life — divorce, redundancy, a death, etc. — and the food is used as a comfort.

However, compulsive eating is more than the kind of 'comfort eating' that most people indulge in now and then. Vast quantities of food can be eaten over long periods of time, or sometimes in a short space of time. The sufferer is almost like an alcoholic — he or she needs his or her fix of food. Soon the initial reason for bingeing is forgotten as compulsive eating becomes a habit and an important part of the sufferer's life.

Compulsive eating may also be interspersed with periods of semi-starvation — a state which may begin as the typical 'yo-yo dieting' of someone trying too hard to lose weight and then giving in and bingeing. A sufferer of this type of alternate binge/starve compulsive eating may either fluctuate in weight or be a fairly average weight as the periods of starvation cancel out the effects of the binges.

If the sufferer is obese (with a BMI of over 30, see page 188), he or she should see a physician and begin a weight reduction programme, as obesity can cause many physical problems and illnesses, including heart disease. This may require close monitoring. Counselling or a self-help group such as Overeaters Anonymous or the Eating Disorders Association local groups are usually vital if the sufferer is to overcome compulsive eating long-term.

Binge/starve compulsive eaters will benefit from similar practical counselling to that for bulimia sufferers. A new idea is that a lack of essential fatty acids in the diet may result in food cravings, but this has yet to be proved.

See also: Section Four - Food for Weight Control, and the Teenage Section in Section Three.

See the Appendix for addresses of useful organizations.

ECZEMA

■ SOMETIMES CALLED DERMATITIS, eczema is an allergic inflammation of the skin, with a red itchy rash which may form small bubbles under the skin. If scratched, these may burst and infection may occur. There may be dry and flaky skin otherwise.

Eczema is a common disease in childhood, with 50% of cases starting before six months of age, but it may start at any time. The severity may change with time and could resolve as the child gets older.

SOLUTIONS

Contact allergy — e.g. to house dust mites, washing powders, clothing, nickel, rubber or pets — is a common cause. These possible allergens should be investigated before dietary intervention.

UK trials have shown that Chinese herbal medicine can have beneficial results with standardized preparations; with impure herbs, however, side effects (including problems with liver and kidney function) may occur, so it is important to work only with an experienced herbal practitioner.

Several studies have shown that foods can provoke symptoms and up to 40% of sufferers could benefit from exclusion diets as explained in the Allergy entry. However, it is often hard to predict which foods may provoke a response, although if increase in itch is noted after eating a certain food, this may indicate it is worth a trial. One or two (or, very occasionally, several) foods may be 'culprit' foods. Any exclusion diet should only be carried out under experienced medical supervision. If any foods are permanently excluded, the nutritional adequacy of the remaining diet needs to be checked.

In breast-fed babies, there may be food from the mother's diet, aggravating the symptoms which may also appear when weaning begins or a switch to cows' milk is made. You should see your dietician for advice. See also Allergies.

FOODS THAT CAUSE ECZEMA

Foods commonly reported to cause problems are milk, cheese and eggs, citrus fruits, food colourings and preservatives, nuts, fish and tomatoes. Eczema sufferers often find that inflammation is reduced if they follow a diet low in saturated fats and high in essential fatty acids.

Evening primrose and fish oils have, in trials, been shown to be effective in minimizing symptoms of both eczema and psoriasis. Some anecdotal evidence exists that zinc supplements may also help. For the address of the National Eczema Society, see the Appendix.

Energy, Lack of, see Fatigue

EYE PROBLEMS

■ GRANNY WAS RIGHT — good eye health really is a lot to do with eating up your carrots. She didn't know why, but we do now — the extremely high beta-carotene content of carrots, which converts to vitamin A in the body — is essential for good eyesight and healthy eye tissue. Beta-carotene is an antioxidant and, for general eye health, it is essential that you get enough of all the main antioxidants in your diet — the carotenoids, vitamin C and vitamin E. Below specific problems and solutions are dealt with in more detail.

* *Night blindness* Nearly always due to lack of vitamin A in the diet. Around 2-3 carrots a day, lightly cooked, should help ease the problem.

* *Blepharitis* (red-rimmed eyes), bloodshot eyes, dull eyes, corner cracks, sties. Often a sign of vitamin B2 (riboflavin) deficiency. Take a daily vitamin B-group supplement and eat plenty of Marmite, offal, nuts, seeds and pulses, as well as

antioxidant-rich foods and plenty of zinc for the immune system, as persistent eye problems are often a sign of being run down. Get adequate sleep. Bathe the eyes in an infusion of eyebright herb (1 teaspoon to 1 cup boiling water).

* Conjunctivitis Can be caused by an infection or allergy and produces red sore, painful eyes. Eat a basic healthy diet high in garlic and onions, which fight infection, and take a daily tincture of echinacea to help quickly boost your immune system. Eyebright bath may also be soothing and helpful.

* Dry eyes, gritty eyes Often a problem with contact lens wearers, but can be triggered by dry atmospheres, lack of sleep, or lack of essential fatty acids in the diet. Eat plenty of oily fish for omega-3s, and try a daily spoonful of linseed (flax) oil, another source of omega-3s. Evening Primrose oil is also useful. All the antioxidant vitamins are important, especially vitamin E, so eat plenty of avocados and walnuts, and other E-rich foods. Try eyebright solution as above.

* Puffy or baggy eyelids Often caused by fluid retention (see entry). Follow the PMS and Diuretic Diet on page 145. Lie with cucumber or potato slices or camomile tea bags (used and cooled) over each eye for 10 minutes each morning.

* Cataracts Very common as people age, but their development can be slowed by a diet that is rich in the antioxidant vitamins C, A and E, and quercetin-containing foods, such as tea, onions and red wine, as well as vitamin B2 (best sources lists, pages 24-7) and a general basic healthy diet. Smoking makes cataracts worse.

FATIGUE

FATIGUE IS A SYMPTOM with many possible causes. Short-term bouts of fatigue may be due to illness, overwork/stress or simply lack of sleep, and the tiredness is the body's way of asking for more rest. In these cases the answer is usually sleep and rest, plus a healthy diet until the fatigue has passed. See also Insomnia and Stress.

Chronic fatigue, sometimes called the 'TATT' or 'tired all the time' syndrome, may be due to an underlying physical cause — for instance, food allergies, anaemia (which is more common in women), ME (which often occurs after a viral illness such as glandular fever and can last for a year or more), underactive thyroid, or possibly even more serious problems such as heart disease or cancer.

It may also be, at least partly, psychologically based, for example linked with chronic stress, depression or boredom. Chronic fatigue should always be investigated by a physician. More detailed advice on dealing with these ailments nutritionally appears under each of the separate headings.

In women, many cases of fatigue are linked to the monthly menstrual cycle or menopause. Tiredness that occurs regularly in the pre-menstrual week or few days and then disappears on day one or two of the period is almost certainly linked to hormonal changes.

Diet itself can cause or exacerbate fatigue. Too much alcohol or caffeine on a regular basis can cause long-term fatigue. A diet that is regularly high in refined carbohydrates, such as sugar, cakes and biscuits, can contribute towards low blood sugar levels, a symptom of which is fatigue.

Crash-type slimming diets, where adequate calories are not consumed, can cause tiredness, as can irregular meals (low blood sugar again) or eating only once a day. Occasionally, vegan and vegetarian diets can cause fatigue through being too low in iron and perhaps the B group vitamins.

SOLUTIONS

To help beat tiredness you should follow a good healthy varied diet, rich in whole foods, complex carbohydrates and nutrients, particularly vitamin B12 (which has been shown in trials to alleviate fatigue when injected), folate and iron, which are responsible for maintaining healthy red blood cells, antioxidant vitamins C and E, the minerals zinc and magnesium, and the essential fatty acids. For best sources of all of these see Section One. The herbal supplement ginseng (either Siberian or Korean) helps some people feel more energetic when taken as a four- to-six-week course at 500 mg a day. Avoid consumption of caffeine while taking ginseng.

You should also take regular exercise (if your health allows), preferably in the fresh air, because tiredness is made worse by a sedentary lifestyle and worse again by stuffy offices and homes which don't get enough air-flow through them. Our bodies need oxygen to function properly; oxygen is supplied in fresh air via our lungs and circulatory systems. These work most efficiently in a fit and exercised body.

Studies have shown that just a 15-minute walk in fresh air can revitalize and refresh and may be exactly what is needed rather than going back to bed. Deep breathing exercises by an open window (in good weather) are also useful for helping to oxygenate the body and clear a fuzzy brain.

FEVER

FEVER — raised temperature (normally considered 39°C/102.2°F plus), usually accompanied by sweating, shivering, aches and pains and sometimes bouts of nausea or diarrhoea — is normally a symptom of some sort of infection, which should be treated according to the advice on page 122.

Most of the symptoms of the fever can be improved with paracetamol, and herbal methods of bringing down a high temperature include use of garlic, ginger and chilli, all of which promote sweating (the body's own natural method of cool-ing the skin and bringing fever down).

Garlic is also a strong antibiotic. A camomile infusion is also useful for controlling the symptoms of fever and a supplement of borage oil (starflower oil), which is a cooling herb and an infection fighter, may also help.

Prolonged sweating means that the body will soon become dehydrated and so anyone with a fever should drink plenty of fluids, preferably diluted lemon or orange juice, perhaps with a spoonful of runny honey added. If the feverish person has lost his or her appetite and is not eating, which often happens, the fluids should also contain a little salt — approximately one teaspoon for every 1 litre / ¾ pint.

The appetite of the feverish person may be whetted by easy-to-eat, tasty or cooling foods, such as ice-cream, stewed fruits, berry fruits, small Marmite sandwiches on white bread, poached egg on mashed potato, and mashed bananas with honey. On the other hand, if the feverish person is feeling chilled and shivery, a little mug of hot soup may be a good idea.

As soon as the patient is eating well again, ensure he or she gets plenty of foods rich in vitamins C and B, which will have been depleted by the illness, as part of the basic healthy diet.

See also Diarrhoea, Infections, and Nausea.

SIX TIPS TO MINIMIZE FLATULENCE

1 Cook food well, particularly pulses, which helps to remove the problem. Canned pulses may be tolerated better than dried ones. Soak all dried pulses well and discard soaking water before cooking thoroughly.
2 Purée foods before eating, e.g. as a side dish or in a soup.
3 Chop food small.
4 Chew food thoroughly, and relax and enjoy your food.
5 Eat slowly and keep the mouth shut. Some excess wind is caused by swallowing air as you eat.
6 Get used to new foods slowly, e.g. if you are beginning to eat more healthily, all the extra fibre in your diet may be too much for you.

FLATULENCE

EXCESS WIND in the digestive system can be both uncomfortable and unsightly — causing a bloated feeling and distension — as well as being noisy and embarrassing. This excess wind, called flatulence, often occurs when gases are formed as the bacteria in the intestines feed on food. Certain foods seem to cause more problems with wind than others. The resistant starches in some high-fibre foods seem to be the worst culprits of all: the peas, beans and lentils of the pulse family, and under-ripe bananas, for example. Bran, dried fruits such as prunes, and members of the brassica family — particularly sprouts and cabbage — are also all foods that cause overproduction of wind for many people. As these foods are all healthy and provide us with much-needed fibre and nutrients, they are best incorporated in the diet using the tips above.

There may be other causes of excess wind. Caffeine, beer, fizzy drinks, high-fat foods, such as cream and pastry, and fresh bread are all known to be culprits.

There may also be an underlying disorder or illness causing the problem. A food intolerance or allergy is likely, or lactose intolerance, coeliac or Crohn's disease. Candida is a fairly common cause, and so is irritable bowel syndrome. These should be investigated by your physician.

For everyday flatulence, relief can be

obtained with an infusion of one of the following herbs: peppermint, camomile, dill, lemon balm, basil or fennel leaves, or a decoction can be made with fresh chopped ginger or fennel seeds. The condition may also be helped with regular servings of live bio yoghurt, as long as lactose intolerance has been discounted. See also Heartburn and Indigestion.

Flu, see Colds and Flu

FLUID RETENTION

■ SURPLUS FLUID IN THE BODY is often mistaken for surplus fat or wind and can result in weight gain of many pounds. The symptoms are a bloated and puffy feeling and visible swelling, especially of the stomach, breasts, face, hands, ankles and feet. Fluid retention is caused by a variety of different things.

Women frequently suffer during times of hormonal change — with PMS, during pregnancy, when on the Pill, or at the menopause. Before a period, a woman can put on as much as 3-4 kilos, much of which will be fluid. The Pill may add this much, too, and the extra fluid tends to stay until the woman comes off that form of contraception. For more detailed advice on fluid retention in pregnancy and the menopause see pages 172 and 178.

Another common cause is a high-salt diet — experts say that up to 4 pounds of surplus fluid may be retained in the body through a typical Western diet high in commercial foods with lots of added salt and salty snacks. Refined carbohydrates such as cakes, biscuits and low-cost white bread may also contribute to fluid retention, so it is wise to cut intake of these right down especially, if female, at vulnerable times such as before a period.

Allergies are another common cause (see Allergies entry). Certain health problems predispose towards fluid retention — heart disease and kidney disorders being the most common — as do certain drugs. In these cases, talk to a physician.

SOLUTIONS

Most cases of fluid retention can be helped by an appropriate diet, such as the PMS and Diuretic Diet on page 145. Salt intake should be kept to a minimum (see list of high-salt foods on page 33) and so should refined starches as above. It is important to drink plenty of plain water as, contrary to popular belief, this doesn't make fluid retention worse but, in fact, allows salt to be excreted more easily.

You should also eat a diet high in potassium-rich foods, such as bananas, tomatoes and whole grains. Potassium works with sodium in the body to balance fluids properly and a high potassium intake is a natural way to help flush out surplus salt.

Some experts also believe that a lack of essential fatty acids in the diet may contribute towards sluggish elimination of fluids, and so it is worth eating plenty of oily fish and pure vegetable oils and perhaps taking a supplement of evening primrose oil for 2-3 months.

Exercise is important in helping to flush surplus fluid out of the body — a swimming session is ideal, or a brisk walk. If you are retaining fluid you will notice that as soon as you have finished the exercise you need to go. Certain types of body massage are also effective.

Avoid anything more than very occasional use of over-the-counter diuretic pills. Misuse of these can affect the correct balance of body fluids and minerals and will eventually make the problem worse. Natural diuretic foods can be incorporated into your diet though — these are most fruits, especially melon and citrus fruits, carrots, salad vegetables including tomatoes, celery, lettuce, watercress, sweet peppers and cucumber, and infusions of dandelion, parsley, lovage, nettle or rosemary.

Food Intolerance, see Allergies

Food Poisoning, see Diarrhoea, Infections, Nausea and Travel Sickness, and Stomach-ache

GALLSTONES

■ MANY PEOPLE HAVE GALLSTONES — some reports put the figure as high as one in three of all women (men are much less likely than women to suffer) but only a minority of those will ever experience problems because of the stones. Pain in the upper right-hand side of the abdomen, which comes on several hours after eating, may be due to stones, which are generally caused by an excess of bile (which helps in the digestion of fats) and cholesterol in the gall bladder that can build up, particularly when the sufferer eats a high-fat diet. Inflammation or pain can occur if the stone tries to leave the gall bladder and becomes lodged in the bile duct. Pain can spread to the back and right shoulder and flatulence is another common symptom.

SOLUTIONS
Gallstones are less common in vegetarians and in people who eat a basic healthy diet of small regular meals, low in saturated fats and sugars and high in fibre, fruit, vegetables, oily fish, folate, magnesium, and vitamin C. A high-fat, low-fibre diet may worsen the pain of gallstones and perhaps predispose to their formation .

One study has shown that gall bladder pain can be overcome by testing for food allergies on an elimination diet. When foods were reintroduced, the foods that most often triggered symptoms were egg, pork and onion.

Gastric Ulcer, see Peptic Ulcer

GLANDULAR FEVER

■ CAUSED BY THE EPSTEIN-BARR VIRUS, glandular fever is a fairly common illness of the teens and twenties, after which it becomes quite rare. Symptoms are enlarged lymph glands (e.g. in the neck and armpits), muscular aches and pains, fever, headache and tonsillitis, tiredness and weakness. Glandular fever usually lasts at least two weeks, but can carry on, with recurring bouts of the symptoms, for a year or more. Some people diagnosed with glandular fever go on to suffer from ME.

SOLUTIONS
To help shorten the duration of glandular fever you need to build up your immune system by, for instance, following the Immune-strengthening Diet on page 143. There is evidence that a diet rich in essential fatty acids can also help, and a daily supplement of tincture of echinacea, 10 drops in 200 ml (7 fl oz) warm water, is a good idea. If the illness has reduced appetite, daily supplements of vitamin B group and vitamin C, both of which are important for the immune system and which are quickly depleted in the body, may be useful. Sensible diet, plenty of rest and gradually building up to a little regular exercise will help to ensure that glandular fever doesn't develop into ME. See also ME.

GOUT

■ A FORM OF ARTHRITIS, gout is caused by the build up of uric acid, a metabolic waste product, in the blood. Gout affects single joints, usually the big toe, and happens when not enough uric acid is passed in the urine, or too much is produced. When the urate level increases, uric acid crystals form, and deposit in the cartilage or joint space, causing inflammation and pain, which can be very severe. Gout sufferers may be at increased risk of insulin resistance and arterial disease.

SOLUTIONS
Treatment is usually by drugs, but the right diet can be helpful. The sufferer should drink plenty of non-alcoholic fluids and avoid becoming overweight. If already too heavy, a sensible weight-loss plan (such as that on page 192) should be followed. However, crash diets and fasting should be completely avoided as these could precipitate an attack. A generally healthy diet rich in vegetables, nuts and fish (including salmon, tuna and trout), and low in rich fatty foods has been shown to be helpful.

Foods high in purines, which may lead to increased uric acid, should be avoided. These are offal, shellfish, sardines, mackerel, whitebait, herrings, anchovies, fish roe and game. Individual tolerance varies, but alcohol often makes gout worse and being teetotal may be advisable.

Some supplements, such as vitamin A and nicotinic acid, may be harmful. Vitamin C is often quoted as helpful but this isn't proven. Quercetin-rich foods, like onions and apples, may help. See also Arthritis.

GUM DISEASE

■ IF YOUR GUMS, OR ANY PART OF THEM, ARE SORE, puffed up, red and inflamed, painful, bleeding (or any of those symptoms) you really need to visit a dentist and get the condition rectified as soon as possible. If you leave it untreated, the condition will most probably worsen and may eventually result in loss of teeth. The most common gum disease is gingivitis, which is most usually caused by insufficient oral hygiene and is often characterized by halitosis and the other symptoms described above.

If the teeth and gums aren't brushed and flossed at least twice a day, layers of plaque (sticky, opaque residues which are

SIX STEPS TO AVOIDING GUM DISEASE

1 Regular dental visits.
2 Twice daily thorough oral hygiene, including flossing.
3 Healthy diet rich in fruit, veg, vitamin C and zinc. Co-enzyme Q10 may help.
4 Avoid long periods of chewing on sweet food, such as toffees.
5 Clean teeth soon after a meal – but leave time after acidic drink or food to allow rehardening of enamel.
6 Avoid lots of sweet, sticky or starchy snacks.

made up of a mixture of food particles and the bacteria contained in the mouth saliva) are left and these then build up on your teeth and gum margins. If left longer, these gradually harden into tartar, which it is not actually possible to remove without going to the dentist. If the tartar isn't removed, infection in the gum margins can easily set in and gingivitis results.

People who usually eat a healthy diet, that is high in fruit and vegetables and whole-foods, and low in sugary and refined foods, may build up less plaque, but this isn't necessarily always the case. Regular tea drinking has been shown to protect against tooth decay. Some people seem more prone to plaque production than others. Research shows that people with gum disease are more prone to both midlife diabetes and heart disease.

However healthy the diet may be, it is nevertheless important to brush the teeth and floss regularly, making sure to brush the gums as well. Very occasionally, bleeding gums may be caused by a vitamin C deficiency. Stress, smoking, drinking alcohol and a poor diet can all possibly result in such a deficiency. Bleeding gums are also quite common in the course of pregnancy.

See also Tooth Decay.

HAEMORRHOIDS

THESE ARE VARICOSE-VEIN-LIKE SWELLINGS of the blood vessels in the wall of the anus, and are usually a result of prolonged constipation, or occasionally chronic diarrhoea or IBS, which may irritate the veins. Straining to pass stools disrupts the support around the tissue, which becomes displaced and congested. Haemorrhoids are not caused by sitting on cold seats or hot radiators! The pressure which builds up can cause the swellings to prolapse or protrude from the anus, when they are known as external (rather than internal) haemorrhoids.

They often occur in people in middle and old age, and may also occur in pregnancy, when blood flow in the lower abdomen may alter, and constipation can be a problem. Haemorrhoids may be painful and a common symptom is bright red blood in the lavatory pan after passing stools. Once symptoms are noticed you should see a physician to check that your problem is caused by piles.

SOLUTIONS

Dietary prevention is similar to that of constipation, with plenty of high-fibre foods, water, fresh fruit and vegetables. A mash of linseeds, available from the health food store, may be helpful.

HAIR LOSS

WHEN HAIR SUDDENLY BEGINS FALLING OUT, hormonal changes are often to blame. After childbirth, during the menopause and during the 'male menopause', hair loss is quite common. In most cases this isn't totally preventable. Other causes of hair loss are hypothyroidism (a medical condition), stress, long-term illness, and large doses of vitamin A. It is also possible that poor circulation in the scalp may effect the hair follicles from which the hair grows. Stress will make this worse by tightening the scalp.

SOLUTIONS

Exercise, relaxation techniques and scalp massage may all help. See Stress and Circulation, Poor for more information. Once hair is lost in male-pattern baldness or menopause, little can be done nutritionally, but a basic healthy diet will help anyone keep their remaining hair in good condition. Hair lost after childbirth or through illness will usually be replaced quite naturally, but, again, a healthy diet will help to ensure this. Adequate iron and zinc intake, and vitamins B group and C are particularly associated with good hair.

HALITOSIS

■ BAD BREATH — OR HALITOSIS — has various causes and successful treatment relies on making the right diagnosis of the cause and then eliminating it. Here we run through the most common causes and suggest appropriate action:

* **Oral infection** Gum disease or tooth decay can cause bad breath. Get the problem sorted out by your dentist and help any necessary healing with plenty of zinc and vitamin C.

* **Poor oral hygiene** Insufficient brushing and flossing will leave particles of food between the teeth and around the mouth, which can smell bad when they decay. Brush and floss at least twice a day, three minutes a time on both.

* **Type of food eaten** Everyone knows how pungent raw garlic is on the breath. Likewise the odour of curried food, alcohol, tobacco and some other foods can linger on the breath. Odours like this can be masked by chewing parsley or mint and, when caused by foods eaten, should disappear within hours. Natural yoghurt eaten every day reduces one of the causes of bad breath – hydrogen sulphide – in 80% of vounteers.

* **Food allergy or intolerance** These can cause bad breath. If you have accompanying symptoms, e.g. bloated stomach, feeling 'off colour', headaches, get your physician to check you over to see if an allergy may be the cause. The solution then is to avoid the item(s) that produce the allergy symptoms (see page 88).

* **Throat or mouth infection** Tonsillitis, sore throat and oral thrush (sore mouth) are often accompanied by halitosis. In most cases, when the infection clears up so will the bad breath. Meanwhile, drink plenty of water.

* **Sinusitis and catarrh** Nasal blockages may cause you to breathe through your mouth and/or to leave your mouth open most of the time. This encourages bad breath by drying out the mouth and lowering levels of saliva, which contains oxygen to keep the mouth fresh. Try a dairy-free diet for 2-4 weeks and see if your sinusitis or catarrh improves. See also Colds and Flu.

* **Sleeping with mouth open** If your bad breath is worst in the morning, it could be that you are sleeping with your mouth open, which encourages bad breath (see previous paragraph). If a nasal problem is causing you to breath through your mouth, get it sorted out by the physician. Also try avoiding dairy produce in the evening (see the previous paragraph on catarrh).

* **Constipation** If you are constipated you may have bad breath, probably because the stored-up waste in the bowel is causing back production of gases which are being eliminated via the breath. If you are constipated, switch gradually to a high-fibre diet, take lots of exercise and drink plenty of water, which will also help to keep the mouth moist.

* **Medication** Some drugs can cause bad breath. If you are taking any medications and can find no other reason for your halitosis, check with your physician and see if perhaps another similar medication could be used instead (if the drug you are taking is long-term). If short-term, it is best to live with the problem for just a few days and chew parsley or mint to sweeten the breath.

* **Predisposition to halitosis** According to experts, some people have higher than normal concentrations of the bacteria which can cause bad breath in the back of their throat and mouth. However careful they are, they may still have bad breath.

Best help is to scrape the area regularly with special tongue scrapers. Mouthwashes are not a good idea as, though they work short-term, long-term they make the mouth drier and encourage the halitosis.

HANGOVER

■ IF YOU'RE GOING OUT for the evening and know you are likely to be drinking more than usual, you can do a lot towards preventing a hangover next morning by taking one or two precautions beforehand.

First, eat a meal and drink some milk. This helps to slow the absorption of alcohol (some of which is absorbed straight through the stomach lining without waiting to go the route of other things that you eat and drink. This explains why we can begin to feel 'tipsy' in a very short time after taking our first drink).

Then drink a glass or two of water, and continue drinking water throughout the evening in between alcohol. This not only helps you to drink less alcohol but helps to stop you dehydrating. Dehydration is the major cause of hangover. Alcohol is a diuretic, which means that you will pass more urine than usual while and after drinking and become dehydrated. When body fluids are too low, we get the classic hangover symptoms of headache, throbbing head, and so on.

When you get home you can do yet more to help prevent that hangover. If you can face it, drink a mug of warm milk, the calcium in which will help you sleep. Alcohol, while probably sending you to sleep well at first, disrupts REM sleep (the deep sleep that we all need in order to feel refreshed) and may cause wakefulness from the early hours. Drink more water before you go to bed — preferably with a soluble vitamin C in it — and keep water by the bed for sipping if you wake in the night.

In the morning, if despite everything you do have a hangover, continue drinking plenty of fluid, preferably water or diluted fruit juice. If you feel queasy, skimmed milk is a good idea. Avoid coffee, particularly strong black coffee, and tea, both of which are also diuretics and will compound the problem. If your hangover has left you feeling a bit jittery and jumpy, the caffeine they contain will also make you feel worse.

You should eat something as soon as you feel up to it — if you can't face anything bigger, a banana is a good idea. This will help boost your blood sugar levels. Low blood sugar is another cause of some of the symptoms of hangover, such as irritability, dizziness and tiredness. 'Hair of the dog' — i.e., another alcoholic drink — is absolutely not a good idea, whatever you have been told. A drink may make you feel temporarily better, but will just compound the problem long-term. It is also the road to addiction. Proprietary preparations for hangover usually contain high levels of alcohol; avoid these

too (check the label).

You can try non-alcoholic herbal remedies such as an infusion of rosemary (a couple of sprigs infused in a cup of boiling water for 5 minutes, strained). Some freshly juiced carrot or mixed vegetable juice may help your liver (which has to process all the alcohol that you drink) to recover. As soon as possible, eat a nutritious meal and then get back to bed for some REM sleep. If hangovers are a common occurrence for you, read the entry on Alcohol Abuse (page 86) and consider ways to cut down your drinking.

KNOW YOUR POISON

Choose your drink carefully. Some drinks are much more likely to cause hangovers than others because of the congeners — the additives — that they contain. Alcoholic drinks are not obliged to list E numbers and the like on their containers and many contain a great deal. The additives that give alcohol colour seem to be the worst culprits in producing hangover. So stick to pale-coloured drinks (vodka is best), followed by gin and white wine. Then follows, in best-to-worst order: lager, beer, cider, whisky, rum, sherry, stout, brandy, red wine and port.

HAY FEVER

■ SEASONAL ALLERGIC RHINITIS, or hay fever, is an allergic reaction to airborne pollens from grass, trees and/or fungi, usually characterized by symptoms including inflammation of the nasal passages, itching or soreness in mouth, nose, throat, eyes, streaming eyes and nose, sneezing and headache.

There are several dietary precautions or remedies that can be followed to minimize the severity of allergic rhinitis. In one recent US study, daily supplements of vitamin C, starting at 500mg and increasing to 2g, were given over six weeks, and volunteers' histamine levels dropped by 40%.

The action of vitamin C is enhanced by the bioflavonoid quercetin, found in rich amounts in red onions, squash, broccoli, courgettes and apples. Other bioflavonoids seem to act as natural antihistamines, so a diet rich in these compounds – most fruits and veg – will help.

Some sufferers also swear by a twice-daily tablespoon of honey from bees local to their area – they believe this acts in a similar way to homeopathy. Lastly, stinging nettle tea has been shown to reduce reaction to pollen. See Allergies.

Headaches, see Migraine and Headaches

HEARTBURN AND INDIGESTION

■ HEARTBURN, which can cause sharp and even severe chest pains, is the result of too much acid in the stomach when a meal is being digested. The excess acid spurts back up into the oesophagus, which connects the stomach and mouth, and the acid causes pain and discomfort, often known simply as indigestion. Heartburn is also a symptom of hiatus hernia, which is more common in people who are very overweight, and may also be a common problem in late pregnancy, when the expanding uterus can literally 'squash' parts of the digestive system.

SOLUTIONS

Whatever the cause, a few simple dietary guidelines can help minimize occurrence and the discomfort caused by heartburn and indigestion. Certain foods are more likely to cause an attack. Both acidic foods, like pickles, sauces and vinegars, and fatty foods, such as fry-ups and pastries, are the most common culprits. Both stimulate the output of acid in the digestive system. Raw vegetables, such as onions, peppers and radishes, curries and chillies, and unripe fruit, are also best avoided, as are alcohol, strong coffee and tea, and fizzy drinks, all of which can cause irritation.

How you eat is also important. Have several small meals rather than one or two large ones; the digestive system will find this easier to handle. Chew food thoroughly, eat slowly and try to relax while eating. After you have eaten, an infusion of fennel or dill or apple mint leaves will help to prevent heartburn. A strategy that works for some is to avoid mixing protein and carbs at a meal (a version of the Hay diet, see page 202).

Lose weight, if necessary, and have a check-up, as there may be another underlying problem that needs attention.

HEART DISEASE AND STROKE

■ CORONARY HEART DISEASE (CHD) is the number one cause of death in the UK and the greatest single cause of premature death in men. It develops when the coronary arteries, which supply blood to the heart, become narrowed by a build-up of plaque (cholesterol and other deposits). This is called atherosclerosis. Blood supply to the heart is reduced and there may be chest pain (angina) and/or irregular heart beat (arrhythmia). In time the arteries may become completely blocked, either by more build-up of plaque and/or by a blood clot (thrombosis), supply of blood to parts of the heart will be blocked and a heart attack will occur. Similarly, a blocked artery that supplies blood to the brain may lead to a stroke.

There are several internationally recognized risk factors for heart disease: old age (most CHD occurs in people aged 70 plus), hereditary factors, diabetes, smoking, heavy drinking, stress, lack of exercise, obesity and abdominal fat, high blood pressure and high blood cholesterol levels. Also men are more likely to get CHD than women, until after menopause when women appear to lose their hormonal protection. The more of the risk factors that you have, the higher the likelihood of your getting CHD.

There is also much recent research into other possible risk factors for CHD. For instance, there is now growing evidence that CHD may also be linked with bacterial infections, particularly those that cause chest infections and gum disease, all of which may be controlled with antibiotics. To reduce risk of contracting infections see advice on page 122 and follow the Immune-strengthening Diet on page 143. See also Gum Disease, Tooth Decay and Bronchitis and Coughs. There is new evidence that a good balance of omega-3 and omega-6 fatty acids is important.

There is also strong evidence that a diet lacking in adequate fruits, vegetables, whole grains and other plant foods is a risk factor in itself, probably because these foods contain the vitamin antioxidants E and C and beta-carotene, the phytochemicals such as flavonoids, and B vitamins, particularly folate and B6, which all now appear to have an important role to play in lowering risk of CHD. Tea – black and green – is an important antioxidant, while coffee is neutral. A diet high in red meat and salt may also be an important risk factor. A recent study by the Imperial Cancer Research Fund found that vegetarians have between 24% and 45% decreased risk of dying from CHD. Other recent research shows that both dark chocolate and tomato juice are rich in special flavonoids that can prevent blood clots.

Preliminary measures to help reduce your risk of CHD are to give up smoking; keep alcohol consumption within safe limits (see page 36); seek ways to reduce high stress levels (see page 134); keep weight below a body mass index of about 26, with a reasonable waist circumference (see page 188) and take regular exercise (latest research says that 11 minutes of aerobic exercise a day will cut the risk by nearly a half). Also eat small regular meals – 'blow-outs' can trigger heart attack by increasing the blood's 'clotting factor'.

If diabetic, sensible management of the condition (see page 105) will help reduce risk of CHD. High blood pressure puts extra strain on the heart and blood vessels (page 95).

■ Cholesterol and heart disease

Cholesterol is a soft, waxy substance that is manufactured mainly in the liver and then circulated in the blood, and is necessary for the smooth running of a variety of bodily functions. The amount of cholesterol that the liver makes may be due to hereditary factors and/or related to the amount of fat, particularly saturated fat, eaten. Cholesterol production and action is also affected by a variety of factors. Some of these seem to involve various aspects of diet, which are discussed below.

There are two types of cholesterol — low-density lipoprotein (LDL) and high-density lipoprotein (HDL). A surplus of LDL in the blood is a major factor in the 'furring' of the arteries and formation of the plaques that lead to atherosclerosis, heart disease and stroke; whereas HDL — often called 'good' cholesterol — actually helps to remove cholesterol from the tissues and delivers it to the liver for excretion. There are various things you can do, nutritionally, to help lower LDL levels, in conjunction with any medical treatments your physician may suggest.

1: You can reduce intake of the types of foods which cause the liver to manufacture more LDL — these are foods high in saturated fats, such as full-fat dairy produce and fatty meat, and those high in trans fats found in many commercial margarines and products. Cholesterol is also found in some foods, particularly offal, eggs, shellfish, meat and dairy produce (see page 19). Intake of high-cholesterol foods may have a small relationship to blood cholesterol levels, but recent research on eggs has shown no detrimental effect on blood fats. For more information about saturated and trans fats, see Section One.

2: You can reduce intake of foods which reduce HDL levels in the blood, therefore lowering the amount available to transport the surplus cholesterol away. Recent research has shown that trans-fats can reduce the amount of HDL by up to 20%. So trans-fats get the 'thumbs down' on two counts and seem to be worse for your blood cholesterol levels than butter. Very high intakes of polyunsaturated fats will also lower HDL levels so, in their case, 'enough' is good, 'too much' is bad. (See page 16 for more information on polyunsaturated fats.)

3: You can eat more of the foods that seem to lower production of LDL, or increase production of HDL and therefore encourage its excretion. The foods which have been promoted as achieving this are:

* Unsaturated fats It is becoming apparent that the healthy approach to fat consumption is to balance intake of the two types of polyunsaturated fats – omega-6s and omega-3s – which can lower LDL, along with a sensible intake of monounsaturated fats, which have been shown in several trials to have a beneficial effect on LDL/HDL balance. Very-low-fat diets (less than 15-20% fat) may actually be inadvisable for some people who are at risk of, or currently with, CHD, research indicates.

* Garlic Its phytochemicals, including allicin, help lower LDL cholesterol.

* Soya While some research has shown that regular intake of soya can lower LDL and reduce heart disease risk, the latest 2006 review of all the studies (Harvard School of Public Health) found no evidence of this and the American Heart Association agrees.

* Soluble fibre Found in greatest quantities in oats, pulses and many fruits and vegetables, can help lower LDL.

* Alcohol The latest overview (University of California, San Francisco 2006) of all the studies conducted over the years on the benefits or otherwise of consumption of red wine, beer, etc, in preventing heart disease has concluded that moderate alcohol intake offers no clear health benefits.

Lastly, your diet can also help to prevent cholesterol from forming the artery-narrowing plaques, and it can help to prevent blood clots from forming. To do this your diet should be rich in oily fish. The omega-3 fatty acids in oily fish, such as salmon and mackerel, will 'thin' the blood and help prevent blood clots. Fish oils also have the effect of lowering blood triglycerides, see below, and slightly lowering blood cholesterol levels.

WHAT ARE ANTIOXIDANTS?

Antioxidants are vitamins, minerals and phytochemicals which help prevent fat from oxidizing. They can prevent the oxidization of food in the storecupboard (for example, when added to fatty foods such as margarine, they can help prevent it from going rancid) and they have a similar role to play in the body. The importance of this is that surplus LDL blood cholesterol needs to be oxidized before it can form the plaques, and so a diet rich in antioxidants can help prevent the furring up of the arteries that leads to atherosclerosis.

The chief antioxidants are vitamins C, E, and beta-carotene, the mineral selenium, and various and numerous phytochemicals such as flavonoids (found in citrus fruits and other fruits), lycopene (found in tomatoes, ruby grapefruits and watermelon), quercetin (found in tea, onions, apples), resveratrol (in red grapes), and the glucosinolates (found in broccoli and greens). Olive oil also seems to make LDL cholesterol more resistant to oxidation, and garlic, too, is an antioxidant.

■ Heart disease and antioxidants

Experts believe that a diet rich in fruits and vegetables, and other antioxidant-rich foods and drinks, may reduce heart disease by up to 20%. For example, regular tea drinking has been shown to cut the risk of atherosclerosis by 50%. One large trial of middle-aged men found those whose had a vitamin C deficiency had a three and a half times greater risk of heart attack.

■ Heart disease and homocysteine

Recent research has found a strong link between raised blood levels of plasma homocysteine and increased incidence of CHD and strokes. More research needs to be done, but it appears clear that low levels of the B vitamin folate predispose to this condition. Other B vitamins, particularly B6, may be involved in homocysteine metabolism and a B-group rich diet may help to protect against, or reverse, this condition. Pulses and green vegetables are rich sources of folate and other B vitamins.

■ Heart disease and triglycerides

Triglycerides are another type of fat found in the blood and evidence suggests that higher than normal levels can also contribute to increased risk of heart disease, particularly in women, diabetics and older people. Levels can be reduced by eating small regular high-fibre meals not too high in fat, by eating oily fish or fish oils and restricting alcohol and sugar intake.

■ Heart disease and supplements

Several large trials have been carried out to see if dietary supplementation, primarily with the antioxidant vitamins C, E and beta-carotene, can help reduce incidence of CHD. Results have been varied (indeed one major review for the WHO found mortality from heart disease increased in smokers who took beta-carotene supplements and another found that 500mg plus supplements of vitamin C thicken artery walls). The message from experts is that it is better to get adequate nutrients from a varied diet high in fruits and vegetables than to rely on supplementation. One reason is that eating natural foods minimizes risk of 'overdosing' on one particular nutrient, another is that it may be an array of different elements that protects (for example phytochemicals working together), rather than just one.

One problem is that there is no definitive amount of any vitamin, nutrient or phytochemical that is known to offer protection, as there are so many variables. However many experts agree that the current RNIs for various nutrients may be too low for optimum protection from diseases such as CHD. While the consensus is that oily fish may help heart health, an analysis (University of East Anglia, 2006) of all the trials on fish oil supplements has found little evidence that they cut the risk of dying of heart disease or stroke.

For more on antioxidants see left and page 24; for supplements see page 146. The Healthy Heart Diet is on page 142.

HERPES SIMPLEX 1

■ COLD SORES are caused by the herpes 1 virus, which is related to the other herpes viruses; genital herpes (simplex 2) and chicken pox (herpes zoster), which may cause shingles later in life. It is not thought that having one form of the virus can make you more likely to get the others. Herpes 1 virus usually produces an initial attack which can make the sufferer quite ill — a cold sore appears, usually around the mouth, and there may be fever, headache, aches and pains and lethargy. The attack can last a week and the sore take up to two weeks to go. The virus then lies dormant in the body and may produce other cold sores in the future (usually with less severe side-effects), particularly if you are run down, stressed, or when your immune system has been weakened for any reason.

SOLUTIONS

By keeping the immune system as strong as possible, the likelihood of frequent recurrence of cold sores is reduced, and if they do appear, they will be milder and of shorter duration. Keeping to a correct diet is quite important in achieving this — you should regularly eat foods which are rich in immune-boosting nutrients zinc, vitamins C, A and E, and the essential fatty acids founds in oily fish, olive and sunflower oil. Best sources of vitamin C are those that are also rich in flavonoids, such as citrus fruit and blackcurrants. Other 'best sources' lists appear in Section One.

You should also take plenty of garlic,

onions, ginger and thyme. Black and green tea are useful for the quercetin and catechins they contain, which have been shown to be anti-viral. Iron deficiency may be linked to cold sores as well; best sources of iron are listed on page 30. There is evidence that the amino acid lysine helps block the herpes virus. Lysine-rich foods are lamb, fish, chicken, milk, eggs and potatoes.

Similarly, the amino acid arginine helps the herpes virus to grow, so cut out arginine-rich foods, including chocolate, nuts, seeds, cereals and raisins if a cold sore seems imminent.

The Immune-strengthening Diet on page 143 is ideal to help keep cold sores away or to reduce their duration if one appears.

HIV, see AIDS and HIV

HYPERACTIVITY

■ ALSO KNOWN AS 'attention deficit hyperactivity disorder' (ADHD), this is a condition which effects up to one in ten children (though most will have only mild or moderate symptoms) and can continue on into adolescence, or even begin then. Its symptoms are disturbed behaviour, such as overactivity and fidgeting, distractibility, impulsiveness, inability to concentrate and aggressiveness.

For the one in two hundred children who do have severe symptoms, life for everyone involved at home, at school and socially can be difficult.

SOLUTIONS

Diet is thought by some experts to play a large part in causing hyperactivity. Diet from weaning onwards should be low in processed and highly refined foods, particularly those containing artificial additives, and drinks high in caffeine and additives, such as cola. Other foods which often seem to cause hyperactivity

are chocolate and juice drinks. In some cases, a supervised elimination diet may be indicated.

The diet should contain adequate amounts of all the necessary nutrients, by ensuring the child receives three good meals a day with plenty of fresh and home-cooked ingredients, especially oily fish, which is rich in omega-3 essential fats, shown to help many cases of ADHD, dyslexia and dyspraxia in children (or omega-3 supplements can be taken). Each hyper-active child should receive personal dietary advice and nutrient supplementation given as necessary.

Supplements found to be effective include zinc, magnesium, vitamin B complex and vitamin E. An address for the Hyperactive Children's Support Group appears in the Appendix. For more information on children's healthy diet and feeding problems, see Section Three.

Hypertension, see Blood Pressure

HYPOGLYCAEMIA

■ HYPOGLYCAEMIA is commonly known as 'low blood sugar'. Hypoglycaemic symptoms include feeling dizzy and/or weak, palpitations and tremor, feeling 'spaced out' and often hungry. Hypoglycaemia can be a problem for diabetes sufferers when the level of insulin in the body isn't matched by correct food intake. Prolonged or extreme physical effort (such as marathon running) without adequate intake of carbohydrate can also result in low blood sugar. To avoid this, runners take sugary drinks along the route and professional tennis players take drinks and eat bananas (a quickly digested source of starch and sugars that will rapidly provide a source of blood glucose).

Poor dietary habits can also result in hypoglycaemia for ordinary people. If meals are skipped, blood sugar levels can dip. This will be compounded if a meal is then eaten that is high in refined carbohydrate, such as sugars and snack foods, which is absorbed rapidly into the bloodstream. The body releases an over-abundance of insulin to cope with this sudden influx and within an hour or more hypoglycaemic symptoms may begin again. Alcohol has a similar effect to sugary foods.

Some people seem more prone to fluctuating blood sugar levels than others. Women may find they suffer more before a period (see Menstrual Problems); caffeine and cigarette smoking may exacerbate the problem. There is also some evidence that a chromium deficiency may be a cause, but chromium is best taken naturally in chromium-rich foods, such as shellfish, cheese, whole grains and pulses.

SOLUTIONS

Hypoglycaemia can be controlled by a sensible and healthy diet (see Basic Healthy Diet, page 53) and by eating 'little and often'. The diet should contain plenty of whole-foods and enough protein, which will release their energy slowly into the bloodstream and thus keep blood sugar levels on a more even keel. Sugary snacks when you are hungry should be avoided. Ideal between-meal snacks are small pieces of half-fat cheese with a rye crispbread, or an apple and a low-fat yoghurt.

For more information on foods for maintaining even blood sugar levels, see Glycaemic Index in Section Four. See also Diabetes.

IMPOTENCE

DIET DOESN'T APPEAR TO PLAY a large part in preventing or curing male impotence (failure to get or maintain an erection), but there are some dietary tips which may help the problem, the most important of which is to eat a diet rich in the mineral zinc. Some research shows that zinc deficiency is linked with a lack of the male sex hormone testosterone and trials have shown a return to potency for men with low zinc levels after supplementation. For a list of the best sources of zinc in the diet, turn to page 31. Zinc supplements are available over the counter and are best taken with vitamin C. It is also wise to avoid caffeine, which can affect absorption of zinc. However, if a male is not deficient in zinc, taking extra is unlikely to be of any benefit.

One alcoholic drink may help relaxation and enhance libido that way, but too much alcohol is associated with loss of libido (by reducing the long-term production of male hormones) and loss of sensitivity in the sexual organs. Long term, a healthy diet low in saturated fats and cholesterol and high in antioxidants and fruit and vegetables (such as the Basic Healthy Diet, page 53) will help maintain potency, as tests have shown that a cause of impotency is blocked arteries to the penis.

A diet rich in garlic will also help to thin the blood and maintain good circulation. Stress is frequently a cause of impotence and in such cases relaxation techniques and the anti-stress diet hints on page 138 may help.

INFECTIONS

AS BACTERIA ARE BECOMING more and more resistant to our usual antibiotic drugs, and viruses are rarely killed by antibiotics in any case, it is important to find natural ways to fight infection. We now know that several foods and herbs do have strong anti-viral, anti-bacterial and anti-fungal effects, and it is likely that in the next few years many more important discoveries will be made in this field.

To ward off infections of the respiratory system, digestive and urinary system and the skin and eyes, and to help minimize the effects of bacterial problems such as food poisoning, a general healthy diet (Basic Healthy Diet, page 53) should be followed, or at times of particular stress or vulnerability, the Immune-strengthening Diet (page 143) can be followed.

Once an infection has set in, try the following:

* **Garlic** and its less powerful but still effective relatives, onion and leek — have been used as infection-fighters for thousands of years all over the world by alternative practitioners. Scientists are now beginning to discover not only that garlic does work, but how it works. Fresh raw garlic can not only kill bugs such as listeria and salmonella but will also kill the new 'superbugs' that antibiotics don't work on any more. Its main active ingredient is allicin, which, sadly, becomes much less potent when the garlic is crushed and then stored before using, or when cooked. Garlic is an expectorant and can help ease symptoms of coughs and colds. Raw garlic can be eaten in salads or dressings, such as pesto and salsa, or high-quality garlic capsules can be taken.

* **Honey** Very useful for skin infections. Rubbed on wounds and burns, it has been shown to heal the skin, leaving minimal scarring, and can also be used to treat ulcers, the fungal infection athlete's foot and the eye infection conjunctivitis.

HERBS TO FIGHT INFECTION

Several herbs have anti-bacterial effects. Thyme is one of the most powerful of the herbal antiseptics. Others are sage and rosemary, which, along with thyme, are best used fresh in cooking and in salads or as an infusion to drink, or can be gargled if sore throat is a problem. Infused mustard seeds also make a good gargle for tonsillitis and throat infections. Oils of peppermint, eucalyptus, lavender and thyme can be used in solution for skin infections.

Internally, honey will help ease coughs and sore throat.

* **Green tea** Has been shown to help kill bacteria when taken as an infusion, and can also be used as a bathing fluid for skin infections.

* **Ginger** Fresh ginger root is thought to be a mild anti-bacterial food which will also help to clear up chesty coughs and colds. Use it grated in meals or infuse for a drink with honey and lemon.

* **Lemon** An antioxidant and antiseptic and, of course, rich in vitamin C (see next paragraph). Taken as juice, with ginger and honey, it is an ideal drink for sufferers of coughs, colds, bronchial problems and flu.

* **Vitamin C** Long talked about as a 'cure' for colds, it is now recognized that lack of C-rich foods can be a factor. For best sources, see page 25. A daily supplement of up to 500mg with added bioflavonoids (phytochemicals which help the vitamin be effective) may shorten length and severity of an infection.

See also entries for Colds, Bronchitis and Coughs, etc.

INFERTILITY

FEMALE INFERTILITY — inability to conceive — may be due to several different medical or physical problems, but diet does play an important role. Regular menstruation and a reasonable body weight are both linked to ease of conception. Women who over-exercise and/or who follow over-restricted diets, which contain neither enough calories nor enough nutrients, may cease menstruation and therefore, at least temporarily, fail to ovulate. A certain amount of body fat, which helps regulate hormone levels, and a Body Mass Index (page 188) between 20 and 25 are important factors in conception. Anorexics and people who exercise a great deal professionally, such as sportswomen and dancers, are frequently unable to conceive; if a sensible diet is followed and less exercise taken, however, periods can usually be restored to normal.

Obesity can also cause infertility, probably by hampering ovulation, so a BMI over 30 should indicate a weight-loss diet. A general basic healthy diet, containing all the nutrients for good health, will help to facilitate conception. New evidence shows that the polyphenols in tea may increase fertility. For more information on pre-conceptual care and on eating for a pregnancy, see Section Three.

Male fertility can be boosted with an adequate intake of zinc-rich foods (see best sources list on page 31) and with a diet high in vitamin C, essential fatty acids and selenium. All males intending to father a baby should eat a general basic healthy diet – preferably organic, as chemical residues may reduce fertility – cut down on alcohol, caffeine and smoking, and get plenty of exercise.

INSOMNIA

INSOMNIA — the inability to 'get a good night's sleep' — is frequently related to psychological symptoms such as stress, anxiety and depression. For more information on these conditions, see the appropriate separate entry. Prescription sleeping pills can be an occasional effective remedy but, used too frequently, the body adapts to them so that they work less well and when you try to do without them, insomnia can be even worse than before. Therefore, natural remedies — of which there are plenty — are a more sensible idea.

SOLUTIONS

Regular exercise is an important factor in good sleep — according to research, a daily walk or other activity in fresh air effects a 50% improvement in sleep patterns. Before bed, a warm bath sprinkled with some calming essential oils, such as lavender or ylang ylang, aids relaxation.

The right diet can do much to help you get a good night's sleep. In general, avoid both over-eating in the evening (which can cause sleeplessness through indigestion) and going to bed hungry, which will keep you awake. The ideal pattern of eating in the evening is to have a medium-sized meal no later than three hours before bedtime, consisting mainly of complex carbohydrates, such as pasta, rice or potatoes, and vegetables, with a small amount of low- or medium-fat protein, such as fish or chicken, eggs, lean meat or low-fat cheese.

Research shows that carbohydrate foods have a calming effect upon the brain, probably because they stimulate the production of a chemical called serotonin, sometimes referred to as the 'happy' chemical, because of its ability to produce a good mood. A low-carbohydrate, high-protein supper, such as a steak and green salad, tends to have a 'stimulating' effect. However, small amounts of protein are important in your evening meal, as they help to provide the amino acid tryptophan which, in turn, converts to serotonin as discussed above.

A small glass of red wine may also help regulate sleep patterns – scientists have found high levels of melatonin, the sleep-regulating hormone, in red wine grapes, especially those used to make Barolo. Before bedtime, it is a good idea to have a small snack or drink rich in both carbohydrate and tryptophan-containing proteins, such as hot milk and a digestive biscuit, a banana, a crispbread and a little low-fat cheese (unless cheese disagrees with you if eaten later in the evening, see the box above right), or peanut butter on bread.

A drink is most easily digested — and milk really is the perfect bedtime drink because not only does it contain tryptophan in the milk protein, it also contains carbohydrate in the form of the milk sugar lactose, and is an excellent source of the mineral calcium, which is some-

FOODS AND DRINKS TO AVOID FOR INSOMNIA

✱ *Caffeine-rich strong coffee and cola drinks*
Cocoa contains caffeine and is best substituted with a malted drink if you prefer that to plain milk. Caffeine is a stimulant and will help to keep you awake.

✱ *Too much alcohol*
One drink may help you to get to sleep, but too much alcohol effects REM sleep and blood sugar levels, which may be an important cause of waking in the middle of the night. Beer contains hops, which are a known sedative.

✱ *'Bad dream' foods*
Some foods, such as cheese and red meat, seem to spark off bad dreams and nightmares in some people. If you think this may be a problem, try eliminating these foods from your diet in the evening.

times called 'nature's tranquillizer'. Insomniacs should ensure they get adequate calcium in their diet (see best sources list on page 29, plus RDA) and also magnesium, which may also be a calming mineral.

There are several herbs which are natural tranquillizers and sleep-inducers. Camomile, lettuce, passion flower, valerian, kava kava and lemon balm all have a reported effect.

IRRITABLE BOWEL SYNDROME

■ ONE IN FIVE OF THE UK POPULATION is said to suffer from IBS, and it affects twice as many women as men. Sometimes called spastic colon, symptoms are abdominal pain, which is related to bowel function, with either constipation or diarrhoea present, and perhaps nausea, wind, bloated stomach, an urgent need to empty the bowels, a feeling of incomplete emptying, passage of mucus and sharp pains in the rectum. These may often be accompanied by depression, fatigue, backache and other symptoms.

The cause of IBS is not certain. One major study found that 10% of cases develop after an acute bout of diarrhoea. Another possible cause is food intolerance, and wheat and dairy produce appear to be two foods strongly associated with IBS. Others are

coffee, potatoes, corn, onion, beef, oats, cheese and white wine. A low-sugar and low-yeast diet may also help. However, virtually any food or drink may provoke an individual response. Intolerances should be investigated with the help of a dietician. See Allergies, page 88.

There is also an association between IBS and psychological factors. One study reported that two-thirds of IBS sufferers have experienced severe stress before onset of symptoms and it may significantly or certainly worsen symptoms for some (see page 134).

SOLUTIONS

During an attack, it is wise to avoid high intakes of tea, coffee, cola, fizzy drinks and alcohol (although some people report that alcohol helps). A prebiotic supplement (fructo-oligosaccharides) plus a probiotic supplement (acidophilus) may help restore normal bowel function, particularly in IBS with constipation.

Aloe vera, slippery elm and evening primrose oil have all been used successfully in some cases. Peppermint tea is anti-spasmodic and fresh ginger tea will help nausea. Long term, a basic healthy diet with regular relaxed meals eaten slowly and thoroughly chewed will help. For IBS with constipation, a high-fibre diet is helpful, but raw bran should be avoided. Soluble fibre — found in greatest quantities in fruits, oats, pulses and linseeds — may help (for a best sources list, see page 14). Fluid intake of 1.75-2.25 litres/3-4 pints a day is recommended.

See also: Colitis. For helpful addresses, see the Appendix.

KIDNEY STONES

KIDNEY STONES are usually made predominantly of calcium (and this is the type we discuss here), which is why it has always been presumed that a low-calcium diet would help to prevent them, but this now appears not to be the case. Men are three times as likely to get kidney stones as women, and it now seems likely that, in fact, a calcium-rich diet can help to prevent the stones, which may be formed when oxalate-rich foods, such as rhubarb, tea, beetroot, spinach, peanuts and chocolate, are eaten. Calcium may interfere with the absorption of the oxalates. It has also been shown that a basic healthy diet, rich in fruits and vegetables and high-potassium foods such as bananas and dried apricots, high in fluids and with not too much meat protein, helps to prevent stones from forming in the first place.

Mastalgia, see Menstrual Problems

ME

MYALGIC ENCEPHALOMYELITIS, also known as ME, chronic fatigue syndrome and post-viral fatigue syndrome, is said to affect 150,000 people in the UK, including children and teenagers, at any one time. It is often described as feeling like a severe hangover, influenza, muscle pain and deep exhaustion (as if having run a marathon) all at once.

It can last for months or even years, is highly disabling and sufferers frequently have to give up work or school.

The diagnosis is often not accepted or recognized by the medical profession. The name myalgic encephalomyelitis is probably a misnomer as it infers chronic inflammation of the brain and spinal cord, and there is no evidence of this in sufferers.

Other symptoms can include sore throat, tender lymph glands, feverishness, poor memory and concentration, abnormal sleep patterns, depression, mood changes and bowel problems, e.g. IBS. Symptoms can vary from day to day, or within the day, and are often worse after exertion.

ME may result from an infection, but sometimes seems to come on for no real apparent reason, or develops in the wake of a stressful event, or there may be gradual onset.

SOLUTIONS

The Immune-strengthening Diet (page 143) may be useful in helping to prevent M.E, otherwise follow a basic healthy diet, including plenty of fresh fruits and vegetables, oily fish and whole grains. Foods rich in potassium may be helpful (see page 32).

Known food intolerances should be avoided. For people with irritable bowel syndrome or other symptoms which may be caused by allergy or intolerance, sufferers may like to try an elimination diet as explained in Allergies, with the help of an experienced dietician.

For some, various dietary supplements seem to help. One trial showed quite significant improvement in symptoms with a regular combination of evening primrose oil and fish oils. Another showed that a course of magnesium injections helped — oral magnesium may also be helpful, as may co-enzyme Q10. Regular moderate aerobic exercise has been shown to improve wellbeing in some sufferers

See also Fatigue. See the Appendix for helpful addresses.

MEMORY, POOR

SLIGHT LOSS OF MEMORY is quite common as we age, and this isn't necessarily a sign of the beginnings of Alzheimer's Disease, although loss of memory, particularly short-term memory, is a symptom of that. Many women report a deterioration in their memory at the time of menopause and others find their memory is worse in the few days before a period, both of which are probably connected to changing hormone levels.

The disorder hypothyroidism also produces loss of memory as one of its early symptoms. If you also have problems with tiredness, constipation and tend to feel cold all the time, it may be worth seeing your doctor to have him check out your thyroid function.

SOLUTIONS

Help your memory to stay in top condition throughout your life with a basic healthy diet rich in the antioxidant vitamins A, C and (especially) E; take plenty of foods rich in B-group vitamins, especially B1.

A recent study showed that people deficient in B1 had poor memories, which were improved with supplementation. (However don't take supplements of B1 alone, you should take the B group together.)

Include in your diet plenty of essential fatty acids found in oily fish, vegetable oils, olive oil, evening primrose oil and linseed oil.

BRAIN BOOSTERS

Supplements of ginkgo biloba are claimed to increase brain capacity and memory and Siberian ginseng is said to have a similar effect. Excess intake of alcohol will impair short-term memory and may impair long-term memory, too, although studies on this are divided.

MENSTRUAL PROBLEMS

PROBABLY THE MOST COMMON COMPLAINT associated with periods is pre-menstrual syndrome, or PMS, the various symptoms of which — such as weight gain, fluid retention, bloating, food cravings, breast pain, tiredness and depression — appear in the 4-10 days before a woman's period begins and disappear a day or two after it has started. These symptoms are caused by changing levels of the hormones progesterone and oestrogen, and all can be helped with dietary intervention and/or supplements.

Heavy bleeding, or menorrhagia, can be a problem from time to time, particularly in the teens and when women near the menopause. If you regularly suffer from heavy periods, you should get checked out by your physician, who may diagnose under-active thyroid, often present when there is also weight gain, dry skin and lethargy. Iron supplements, taken with plenty of vitamin C, may be needed to correct iron-deficiency anaemia.

Painful periods (dysmenorrhoea), with or without heavy bleeding, can be eased through exercise, such as walking and yoga, extra EFAs, and supplements of calcium and magnesium. The herb meadowsweet is a natural analgesic and foods high in tryptophan may help pain by producing a calmer mood.

Absence of periods (amenorrhoea) is usually a sign of pregnancy, which is the first option to get checked out. Other reasons are stress, over-exercise, and under-eating. Any woman who loses a lot of weight quickly, goes on a crash diet or, for any other reason, doesn't eat enough risks amenorrhoea. Prolonged amenorrhoea can result in osteoporosis and possible infertility. Periods will usually return if lifestyle and eating habits return to normal. Periods can also cease due to the effects of diabetes or an over-active thyroid.

SOLUTIONS

The basic healthy diet is a good starting point for eating on most days of the month. It contains all the nutrients you need for healthy periods in the right balance. These are: enough calories to maintain a reasonable body weight; and enough essential fatty acids, B and E vitamins, iron, zinc, calcium and magnesium to keep the female hormone system functioning well.

However, to alleviate — or even help to prevent — the PMS symptoms, or whichever ones you may get, a little further dietary modification may be necessary.

* Watch the salt Fluid retention is a natural occurrence before a period, accounting for up to 3.25 kg / 7 pounds of extra weight, so watch your intake of salt (see the list of high-salt foods on page 33) and refined carbohydrates to minimize fluid retention, stomach bloating and breast tenderness. You should also eat plenty of potassium-rich foods, which have a role in fluid elimination. See also Fluid Retention, page 113.

* Avoid caffeine for problems with breast tenderness, particularly in the week pre-period.

* Eat extra vitamin B-rich foods including yeast extract, whole grains and dark green leafy vegetables. The vitamin B group is important for healthy nerve functioning and is depleted when we are under stress. Vitamin B6, in particular, has been found to be important in minimizing PMS because it helps to break down oestrogens. Controlled trials of its use have indicated that supplements up to 100mg a day may help. Women wishing to increase their B6 intake through food should eat wheatgerm, pulses, whole grains, oily fish, bananas and poultry (see the best sources list, page 26).

* Eat more essential fatty acids particularly those found in oily fish first, and in plant oils, nuts and seeds, and in supplements of evening primrose oil, linseed oil and starflower oil. The EFAs are particularly useful in helping to prevent breast tenderness (mastalgia). One research study showed that two-thirds of women with pre-menstrual breast pain had lower levels of EFAs than other women. Vitamin E appears to have a similar effect.

* There is some research to show that extra calcium and magnesium in the diet can help ease PMS — 1 g of calcium and 500 mg of magnesium a day may be the optimum level – as can the herbal supplement agnus castus, Kava kava helps menstrual pain.

* Food cravings in the week before a period can be controlled by following the tips in the Hypoglycaemia (low blood sugar) entry and by avoiding alcohol. Low moods and depression can be alleviated by a diet that is high in complex carbohydrates, such as whole grains and pulses, and by eating tryptophan-rich foods (see Insomnia), which produce the mood-lifting chemical serotonin. Bananas are a particularly ideal food before a period as they are quite high in serotonin, potassium, vitamin B6 and complex carbohydrate.

* Constipation can be a problem before a period — follow all the advice under the separate entry.

* For undue tiredness see the separate entry on Fatigue; however, tiredness will be reduced to a minimum in most cases by following the other tips in this entry.

* Iron deficiency could also be a problem if periods are heavy (see page 126).

* Drink plenty of fluids, preferably natural water, before a period (this will not make fluid retention worse) and cut down on consumption of both caffeine and alcohol.

* PMS is often helped by solving any food allergy or intolerance problems; for some an 'anti-candida' diet may help.

See the PMS and Diuretic Diet on page 145.

MIGRAINE AND HEADACHES

■ COMMON MIGRAINE — a severe throbbing headache, which is often one-sided and may be associated with nausea, vomiting and aversion to bright lights or noise — affects one in ten of the population and is twice as frequent in women. First attacks usually occur between childhood and early adulthood, with 90% first occurring before the age of 40, although menopausal women sometimes experience a first attack at this time, probably because of reducing levels of the hormone oestrogen. In women, attacks may also occur more frequently pre-menstruation and less frequently during pregnancy.

Classic migraine, which affects 20% of sufferers, includes all the above symptoms but also aura, which may include flashing lights, split- or half-vision, blind spots and mood changes before the attack begins.

Research indicates that there are very many triggers for migraine. In general, skipping meals and any crash or severe diets are to be avoided as they can cause hypoglycaemia (low blood sugar), which may precipitate an attack.

Individual foods can also be culprits. Cheese contains tyramine, which may trigger attacks. Caffeine over-consumption, or even withdrawal, may well set off a reaction. Bread and cereals have been shown to cause headaches in some, probably due to the gluten. Red wine contains phenolic flavonoids which can cause migraine. Many other foods can start a migraine and this is thought to be due to allergy or food intolerance. Interestingly, according to one recent US study, chocolate doesn't play a significant role in triggering migraine.

The mechanism by which a particular food triggers a migraine is not yet fully understood, but trials have shown that up to 70% of migraines in adults may be caused by various foods. Another trial in children has shown that, if the trigger foods can be avoided, other known triggers for migraine, such as perfume and cigarette smoke, no longer provoke a migraine. In view of this, if other typical allergic symptoms are present, such as urticaria or irritable bowel syndrome, then an elimination diet as explained on page 89 in the Allergy entry may be a good idea.

Regular meals, adequate fluid intake and plenty of foods rich in magnesium (see best sources list on page 32) and oily fish are all thought to help prevent migraine. One US study found that fish oil supplements halved the number of attacks and reduced severity. Another study shows that feverfew helps 3 out of 5 people.

Other headaches

Headaches can be caused by many factors, including eye problems, hangover, allergy, catarrh, infection, high blood pressure, stress and hypoglycaemia. Check out the different entries for all these. Other causes can be poor posture, dehydration, and a diet that is high in protein and low in carbohydrate. See the Basic Healthy Diet on page 53 for information on improving the balance of your diet. Persistent headache or migraine should be checked by your physician.

See the Appendix for helpful addresses.

MOUTH ULCERS

SMALL PAINFUL ULCERS inside the mouth are a common occurrence and it is often not at all easy to pinpoint the exact reason for a flare-up. However, certain food intolerances may cause them and can be a symptom of coeliac disease — see Allergies. Dairy products, wheat, strawberries, Marmite, tomatoes, and even oranges may be to blame.

NATURAL REMEDIES FOR MOUTH ULCERS

✳ Eat some natural bio yoghurt: high in acidophilus bacteria, every day. Keep it in the mouth as long as you can — these 'healthy' bacteria may clear the ulcer up more quickly.

✳ Put honey (set, not runny) on the ulcer — honey is antiseptic, soothing and healing, and will stay in place for longer than most of the gels that are sold for ulcers.

✳ Eat plenty of garlic, also an antiseptic. Try opening a garlic capsule and dabbing the contents on the ulcer.

✳ Sage leaves are said to heal ulcers — crush a leaf lightly and dab it on to the ulcer directly, or make a strong infusion and, when cool, use as a mouthwash.

✳ The herb echinacea is also said to help — use tincture of echinacea to dab on the ulcer, or dilute in warm water and use as a mouthwash.

SOLUTIONS

People who are run-down or recovering from illness, or are under great stress, may be much more likely to get mouth ulcers. Try the Immune-strengthening Diet or the anti-stress diet hints on pages 143 and 138.

A diet that is low in vitamins, minerals and other nutrients, and high in junk and processed foods, may also be a factor. Follow the Basic Healthy Diet on page 53 and include plenty of antioxidant-rich foods, which include the vitamins C and E and the carotenoids. These work to help ensure mucous membrane health.

Acid foods in general will be painful to eat while you have an ulcer — avoid things like ketchups, vinegar, pickles, chutneys, French dressing, citrus fruits, tomatoes, and so on, until the ulcer has gone.

Regular consumption of cranberry juice has been found helpful in the prevention of mouth ulcers.

Some ulcers may be caused by a foaming agent in toothpaste – sodium lauryl sulphate (check the label).

MUSCULAR PAIN AND RHEUMATISM

MUSCULAR PAIN can be caused by any activity you are not used to — e.g. a cycle ride, if you haven't cycled for years, will cause a build-up of lactic acid in the used muscles and result in them aching, a result which can be minimized by doing stretching exercises on the used muscles immediately before and after the activity. Another prevalent muscular pain is cramp, and a further common cause of aching muscles, particularly in the neck, shoulders and back, is stress anxiety or tension.

Muscular pain can also be associated with various other conditions, or called by various other names and sometimes this involves what people often term 'rheumatism'. Rheumatism isn't, in fact, a real medical condition, but a blanket term used to cover all kinds of aches and pains in the joints, muscles, ligaments and tissue. There may be local tender spots or pain, inflammation, 'shooting' pains up limbs, stiffness and, perhaps, swelling and general discomfort. Associated syndromes are polymyalgia, fibrositis, repetitive strain injury, tendonitis, ankylosing spondylitis, housemaid's knee, tennis elbow, and so on! Aches and pains associated with tiredness, fever, weakness and a general feeling of being unwell may, in fact, be rheumatoid arthritis. Joint pains may be osteoarthritis. See also the Arthritis entry.

SOLUTIONS

There is no guaranteed diet that you can follow to prevent muscular aches and rheumaticky problems, but the Basic Healthy Diet on page 53 is a good starting point, including plenty of essential fatty acids, which are known to help inflammation. Selenium, vitamin E, evening primrose oil and cod liver oil may also be of help. Take extra selenium in the form of foods rich in the mineral (see best sources list on page 31), and vitamin E, evening primrose oil and cod liver oil may be taken as daily supplements. Any chronic or acute joint or related pain with no obvious cause should be discussed with your physician.

NAUSEA AND TRAVEL SICKNESS

■ NAUSEA, a feeling of queasiness or sickness which may or may not result in vomiting, can have various causes. A food allergy could be the cause (see Allergies). Frequent bouts of nausea which don't seem to have a cause may be a food intolerance (see also Allergies). In women, nausea is a fairly common side-effect of PMS and can often be relieved by a small low-fat, high-protein snack such as a spoonful of cottage cheese. It is also common in pregnancy, see the Pregnancy feature in Section Three (page 172).

If the problem is food poisoning, nausea will soon be followed by vomiting and diarrhoea. Drink plenty of orange juice diluted with water and avoid food until the vomiting is over. Another likely cause of nausea, especially in children, is the onset of an infection. Again, plenty of fluids should be taken and food ignored until the child feels like eating again. Stress and worry can cause feelings of nausea, often associated with appetite loss. Eat small meals or take nutritious drinks until appetite returns and see page 175.

Travel sickness is a type of nausea that happens because of the motion of travelling. One of the best cures for this is fresh ginger — some tests have shown it to be more effective than travel sickness pills from the chemists. Try an infusion of grated ginger root half an hour before travelling and eat a little crystallized ginger as you travel. To settle the stomach before bed after a day of travelling, a small glass of ginger wine may be a good idea. Peppermint alleviates nausea — a few peppermint sweets will help, or peppermint tea.

Any unexplained nausea lasting more than a day should be checked out with your physician.

Nervousness, see Anxiety

Nettle Rash, see Urticaria

NEURALGIA

■ NEURALGIA is a blanket term for nerve-related pain in any part of the body and can include pain from trapped or compressed nerves, as in a slipped disc or, sometimes in late pregnancy, damaged nerves due to illness such as MS, viruses such as shingles, and the sometimes long-term pain that can carry on after the acute stage of shingles.

SOLUTIONS
The health of the nervous system is dependent, at least partly, on a healthy diet with adequate supplies of all nutrients, particularly the B vitamin group and vitamin E. Check out best sources on pages 22–33, and follow the Basic Healthy Diet on page 53, including plenty of essential fatty acids. Omega-3 fats, combined with a diet low in saturated fat, have been shown to help MS sufferers. In one trial, high doses of vitamin E cured post-shingles nerve pain in almost three-quarters of cases. The herbs meadowsweet and camomile are said to ease the pain of neuralgia. Both can be taken as an infusion. Cannabis has been shown to be very beneficial for MS and other pain, but its use is still illegal in the UK.

Night Blindness, see Eye Problems

NOSEBLEED

NOSEBLEED may be a symptom of high blood pressure — if you have a nosebleed it is wise to see your physician and get this possibility checked out. Dietary advice similar to that for people with high blood pressure may be of use in preventing recurrence. The tannin in tea is said to help prevent nosebleed. Tea can be used as a drink and cold tea bags or cotton wool soaked in tea can be used as a poultice over the nose to help stop bleeding. Nettle tea may have a similar effect.

Osteoarthritis, see Arthritis

OSTEOPOROSIS

OSTEOPOROSIS causes over 200,000 bone fractures a year in the UK. It affects approximately 75 million people in Europe, Japan and the USA, including one in three women aged 50 plus, and one in 12 men. It can affect all ages, but is most common in post-menopausal women, due to reduced levels of oestrogen in the body after the menopause, which causes acceleration of loss of calcium and other minerals from the bones.

Osteoporosis is sometimes called 'brittle bone disease', but that really is a misnomer — the condition happens when skeletal bone loses its substance and density, becoming thinner, more fragile, more porous, and therefore much more at risk of fracturing. People with the condition are sometimes unaware that they do have low bone density until they suffer a fracture, which is why it is often referred to as 'the silent disease'.

Areas commonly affected are the hips, spine and wrists, and it can cause severe back ache, pain and disability, as well as loss of height — up to 12.5 cm (5 inches) — and may cause spinal curvature, known as 'dowager's hump'. Once bone density is lost, as yet there is no complete cure, although progress is being made — for example the drug alendronate sodium is claimed to rebuild bone at all affected sites and reduce the risk of fracture.

Still, the best method of dealing with osteoporosis is in prevention — particularly by building strong large bones. The human skeleton is a dynamic structure which is constantly changing. A child's skeleton is totally rebuilt every two years, and an adults every 7-10 years. When the bones stop growing in length (which happens by the late teens in most people), they still increase in density until about 30-35, when 'peak bone mass' is reached. After this time, bone mass should be maintained by sensible precautions, including correct diet.

Maximizing the amount of bone in your body may mean that in later life, even if bone thinning occurs, enough bone density may be retained to prevent fractures. After the early thirties, there is a natural slow reduction of bone density in most people — about half a percent per year in both sexes, caused when the body loses more bone than it can replace. At menopause, and for the next five or so years after, there is a marked increase in the rate of bone loss (without intervention, see below), estimated at an average total loss of 15%. After this, bone loss slows down again.

■ Factors which will help to achieve and maintain your peak bone mass :

Calcium intake
Calcium is the major component of bone, and adequate amounts in the diet from birth are vital in order to reach peak bone density in adulthood. However, there is considerable debate over the optimum level to prevent osteoporosis. In the UK, the National Osteoporosis Society recommends higher levels of calcium intake than the amounts laid out in the Department of Health guidelines (see page 28). The NOS suggestions are 1,000 mg for men aged 20-36 and women aged 20-45, and 1,500 mg for women over 45 unless on HRT, and for men over 60. One US trial found that with 1,200-1,500mg daily intake (including a 500mg supplement), older people suffered 50% less fractures.

Adequate vitamin D is needed in order for calcium to be absorbed from foods. The best form of calcium supplement is calcium citrate malate.

Magnesium intake
Calcium works together with magnesium in the formation of bone, so adequate intake of magnesium is as important as calcium. There is evidence that the mineral boron may reduce loss of calcium and magnesium, as well as increasing oestrogen and testosterone in the body.

Essential fatty acid intake
The EFAs — found in fish and vegetable oils and evening primrose oil, for example — are now thought to be of some importance in helping build and maintain bone mass by assisting calcium absorption and delivery of calcium to the bones.

Intake of fruit and vegetables
Bone health and maintenance may also be affected by a range of other nutrients, including vitamin C and potassium, found in excellent quantities in fruit and veg. These may also help being alkaline-forming, which seems to favour bone mass retention. New research suggests that eating onions may offer bone protection. Scientists have found that a peptide in onions slows bone loss in animals, and the same result would be likely in humans.

Maintenance of reasonable body weight
Thin people are more prone to osteoporosis than people with a sensible body mass index (or, indeed, than overweight

people, although excess weight is not a sensible way to prevent osteoporosis as it involves so many other health risks). This is because thin people may have lower levels of the hormone oestrogen, which helps to prevent bone loss, and because they have less weight to carry around, thus minimizing the beneficial effects of weight-bearing exercise, see below.

Also, if diet is seriously inadequate, menstruation may become infrequent, or cease completely and this will have a similar effect to early menopause, (see below).

Weight-bearing exercise

Regular exercise which involves using the body's own resistance or weight, (or any other type of weight) is an important factor in building and maintaining bone. Walking, dancing or step exercising is weight-bearing exercise for the legs (but not the arms), tennis is a weight-bearing exercise for the racket-holding arm (in tests, players' playing arms have significantly more bone than the non-playing arms). Swimming is a non-weight-bearing exercise.

Weight-bearing exercise should be carried out regularly in moderate amounts as excessive exercise may actually make osteoporosis more likely, not less (see Anorexia, Menstrual Problems).

Hormone replacement therapy

One of the major benefits of HRT for women of menopausal age is that the accelerated bone loss at this time, due to marked decrease in the body of the hormone oestrogen, can be largely prevented. Oestrogen replacement can reduce bone loss to pre-menopausal levels and therefore reduce fracture rates. Any woman considering HRT should see her physician to discuss the possibilities.

Soya-rich diet

A high-soya diet has frequently been suggested as a way to strengthen bones and prevent bone loss associated with the menopause. This is because soya beans are rich in isoflavones – plant estrogens (see page 35). However, recent research has cast doubt on this and the latest advice from the UK's Food Standards Agency (2006) is: 'It is not clear if phytoestrogens in food or dietary supplements can reduce menopausal symptoms (including osteoporosis) because the current scientific evidence is conflicting. More research is needed....' However, replacing some animal protein (e.g. red meat) with the vegetable protein of soya and other pulses may be a good move even so – as we see overleaf, high animal protein intake may be detrimental to bone health. Also, soya is high in calcium.

■ Factors which may have a detrimental effect on your peak bone mass:

Inadequate intake

Inadequate intake of all the correct nutrients and/or calories (see above.)

Sedentary lifestyle

Osteoporosis is on the increase worldwide not only because the numbers of older people are increasing but because of our sedentary lifestyles. Look at ways to build more mobility into your life, particularly weight-bearing exercise (above).

High-salt diet

A diet high in sodium causes increased excretion of calcium in the urine, and the higher the salt intake the greater the risk of osteoporosis, research shows.

Alcohol intake

Heavy drinkers and alcoholics often suffer from low bone density. This may be because alcohol reduces absorption of calcium, a direct effect of alcohol on the bone, or through general malnutrition. However, one study has shown that drinking alcohol within DoH guidelines has no detrimental effect and may even have a beneficial effect on bone density.

It is possible to find out your risk of osteoporosis and fracture with a simple low-dose x-ray to measure your bone density. This is called a DXA scan and is becoming more widely available.

For more details, contact the British College of Naturopathy and Osteopathy or the NOS (for addresses, see the Appendix).

Cigarette smoking

Heavy smokers are more at risk. The longer you smoke, and the more you smoke, the higher the amount and rate of bone loss. The WHO cites double the risk.

Excess protein

Too much protein — particularly animal protein — in the diet can increase calcium excretion. However, one study showed that in a high-protein diet more calcium is absorbed to 'make up for' the extra calcium excreted, so perhaps excess protein may only be a problem if overall calcium intake is low. Thus it is wise to limit protein intake to no more than the RNIs listed on page 20, unless advised otherwise by your dietician or physician. Milk is an interesting food in this debate — it is one of the best sources of calcium, but is also a good source of protein. However, the lactose (milk sugars) it contains help calcium to be absorbed and so, despite its protein content, it still is an excellent source of easily absorbed calcium.

Caffeine intake

Caffeine — found in coffee, tea, chocolate, cocoa and cola drinks, as well as some food supplements such as guarana — increases calcium excretion in the urine, therefore it is wise to limit intake of these, especially for individuals who may be at high risk of osteoporosis (see box). One major Norwegian study found that drinking more than nine cups of coffee a day almost doubled the risk of hip fracture in women — but, interestingly, not in men, and in the USA, teenage girls with the highest consumption of fizzy drinks were found to suffer 300% more fractures than those who avoided them.

Intake of foods high in phytates and oxalates

Raw wheat bran, spinach, rhubarb, chocolate and tea should be limited because the phytates or oxalates they contain hinder calcium absorption.

High phosphate intake

Diets high in phosphate-containing items such as fizzy drinks, soft drinks and processed foods will limit calcium absorption.

Other factors, which may be unavoidable, can effect bone density and the likelihood of developing osteoporosis. These are: early menopause, early hysterectomy, long-term use of cortisteroids, irregular or infrequent periods (see Menstrual Problems, Anorexia), low body weight due to natural tendency, lack of sunshine and therefore of vitamin D, diseases such as hyperthyroidism and coeliac disease, race (Caucasians and Asians have much greater risk of osteoporosis than black people) and genetic tendency — i.e. a family history of osteoporosis.

Calcium - to supplement or not?

As we've seen, an adequate intake of calcium is vital, especially in childhood and youth, in order to reach 'peak bone mass'. Yet, according to the WHO, data appears to show that optimum levels are not being met. In two separate trials, youngsters who received calcium supplementation achieved greater gain of bone mass than those who received none, and the WHO report suggests that intake of 1,000-1,600 mg a day appears to be optimal for children and young adults between the ages of 2 and 30. Other organizations, including the UK's NOS suggests that intake for people with osteoporosis should be 1200mg a day. Levels such as this may not be easy to obtain through diet without consuming too many calories and so supplementation with calcium tablets may be advisable, especially if several of the risk factors are present. However, exactly what level of supplementation is necessary, and for how long, will continue to be debated.

Little data is available on the effects of supplementation for pre-menopausal adult women or males, but several studies have been carried out on the effects of extra calcium for post-menopausal women. Calcium supplementation has been shown to reduce bone loss and fracture, but the benefits appear to be greatest after the first five years beyond menopause. In the five-year period following menopause, calcium supplementation by itself doesn't seem to slow bone loss. In elderly people, both calcium and vitamin D supplements appear to retard bone loss and reduce the incidence of hip fractures.

PALPITATIONS

WHEN THE HEARTBEAT can be easily felt by a hand placed over the heart, and when the beat feels abnormal (very fast, for instance) and can be heard by the sufferer, the term palpitations is usually used. Sudden panic, fear or nerves are very usual causes of palpitations — the adrenaline released at this time causes a sudden rise in blood pressure, with the palpitations as an immediate result. See Anxiety, and Stress.

SOLUTIONS

Find the cause of the nervousness and ensure adequate supplies of the vitamin B group within your diet. People of a nervous disposition, likely to experience palpitations, should cut down on caffeine in coffee, colas, chocolate and tea, as this will exacerbate the problem.

Another likely cause of palpitations is low blood sugar or hypoglycaemia. Eat little and often and never go for long periods without food. Eat a basic healthy diet and don't eat very large meals, which can in themselves cause palpitations because the blood supply is diverted to the stomach and digestive system to cope with the amount of food.

Anaemia can cause palpitations. If you also feel tired, are pale, weak and generally lethargic, check with your physician that you are not anaemic.

PEPTIC ULCER

A PEPTIC ULCER — either gastric (when in the stomach) or duodenal (when in the duodenum or upper intestine) — is an open sore on the wall of the stomach or intestinal muscle, where the protective lining has worn away, made worse by the acid secretions in the stomach which aid breakdown of food. Peptic ulcers occur in about 10% of the population, are more common in men and also have a hereditary factor.

It is now known that ulcers may often be caused by the bacterium Helicobacter pylori (especially duodenal ulcer), which is passed on through contact (e.g. between family members). Presence of this bacterium needs diagnosing by a medical specialist and treating with suitable antibiotics. Rarely, an ulcer may become so deep that it perforates the stomach or intestinal wall, which is a serious condition requiring immediate medical treatment.

Symptoms of a peptic ulcer are upper abdominal pain and perhaps nausea, which comes and goes, is triggered by particular foods, and is often worst at night.

SOLUTIONS

Medicines that neutralize the stomach acids will take away the pain. Trigger foods are frequently spicy foods, high-fat foods and very rich foods, very hot or very cold foods, alcohol, tea and coffee (including decaffeinated), and too many sweets and chocolates. Smoking and some drugs, such as aspirin, can also cause peptic ulcers. Stress increases acid secretion.

A suitable diet for helping to prevent peptic ulcers is one high in fibre, wholegrains and fresh fruit and vegetables, and with adequate essential fatty acids. Small frequent meals and avoidance of late-night eating, as well as chewing slowly and thoroughly, are also helpful. There may be slight continual blood loss from an ulcer, which may result in anaemia, so a diet high in iron-rich foods may be important once an ulcer is formed.

Eradicating the Helicobacter bacterium significantly reduces peptic ulcer recurrence and essential fatty acids are thought to play a role in this by inhibiting the bacteria. EFAs also help by helping to keep the correct balance of mucus and acids in the stomach. Also, cranberry juice has been shown to block the action of H. Pylori in the stomach.

Post-viral Fatigue Syndrome, see ME

PMS (pre-menstrual syndrome), see Menstrual Problems

Respiratory Problems, see Bronchitis and Coughs, and Asthma

Rheumatism, see Muscular Pain and Rheumatism

Rheumatoid Arthritis, see Arthritis

Shingles, see Herpes Simplex 1

Sinusitis, see Colds and Flu

SKIN, DRY

DRY, FLAKY SKIN with no other symptoms (such as rash, redness, swelling or itching) is a common complaint, and even people who have oily or normal skin in youth and young adulthood may suffer from dry skin as they get older, which may wrinkle more easily.

SOLUTIONS

To help maintain the skin's natural moisture balance, eat the Basic Healthy Diet (page 53) with adequate essential fatty acids from vegetable oils, fish oils, linseed, evening primrose oil and so on. Don't try to follow a diet too low in fat, e.g. a fat-free diet, as we all need some fat in our diets. Any diet providing less than 20% of its total calories as fat may result in dry skin. Don't try to maintain too low a body weight, either.

Get adequate vitamin E in your diet (for best sources list, see page 24) or supplement your diet with natural-source vitamin E (alpha or a-tocopherol, as opposed to synthetic vitamin E, alpha-dl tocopherol) capsules and, in addition, use 2-3 of these every night on your skin as a 'night cream' — split the capsules carefully and smooth the oil into the dry areas. Once a week or so, make a face mask of ground oats and vitamin E or EPO or linseed oil and spread it gently on your dry patches (or face). Leave for 15 minutes then rinse this off gently with soft water.

Get plenty of all the antioxidants in your diet — vitamins A and C as well as E, and the minerals selenium and zinc. These help to fight the free radicals which form in our bodies as a result of stress, pollution, illness and various other reasons, and contribute to the ageing process. Selenium is also an anti-inflammatory. For best sources of all these, see pages 22-33. For more information on the many different kinds of natural antioxidants, see Section One, page 24.

Drink about .75-2.25 litres (3-4 pints) of water a day for your skin's health and spray your face regularly with a water spray. Psoriasis – patches of thick red, perhaps scaly skin – can be helped with the essential fat EPA, found in oily fish. Have one 150g portion several times a week.

See also Eczema.

Spots, see Acne and Spots

STOMACH-ACHE

ABDOMINAL PAIN is a symptom of many different conditions and illnesses. Upper abdominal pain (around and just below the breastbone and to either side of the lower ribcage) may be caused by heartburn and indigestion, hiatus hernia, peptic ulcer, gallstones or infection. Central abdominal pain (around the front and sides of the waistline) may be caused by food poisoning (see Diarrhoea), constipation, irritable bowel syndrome, diverticulitis, appendicitis (see your doctor immediately), ulcerative colitis or Crohn's disease (see Colitis). Lower abdominal pain may be caused by flatulence, constipation, cystitis or menstrual problems. General stomach-aches may also be a symptom of allergies, anxiety, coeliac disease and stress, or, rarely, cancer of the stomach, colon or bowel, or elsewhere within the body. Stomach-ache which cannot be explained and which persists longer than a few days or so should be investigated by your physician.

SOLUTIONS

Mild bouts of stomach-ache caused by everyday problems such as indigestion, flatulence or over-indulgence can usually be eased somewhat by taking herbal infusions of basil, dill, fennel or peppermint.

STRESS

WHEN THE BODY IS UNDER STRESS, particularly long-term stress, such as found in people with demanding jobs or perhaps long-term domestic problems or illness, it needs careful handling nutritionally in order both to minimize the stress and ensure that nutrient requirements are met. Stress tends to deplete the body of certain vital nutrients, and anyone under long-term stress should either be extra careful to incorporate plenty of these into the diet with the right foods, or take supplements. The vitamin B group is largely responsible for smooth running of the nervous system and, as the B group is water-soluble and cannot be stored in the body for long, chronic stress will soon severely deplete it. The same applies to vitamin C, which most experts believe a stressed person will needed in much greater quantities than the RNI of 40 mg a day — 200 mg is probably appropriate.

The minerals zinc (which helps strengthen the immune system) and magnesium (excreted in greater amounts from the body when under stress) may need to be supplemented, or zinc- and magnesium-rich foods incorporated into the diet (for best sources lists, see pages 22-33). Bodies depleted of vitamins B and C and zinc are also at increased risk of getting endless minor infections, colds, coughs, cold sores and so on, because these are the nutrients that help to protect the immune system and that is why so often stressed-out people complain that they are 'run

SYMPTOMS OF STRESS

Stress can have many other physical symptoms, such as eating disorders, fatigue, migraine, heartburn, impotence, insomnia, irritable bowel syndrome, memory problems and muscular pain — see individual entries for all of these. Turn to page 138 for the Anti-stress diet tips. See also Anxiety, Depression.

down'. The Immune-strengthening Diet (page 143) will help in this case.

Stressed people may turn to alcohol or smoking — both make the nutritional problems worse as they also deplete the body of B and C vitamins and can hinder absorption of others. Caffeine drinks increase the adrenaline generated at times of stress and so are best avoided.

The better (food) way to tackle stress relief is to eat plenty of complex carbohydrates, such as pasta and whole grains, which will assist the brain to calm down by helping to release the chemical serotonin. New research also indicates that oily fish can block the production of the enzyme that makes us tense under pressure. Long-term stress, and the higher levels of adrenaline it produces, raises the level of fats and cholesterol in the blood. This can be a contributing factor in increased risk of circulatory and heart diseases. Blood cholesterol and fats can be reduced by regular aerobic exercise such as walking, which, happily, will also reduce stress. For a Healthy Heart Diet, see page 142.

Stroke, see Heart Disease and Stroke

SUNBURN

■ THE BEST WAY TO TREAT SUNBURN is to avoid it — by building up to periods in the sun very gradually, by wearing sun-protection factor and by wearing suitable clothing. There are also dietary means by which you can lower the risk of sunburn even when exposed to the sun. It is well documented that carotenoids — the orange pigment found in carrots, sweet potatoes and dark leafy greens — offer protection against the harmful ultraviolet rays of the sun.

In early summer, or before going to a sunny climate, you can give yourself added protection by eating a large portion of carrots every day and including a selection of beta-carotene-rich vegetables and fruits in your diet for two weeks before exposing yourself to strong sun. There are also carotenoid supplement capsules. Extra carotenoids may make your skin look slightly orange, which is evidence that they are working to protect your skin. HOWEVER, it is important not to exceed stated doses for supplements or to eat more than normal quantities of carrots as carotene toxicity can occur.

Recent research also indicates that essential fatty acids may also offer protection against sunburn. Volunteers took fish oil capsules for three months, by which time their sun-protection factor increased by a factor of three. It isn't clear yet whether it is only the essential fatty acids (omega-3s) in oily fish that achieve this result or whether the same benefit would be gained from eating other EFAs, such as are found in evening primrose oil, sunflower and olive oil. It is possible that the high vitamin D content of oily fish may play a part, as vitamin D is also produced by the action of sunlight on the skin. But as the EFAs are essential to health in so many ways, with few drawbacks, and many of us don't get enough, it will do no harm to increase intake before exposure to sun.

A diet rich in all the antioxidants is also thought to be important in helping to protect the skin. If you do have sunburn, again eat a diet rich in the antioxidants, which help to fight the free radicals released when the skin is damaged.

Also take plenty of zinc-rich foods, as zinc is important to the healing process. Drink plenty of fluids, as sunburn causes dehydration, and a vitamin E-rich oil applied to the skin will help. Alternatives are aloe vera gel, lavender oil diluted in a base, or, for slightly worse burns, tea tree cream.

Sunburn accompanied by fever, nausea or delirium should be attended by a physician.

Tension, see Stress

Thrombosis, see Heart Disease and Stroke

Tiredness, see Fatigue

TONGUE, SORE

A SORE TONGUE, which is smooth and bright or fiery red, may be caused by a type of anaemia due to deficiency of vitamin B12 and sometimes iron and folate, or a vitamin B2 or B6 deficiency. Other symptoms such as tiredness may also be present, and your physician should make a diagnosis and then supplement your diet as necessary.

SOLUTIONS

A well-balanced nutrient-rich diet, such as the Basic Healthy Diet (page 53), should prevent this type of problem from occurring. A sore tongue accompanied by furring and, possibly, bad breath is probably caused by oral thrush, which may be linked with vaginal thrush (see Candida) and may also be present after being treated with antibiotics. Regular spoonfuls of live bio yoghurt containing the bacteria acidophilus may help.

Ulcers on the tongue may be a symptom of coeliac disease, but can also be due to allergies or food intolerances, or possibly sensitization to substances used in dental treatment. See also Mouth Ulcers. Occasionally, sore tongue may be caused by a severe protein malnutrition, but this should be diagnosed professionally.

TONSILLITIS

TONSILLITIS is an infection of the tonsils at the back of the throat. Tonsils become infected as a 'first line of defence' against infection going down to the chest. Infections are more likely to take hold in someone who has lowered resistance or immunity, perhaps through overwork or stress of another kind, or perhaps through a diet deficient in the necessary vitamins, minerals and so on, which we need to maintain a healthy immune system.

At times of stress, our bodies need more of these nutrients, so poor diet and stress together can be a 'double blow' to the immune system, and can easily be followed by an infection such as tonsillitis. See Infections.

SOLUTIONS

Sore throat can be eased with drinks of honey and lemon juice diluted in warm water. Lemon contains vitamin C, which is an antioxidant, and honey is a known antiseptic soother. Gargles of infused sage leaves are said to help cure tonsillitis and a drink of infused meadowsweet tea will lessen the pain.

When tonsillitis is bad, it is hard to eat a normal diet because swallowing hurts — soft foods, such as soups, purées, eggs, ice-cream and custards are, therefore, ideal. To avoid repeated bouts of tonsillitis and other similar throat infections, try the Immune-strengthening Diet on page 143.

TOOTH DECAY

DENTAL CARIES are caused when the teeth become coated with plaque (a combination of food particles and bacteria). If the plaque isn't removed, the bacteria break it down and acid is formed, which may eventually dissolve the tooth enamel and eventually cause tooth decay. Tooth decay can nowadays largely be avoided.

TOOTH DECAY IN CHILDREN

Children's teeth are particularly prone to decay, but the mineral fluoride is an important preventer. Tap water usually has fluoride added, as does toothpaste. Fluoride tablets can be bought if water isn't fluoridated. It is also important that children should get enough calcium (from which teeth are mainly formed) and magnesium, which works with calcium, as well as vitamin A. For best sources of all these, see pages 22-33.

SOLUTIONS

Regular brushing of teeth and flossing thoroughly, preferably soon after every meal and snack, removes the plaque before bacterial action can begin, though research shows that, after an acidic meal or drink, cleaning should be delayed to allow the tooth enamel to re-harden. Diet is also important. Sugary foods are quickly attacked by the bacteria and acid is soon formed. Refined carbohydrates are also major offenders, as their residues appear to cling to the teeth readily. Any sweet or sticky food which remains in the mouth for a long time is particularly bad in this respect.

Poor dietary habits, such as frequently sucking sugary or fruit drinks through straws, will contribute to decay. Some 'healthy' foods, such as dried fruits and fruit juices, produce plaque just as much as confectionery and fizzy drinks do. However, it has been shown that regular tea drinking inhibits plaque formation and protects against tooth decay.

If you can't clean your teeth straight after eating or drinking something, eat a small piece of hard cheese and chew it thoroughly, as this helps to stop the formation of acid. Chewing on sugar-free gum also helps, as it increases saliva production and this, in turn, helps to disperse the acids.

Thrush, see Candida

Travel Sickness, see Nausea and Travel Sickness

Ulcer, see Peptic Ulcer

Ulcerative Colitis, see Colitis

■ URTICARIA IS A SKIN RASH with, often, large red raised, very itchy patches and, perhaps, areas of white, resembling that of a nettle sting. The rash may last for several hours or days and there may be other symptoms, such as nausea or fever. There are several different causes, of which food allergy is one. Shellfish and strawberries are frequently linked with the condition, but there are several non-food causes which trigger the rash, for example, heat, insect bites, drugs or hot sun.

URTICARIA (HIVES OR NETTLE RASH)

SOLUTIONS

Dietary treatment is to avoid the food(s) known to cause problems. In acute cases it is often possible to pinpoint the cause — otherwise an elimination diet may be the answer (see Allergies). Other reported methods of control are using an 'anti-candida diet' (see page 141) or a diet low in food additives and salicylates, including avoiding aspirin.

■ VARICOSE VEINS are veins (most often to be found in the legs) that have become dilated with blood because the system of valves which ensure that the blood is pumped back to the heart through the veins has become weakened. The problem is about four times more common in women than it is in men and it does frequently seem to be hereditary. It quite often starts in pregnancy and is also much more usually to be found in people who are significantly overweight or, more particularly, obese.

VARICOSE VEINS

SOLUTIONS

A basic healthy diet, avoidance of too much weight gain at any time, but especially during pregnancy (see Section Three), and a regular programme of exercise for healthy circulation, will all help to prevent varicose veins.

There is also some evidence that bioflavonoids called rutins, found in vitamin C-rich fruits and vegetables, act to strengthen the veins, so make sure that your diet regularly includes plenty (for best sources of vitamin C, see page 25). The supplement horse chestnut may also help.

Vomiting, see Nausea and Travel Sickness

■ MINOR WOUNDS, BURNS AND GRAZES are best thoroughly cleaned and left to heal naturally. Small cuts can be pulled together with a micropore tape, which will also stem the bleeding. Excessive bleeding may possibly be a sign of a deficiency in vitamin K — the vitamin which helps the blood to clot. Vitamin K is found in leafy green vegetables. Wounds are helped to heal with a diet rich in zinc and vitamin C. Honey is a gentle and effective antiseptic when applied to inflamed grazes, cuts or burns. Vitamin E is said to help wound healing and minimize scarring. Vitamin E capsules can be broken and the oil massaged into healing wounds, and it may be a good idea to get extra vitamin E in the diet, in the form of vegetable oils, nuts and seeds (see best sources list on page 24).

WOUNDS, CUTS AND GRAZES

DIETS FOR PARTICULAR CONDITIONS

The diets that follow are examples of the type of eating that can be used to help prevent or alleviate the specified conditions. They should be used in conjunction with the advice in the preceding Ailments and Solutions section and, where appropriate, should be discussed with your physician or dietician. They are not intended to replace any diet that you may be following on medical advice and are for general guidance only.

To begin with, below we set out some quick hints on using diet to help you cope with times of high stress in your lives. Recipes for the dishes that are capitalized are to be found in Section 5.

Quick dietary hints for anti-stress

■ Shopping guide

Star foods: pulses, nuts, seeds, leafy green vegetables, fish, liver, yeast extract, milk, brown rice, fresh fruit.

Foods to choose:

In general — complex carbs, especially whole grains and wholewheat pasta.

■ Rich in vitamin B group — yeast extract, whole grains, nuts, seeds, meat, low-fat dairy produce, tuna and other fish, lentils and other pulses, liver, leafy green vegetables.

■ Rich in vitamin C — citrus fruits, kiwi fruit, strawberries, blackcurrants, red peppers, leafy greens, mange-tout peas, melon.

■ Low-fat protein sources (preferably non-meat) — low-fat dairy produce, pulses, Quorn, white fish, shellfish, tofu.

■ Rich in zinc — oysters and shellfish, liver, wheatgerm, seeds, nuts, lamb, beef.

■ Rich in calcium — low-fat dairy produce, pulses, nuts, seeds, leafy greens, canned fish, fortified soya milk and yoghurt.

■ Rich in magnesium — nuts, seeds, lentils and other pulses, bulgar wheat, brown rice, pot barley.

Notes

✱ Daily supplements of vitamin B group and C may be taken.

✱ To drink — water, low-fat milk, fresh fruit and vegetable juices, camomile tea, lemon balm tea.

✱ Snacks — yeast extract on wholemeal bread; nuts, seeds, low-fat fromage frais and yoghurt, tuna pâté on rye crispbreads, fresh fruit dressed with yoghurt.

Anti-arthritis diet

May help to prevent or ease the symptoms of all types of arthritis.

■ Shopping guide

Star foods:

mango, sweet potatoes, kale, cantaloupe melon, spinach, broccoli, sunflower seeds and oil, walnuts, tuna, salmon, sardines and all fish.

Foods to choose:

■ High in fish oils — mackerel, herring, salmon, trout, tuna.

■ High in vitamin C — blackcurrants, kiwi fruit, strawberries, raspberries, mango, nectarine, peaches, pawpaw, cantaloupe melon, spring greens, kale, Brussels sprouts, cabbage, broccoli, mange-tout, spinach, sweet potatoes.

■ High in vitamin A (beta-carotene) — carrots, squash, sweet potatoes, chard, spinach, kale, greens, broccoli, mango, cantaloupe melon.

■ High in vitamin E — sunflower oil, polyunsaturated spread, sunflower seeds, corn oil, pine nuts, sweet potatoes, avocado, muesli, tuna, salmon, chickpeas, Brazil nuts, hazelnuts, almonds, spinach.

■ High in selenium — walnuts, lentils, tuna, squid, liver, sardines, sole, cod, swordfish, salmon, prawns, mussels, pork, wholemeal bread.

■ Anti-inflammatory — ginger, apples, garlic.

Foods to avoid:

Those high in saturated fat, e.g. full-fat dairy, fatty cuts of red meat (limit red meat anyway).

■ Members of nightshade family (only if found to aggravate symptoms) — potatoes, tomatoes, aubergines and peppers.

■ Coffee.

■ Alcohol.

Notes

* A minority of arthritis sufferers report a negative reaction to dairy products, wheat, corn, citrus fruits and nuts, but many other arthritis sufferers can eat these foods with no problem; they all provide valuable nutrients.

* You may like to take a daily supplement of omega-3 fish oils, cod liver oil and/or evening primrose oil.

* People on steroids should include plenty of calcium- and iron-rich foods in their diet.

* Use sunflower oil in cooking.

* To drink — water, tea, herbal tea, fruit juices, milk or calcium-enriched soya milk.

* Have daily 1 tbsp of sunflower seeds.

* Snack ideas: raw carrot, handful of Brazil nuts, almonds or hazelnuts or mixed nuts, slice of wholemeal bread with sunflower spread and honey.

ANTI-ARTHRITIS DIET

DAY ONE

Breakfast

muesli with skimmed milk, peach juice
wholemeal bread, sunflower spread, honey

Lunch

Lentil and Coriander Soup, white bread roll
mango and low-fat yoghurt

Evening

Salmon and Broccoli Risotto
large green salad, slice of cantaloupe melon

DAY TWO

Breakfast

porridge with skimmed milk and honey
mango juice
slice of wholemeal bread with sunflower
spread and low-sugar jam or honey

Lunch

Hummus, pitta bread, salad of avocado and
leafy greens with pine nuts

Evening

pork chop fillet with kale, carrot and sweet
potato, Stir-fried Fruit Salad

DAY THREE

Breakfast

As Day 1

Lunch

Spinach, Parsley and Garlic Soup
French bread with sunflower spread
slice of cantaloupe melon with ginger

Evening

Sardines with Redcurrant Glaze
green salad
Peach and Banana Fool

DAY FOUR

Breakfast

Sheep's-milk yoghurt
strawberries or kiwi fruit
handful of mixed chopped nuts

Lunch

tuna and avocado sandwich on wholemeal
bread, small mango

Evening

Spiced Chicken and Greens
brown rice, broccoli, apple

DAY FIVE

Breakfast

As Day 1

Lunch

soup of butternut squash simmered with
onion and stock
rye bread with small portion of low-fat
cheese, apple

Evening

Herring Fillets with Ginger and Coriander
spinach, couscous

DAY SIX

Breakfast

As Day 2

Lunch

Seafood and Tropical Fruit Salad
2 rye crispbreads with sunflower spread
fruit bio yoghurt

Evening

Almond, Chickpea and Raisin Pilaff
mange-tout peas, Raspberry Gratin

Anti-cancer diet

May offer protection against some cancers and may help to control cancer growth. See also page 96.

■ Shopping guide

Star foods:

tomatoes, broccoli, Brussels sprouts, watercress, carrots, sweet potatoes, grapes, cherries, strawberries, citrus fruits, olive oil, oily fish, garlic, Brazil nuts, tuna, whole grains, soya and other pulses.

Foods to choose:

■ All starchy high-fibre foods, including whole grains, root vegetables, various pulses, bread, breakfast cereals, pasta.

■ All fruits, especially cantaloupe melon, mangoes, apricots, oranges, pawpaw, peaches, nectarine, citrus fruits, berry fruits, cherries, grapes, apples, pomegranates.

■ All vegetables, especially broccoli, Brussels sprouts, kale, spring greens, watercress, carrots, sweet potatoes.

■ Nuts, seeds, oily fish, garlic, Oriental mushrooms (fresh).

■ Low-saturated-fat, non-meat sources of protein — such as various pulses, Quorn, tofu, skimmed milk, low-fat yoghurt, cottage cheese, soya milk, soya yoghurt, fish and seafood, various nuts and seeds.

Foods to avoid or cut down on:

■ Saturated fats and meats, especially char-grilled, barbecued and well-done meats.

■ Salt-cured, pickled and smoked foods of all kinds.

■ Alcohol.

Notes

* Keep weight at a reasonable level.
* To drink — a glass of red wine or red grape juice daily, green tea, water, fresh fruit and vegetable juices, skimmed milk.
* Snack ideas — fresh fruit, nuts, seeds, dried fruits, bread, raw carrots with hummus, soya yoghurt, sesame seed bar.

ANTI-CANCER DIET

DAY ONE

Breakfast
Weetabix with soya milk, grapes
wholemeal bread with sunflower spread and honey

Lunch
Carrot and Orange Soup
wholemeal bread, Brazil nuts

Evening
Salmon and Broccoli Risotto
mixed salad with tomatoes included
cantaloupe melon

DAY TWO

Breakfast
bio yoghurt or soya yoghurt
strawberries and lemon
muesli with added chopped nuts
fresh orange juice

Lunch
salad of drained tuna in oil, avocado,
tomato, crushed garlic and tofu mayonnaise
wholemeal bread, peach

Evening
Winter Squash with Lentils and Ginger
baked potato, Brussels sprouts
Mango Filo Tart

DAY THREE

Breakfast
pink grapefruit
wholemeal bread with sunflower spread and
honey, yoghurt

Lunch
Marinated Shiitake Mushrooms
wholemeal bread and sunflower spread
banana and low-fat fromage frais with
brown sugar

Evening
Pasta with Olives and Sardines
tomato and watercress salad
plateful of grapes or cherries and fresh nuts

DAY FOUR

Breakfast
muesli with extra chopped nuts and
dried apricots
skimmed milk or soya milk
grapes or cherries, fresh orange juice

Lunch
Spinach, Parsley and Garlic Soup
rye bread with tofu pâté

Evening
Chickpea, Almond and Raisin Pilaff
broccoli, kale
compote of summer fruits

DAY FIVE

Breakfast
Shredded Wheat
1 tablespoon sunflower seeds
skimmed milk or soya milk
strawberries or orange

Lunch
salad of grated carrot, hazelnuts and half-fat
Cheddar on a bed of watercress with olive oil
vinaigrette, wholemeal bread

Evening
Potato and Mediterranean Vegetable Bake
peas and lettuce, cantaloupe melon

Anti-candida diet

May help to prevent or minimize symptoms of gut dysbiosis (candida, thrush). See also page 99.

■ Shopping guide

Star foods:
live yoghurt, garlic, oysters, green vegetables, peppers, mange-tout peas.

Foods to choose:
■ Zinc-rich foods — wheatgerm, calves' liver, oysters, cocoa powder, pumpkin, beef, crab.
■ C-rich foods — broccoli, sweetcorn, most salad leaves, spinach, tomatoes, chillies, peppers, leafy greens, sprouts, mange-tout peas, blackcurrants, kiwi fruit, strawberries, citrus fruits, pawpaw.
■ Garlic
■ Live yoghurt

Foods to avoid:
■ All yeast-containing (raised) bakery goods, e.g. breads, buns, all leavened breads.
■ All fermented drinks — beers, wines, sherries, spirits.
■ All alcohol-containing products, e.g. some medicines (check label).
■ All vinegars, including malt and wine vinegars, and foods containing these — e.g. pickles sauces, relishes.
■ All cheeses.
■ All malted drinks, malted cereals and sweets.
■ Mushrooms and fungi of all kinds.
■ Nuts and seeds may also be yeasty or carry moulds and so you may also like to avoid these, see note below.
■ Soy sauce.
■ Vitamin B supplements and brewers' yeast tablets, unless they are labelled 'yeast-free'.
■ Canned, packeted or frozen fruit juices (home-squeezed is fine).
■ Dried fruits.
■ Sugars, syrups and high-sugar products.
■ Vegetarians and vegans should not avoid nuts and seeds, but preferably use cashews and pine nuts (which tend to be tolerated better) in preference to other types of nuts.

Notes
* You may like to take a daily supplement of the pre-biotic fructo-oligosaccharides (from chilled cabinets of some health-food shops and by mail order) and pro-biotics containing lacto-bacillus and bifidobacteria. You can eat several portions a day of live yoghurt containing the pro-biotic bacteria too, which will help boost levels.
* To drink — water, herbal teas, skimmed milk or semi-skimmed milk (drink at least 200 ml / 7fl oz a day), fresh fruit and vegetable juices, cocoa made with skimmed milk and artificial sweetener.
* Snack ideas — live yoghurt, rye crispbread with hard-boiled egg; pitta with hummus.
* Breakfast every day - live bio yoghurt, orange or kiwi fruit, home-made muesli with no dried fruits.

ANTI-CANDIDA DIET

DAY ONE
Lunch
Country Pea Soup, Tzatziki, soda bread
Evening
Rice and Beans, with hard-boiled egg chopped on top, broccoli

DAY TWO
Lunch
Cannellini Bean and Basil Spread
Ryvitas, banana, green salad
Evening
Pork, Onion and Pepper Kebabs
brown rice, tomato salad

DAY THREE
Lunch
Spinach, Parsley and Garlic Soup (omit Parmesan and swirl in some yoghurt instead) chapati
Evening
Potato and Mediterranean Vegetable Bake
Mango and Peach Booster

DAY FOUR
Lunch
Skordalia, soda bread
mixed salad with olive oil and lemon dressing
Evening
Avocado and Turkey Tortillas
apple, pecan nuts

DAY FIVE
Lunch
Hummus, pitta bread
Roast Tomato, Garlic and Pepper Soup
Evening
Baba Ganoush, with crudités
Spanish-style Baked Trout with Chard
mange-tout peas

Healthy heart diet

May help to reduce the risk of heart disease and maintain a healthy circulatory system.

■ Shopping guide

Star foods:

all fruits and veg, especially citrus, apples, blackcurrants, mango, cantaloupe melon, carrots, squash, sweet potatoes, broccoli, leafy greens; oily fish, garlic, oats, pulses, whole grains, nuts and seeds, olive oil.

Foods to choose:

■ Rich in vitamin C and flavonoids — citrus fruits, blackcurrants, melon, berries, red peppers.

■ Rich in carotenoids — squash, carrots, tomatoes, sweet potatoes, chard, spinach, kale, cabbage, broccoli, peas.

■ Rich in vitamin E — wheatgerm oil, sunflower oil, polyunsaturated spread, sunflower seeds, corn oil, sweet potato, avocado, pine nuts, muesli, chickpeas, tuna, salmon, squash, spinach, kale, Brazil nuts, hazelnuts, almonds.

■ Rich in folate — yeast extract, liver, pulses, cereals, muesli, leafy vegetables.

■ Rich in vitamin B6 — wheatgerm, fish, pulses, nuts, chicken, potatoes.

■ Rich in selenium — walnuts, lentils, sunflower seeds, wholemeal bread, tuna, sardines, salmon, swordfish, cod, sole.

■ Rich in monounsaturated fatty acids — olive oil, rapeseed oil, groundnut oil

■ Rich in soluble fibre — oats, pulses, many fruits and vegetables.

■ Rich in omega-3 oils — salmon, mackerel, herring, sardines, trout, fresh tuna.

■ Phytochemicals — watermelon, pink grapefruit, onions, broccoli, Brussels sprouts and many more fruits and vegetables, garlic, soya, wine and beer, tea.

Foods to avoid or limit:

■ Too much alcohol (limit).

■ Trans fats and saturated fats.

■ High-cholesterol foods (limit)

■ High-calorie snacks (to avoid obesity).

■ Salt and salt-rich foods.

Notes

✳ Avoid smoking.

✳ Supplements of vitamin E, selenium, garlic oil, may be taken.

✳ To drink — water, fruit and veg juices, soya milk, skimmed milk, tea, green tea.

✳ One or two alcoholic drinks a day, especially red wine, are allowed.

HEALTHY HEART DIET

DAY ONE
Breakfast
muesli
calcium-enriched soya milk, pink grapefruit
Lunch
Roast Tomato, Garlic and Pepper Soup
Oatbread, Rouille
Evening
Pasta with Broccoli and Anchovies
large mixed salad
Peach and Banana Fool

DAY TWO
Breakfast
porridge made with skimmed milk
glass of fresh orange juice
slice of wholemeal bread with sunflower
spread and marmalade
Lunch
Smoked Mackerel Pâté Salad
Oatbread, apple
cantaloupe or watermelon
Evening
Potato and Mediterranean Vegetable Bake
peas
strawberries and low-fat fromage frais

DAY THREE
Breakfast
As Day 1, but with melon
Lunch
Lentil and Coriander Soup
Oatbread, banana
Vegetable Cup
Evening
Spanish-style Baked Trout with Chard
broccoli, blackberry ice

DAY FOUR
Breakfast
As Day 2
Lunch
Thai Salmon Salad, Oatbread
Evening
Winter Squash with Lentils and Ginger
kale or Brussels sprouts, apple

DAY FIVE
Breakfast
As Day 3
Lunch
Spinach, Parsley and Garlic Soup
Oatbread, Hummus
Evening
Sardines with Redcurrant Sauce
potatoes mashed with olive oil
Stir-fried Fruit Salad

Immune-strengthening diet

Helps to strengthen the immune system generally and fight against disease and infection.

■ Shopping guide

Star foods:

leafy greens, sweet potatoes, Brazil nuts, walnuts, sunflower seeds, tuna, broccoli.

Foods to choose:

■ Rich in vitamin C — citrus fruits, black-currants, berries, melon, red peppers, leafy green vegetables, broccoli.

■ Rich in zinc — nuts, seeds, wheat-germ, Quorn, All Bran, beef, oysters, crab, lamb, pork, pot barley.

■ Rich in vitamin A (beta-carotene) — carrots, squash, chard, sweet potatoes, spinach, kale, leafy green vegetables, mango, cantaloupe melon, broccoli, tomato.

■ Rich in vitamin B group — whole grains, yeast extract, meat, nuts, seeds, low-fat dairy produce, tuna, other fish, lentils and other pulses, leafy green vegetables.

■ Rich in vitamin E — wheatgerm oil, sunflower oil, polyunsaturated spread, sunflower seeds, corn oil, pine nuts, sweet potato, avocado, muesli, chickpeas, Brazil nuts, hazelnuts, almonds, squash, kale, salmon, tuna.

■ Rich in selenium — Brazil nuts, walnuts, lentils, tuna and other oily fish, swordfish, cod, sole, mussels, wholemeal bread, sunflower seeds.

■ Rich in antioxidants — garlic, thyme, onions, ginger, black and green tea.

Foods to avoid:

■ Low-nutrient foods
■ Alcohol
■ Also avoid smoking

Notes

✱ You may take supplements of zinc and echinacea.

✱ To drink — water, fruit and vegetable juices, yeast extract, cocoa, green tea, black tea, herbal tea.

✱ Snack ideas — walnuts, sunflower seeds, wholemeal bread, hazelnuts, pine nuts, almonds, Brazil nuts, yoghurt, pesto on bread.

IMMUNE-STRENGTHENING DIET

DAY ONE
Breakfast
pink grapefruit
muesli with extra nuts and seeds
1 dessertspoon wheatgerm
Lunch
Tzatziki and wholemeal pitta bread
Spiced Lentils and Mixed Green Vegetables
carrot juice
Evening
Scallops and Mussels in the Pan
Stir-fry of green beans, broccoli and baby corn, cantaloupe melon

DAY TWO
Breakfast
boiled egg, wholemeal bread
Brazil nuts, almonds and sunflower seeds
freshly squeezed orange juice
Lunch
Panzanella with extra garlic
bio yoghurt with banana
Evening
Seafood Risotto with Ginger
salad of Cos, watercress and rocket
Summer Fruit Compote

DAY THREE
Breakfast
As Day 1, but with melon
Lunch
Warm Broccoli, Red Pepper and
Sesame Salad, rye bread
Evening
Speedy Herbed Swordfish
sweet potato
stir-fried shredded kale
Watermelon Refresher

DAY FOUR
Breakfast
As Day 1
Lunch
Salad of Tuna, Avocado and Tomato
wholemeal pitta, orange
Evening
Pork, Onion and Pepper Kebabs
quinoa, mango

DAY FIVE
Breakfast
As Day 2
Lunch
Squash, Potato and Butter Bean Soup
rye bread, berry fruits
Evening
Tiger Prawns with Rice Noodles
Spinach, Broccoli and Walnut Stir-fry
Citrus Granita

Anti-osteoporosis diet

May help to protect bones against osteoporosis. See also page 130.

■ Shopping guide

Star foods:

low-fat dairy produce, such as skimmed milk, low-fat yoghurt, low-fat fromage frais and cottage cheese; leafy green veg, nuts, pulses, soya, wheatgerm, fish, white bread, whole grains.

Foods to choose:

■ Sources of calcium — low-fat dairy produce, pulses, tilapia fish, canned sardines, pilchards, prawns, fortified soya products, e.g. calcium-enriched soya milk, calcium-enriched soya yoghurt; white bread, white flour, seeds and nuts.

■ Sources of magnesium — nuts, seeds, pulses, bulgar wheat, Shredded Wheat, brown rice, lentils, pot barley, Ryvita.

■ Sources of vitamin D — sunlight, cod liver oil, oily fish, margarine, fortified breakfast cereals, eggs.

■ Sources of zinc — wheatgerm, liver, fish, shellfish, seeds, nuts, lamb, beef.

■ Sources of folate — yeast extract, chicken livers, pulses, fortified breakfast cereals, muesli, nuts, broccoli, Brussels sprouts, kale, leafy green vegetables.

■ Sources of B6 — wheatgerm, fish, pulses, nuts, chicken, potatoes.

■ Sources of potassium — soya beans and other pulses, dried apricots, dried figs, tomatoes, potatoes, many fruits and vegetables.

■ Sources of essential fatty acids — vegetable, seed, nut and grain oils, seeds, nuts and whole grains.

Foods to avoid:

■ Those high in sodium.

■ Those high in alcohol.

■ Excess animal protein.

■ Caffeine — e.g. strong coffee, tea, colas, guarana drink.

■ Foods rich in phytates and oxalates — raw wheat bran, spinach, rhubarb, chocolate and tea.

■ Fizzy drinks, soft drinks, processed foods.

Notes

✱ To drink — 2 glasses of soya milk a day may help to prevent osteoporosis, but use calcium-enriched soya milk. Also drink at least 450 ml (¾ pint) in total low-fat dairy or calcium-enriched soya milk a day.

✱ You may like to use a daily supplement of cod liver oil for vitamin D, or a combined calcium, magnesium and vitamin D supplement.

✱ Snack ideas — dried figs and apricots, nuts, seeds, yeast extract on white bread, fresh fruit.

ANTI-OSTEOPOROSIS DIET

DAY ONE
Breakfast
baked beans on toast
glass of skimmed milk or soya milk
glass of fresh orange juice
Lunch
Smoked Mackerel Pâté Salad
ciabatta roll, mixed salad
Evening
Rice and Greens, with extra Parmesan (use extra broccoli instead of the spinach)
bio yoghurt, Stir-fried Fruit Salad

DAY TWO
Breakfast
muesli with 1 dsp wheatgerm and extra nuts, seeds and dried fruit, skimmed milk, glass of fresh orange juice, white bread with sunflower spread and honey
Lunch
Squash, Potato and Butter bean Soup
25 g (¾ oz) Brie, wholemeal bread, tomato
Evening
grilled tilapia fish, broccoli
green lentils with herbs, new potatoes

DAY THREE
Breakfast
Shredded Wheat, cantaloupe melon, white bread with sunflower spread and marmalade
Lunch
sardine and salad sandwich on brown bread
low-fat yoghurt or calcium-enriched soya yoghurt , Summer Fruit Compote
Evening
Potato Gnocchi with Cheese and Cauliflower kale

DAY FOUR
Breakfast
As Day 2
Lunch
Feta and Pepper Spread, Ryvitas
sunflower seeds
ready-to-eat dried apricots
Evening
grilled lamb, onion and green pepper kebabs
Tabbouleh
large bowl of mixed salad, ice-cream

DAY FIVE
Breakfast
porridge made with skimmed milk, honey
white bread with sunflower spread and marmalade, orange
Lunch
Thai Salmon Salad, low-fat fruit yoghurt
Evening
Pasta with Chicken Livers
1 tablespoon extra Parmesan cheese
salad of Cos lettuce and watercress

PMS and diuretic diet

May help reduce symptoms of pre-menstrual syndrome and help to reduce fluid retention at any time.

■ Shopping guide
Star foods:

For minimizing fluid retention, these are some naturally diuretic foods: asparagus, melon, citrus fruits, salad vegetables particularly celery, cucumber, watercress, lettuce, tomatoes, sweet peppers, carrots, tomato juice, carrot juice, mixed vegetable juice.

For helping other symptoms of PMS: all whole foods, fresh fruits and vegetables, especially pulses, pasta, bananas, nuts, seeds, grains.

Foods to choose:

■ Rich in potassium — bananas, toma-toes, onions, potatoes, whole grains.

■ Rich in vitamin B6 — wheatgerm, pulses, whole grains, oily fish, bananas, poultry.

■ Rich in vitamin E — most vegetable oils, various nuts and seeds, avocados, tuna, salmon, sardines, brown rice, asparagus.

■ Rich in essential fatty acids — vegetable oils, fish oils, nut and seed oils, grain oils, oily fish, nuts, seeds and whole grains.

■ Rich in calcium — low-fat dairy produce, dark leafy greens, canned fish, seeds, nuts.

■ Rich in magnesium — nuts, seeds, lentils and other pulses, bulgar wheat, brown rice.

Foods to avoid:

■ Salt and all salty foods

■ Alcohol

■ Sugary snacks

■ Caffeine

■ Refined starches — e.g. cakes, biscuits, soft white bread

■ Notes

✱ To drink — water, low-fat milk, vegetable juices, fruit juices, herbal teas (some herbal teas, such as nettle, parsley and dandelion, may help minimize fluid retention).

✱ Supplements of evening primrose oil, linseed oil, calcium/magnesium may be taken daily.

✱ Snack ideas — nuts, seeds, low-fat yoghurt, low-fat fromage frais, fresh fruit.

✱ Small main meals and plenty of in-between snacks are the key to managing PMS symptoms — i.e., eat little and often.

PMS AND DIURETIC DIET

Breakfast every day
low-fat natural yoghurt
handful of no-added-sugar-or-salt muesli, with extra nuts and seeds
dessertspoon of wheatgerm sprinkled on top
selection of fresh fruits chopped over, preferably including melon, one citrus fruit and some banana

DAY ONE
Lunch

small slice of wholemeal bread
salad of cooked asparagus, avocado, tomato, sliced onion and tuna in water or oil, well drained, tossed in a little sunflower seed oil and lemon juice

Evening

Rice and Beans, slice of melon
Vegetable Cup

DAY TWO
Lunch

large salad, including celery, watercress, lettuce, tomato, cucumber and onion tossed in dressing as Day 1
small slice of wholemeal bread with sunflower spread, Hummus

Evening

Spanish-style Baked Trout with Chard
carrot or orange juice

DAY THREE
Lunch

Warm Broccoli, Red Pepper and Sesame Salad
Banana and Strawberry Smoothie, apple

Evening

Spiced Chicken and Greens
carrots, Vegetable Cup

DAY FOUR
Lunch

Carrot and Orange Soup
Crudités with Feta and Pepper Spread

Evening

Chickpea and Vegetable Crumble
Watermelon Refresher

DAY FIVE
Lunch

small slice of wholemeal bread
Cannellini Bean and Basil Spread
large mixed salad as Day 2
orange

Evening

Salmon and Broccoli Risotto
Vegetable Cup
handful of dried apricots and sunflower seeds

Food supplements — clever aids to health or a waste of money?

We spend over £280 million pounds a year in the UK alone on vitamin, mineral and food supplements — more than we spend on any other over-the-counter health products except headache remedies – and that is excluding mail-order and health-food shop sources.

The most popular supplements are fish oils, multivitamins, evening primrose oil, single vitamins, and garlic, but literally hundreds of different products exist in varying combinations, and new products are appearing all the time. Here we look at whether supplements are worth the expense.

Vitamin and mineral supplements

Various types of vitamin and mineral supplement are regularly prescribed by doctors, for good health maintenance, disease prevention and cure. For example, iron supplements are often prescribed for anaemia; folate for early pregnancy, vitamin D for the elderly, vitamin B12 for vegans, and so on. Obviously, then, supplements ARE a necessary and important part of staying healthy — at least, for some of us... occasionally.

Many more vitamin and mineral supplements are, however, sold direct to the consumer who, in buying them, is making his or her own diagnosis about his or her state of health and nutritional needs. About 12 million consumers take supplements regularly, on a permanent basis, as 'health insurance'... but is this wise or necessary?

Most doctors and qualified nutritionists will say that, if you eat a basic healthy diet (such as that on page 53) and are in good health, supplements of vitamins and/or minerals are often a

waste of money. They will say that if you are not in good health or there is any other reason why you think you should take a supplement, then a visit to your physician will confirm or deny that (and if you need supplements you will be offered a prescription).

They will say that supplementing without professional advice can cause as many problems as it may cure — for example, through overdosing, toxicity, creating nutritional imbalances or through encouraging the false idea that it doesn't matter how unhealthy your diet is as long as you take vitamin pills. They may say that you can't transfer all the nutritional benefits of food into manufactured pills. They might even quote trials which have shown that sometimes supplements intended to help beat disease may actually have the reverse effect.

Other nutritionists and complementary practitioners will argue that the current RNIs for vitamins and minerals are too low, offering only protection against the deficiency diseases, such as rickets (lack of vitamin D) and scurvy (lack of vitamin C); that for optimum health and protection against disease, much larger amounts of several of the vitamins and minerals are needed; that these amounts are difficult to obtain through an average healthy diet and that supplementation is often the only option.

Here we look at these points of view in more detail.

■ Are the recommended daily amounts too low for people in normal health?

At certain times and in certain situations, you may need more than the RDAs or RNIs (see pages 22-33) and sometimes it IS hard to get your needs from diet. For example, a woman with iron-deficiency anaemia brought on by heavy periods will almost certainly need iron supplementation to bring her back to a suitable level. Someone who smokes and drinks heavily may well be short of vitamins B group and C and may well need supplements, as another example. The chart overleaf lists some typical uses for the main vitamin and mineral supplements.

However, it is extremely hard to find a definitive answer as to whether or not someone in reasonable health with no illness or deficiency would benefit from any extra supplements. There is much anecdotal evidence that supplements help people to feel better. For example, someone prone to several colds each winter may begin to take supplements of vitamin C and zinc daily, have no colds, and claim that the supplements did the trick. There is certainly convincing evidence that supplements of vitamin C of at least 1g daily (much greater than the UK RNI of 60mg) can help to minimize severity and duration of colds. There is also good evidence that high doses of vitamin B6 can help with menstrual problems. However, the people who may well benefit most from vitamin and mineral supplements — the elderly and the poor, both of whom have lower levels of intakes of many nutrients, are least likely to be able to afford them.

The consensus is that once your body has its optimum amount of the vitamins and minerals, taking any extra is at best a waste of time and at worst could be toxic.

■ Can high-dose supplements help prevent the major diseases?

For people with more serious problems, such as CHD or cancer, trials to show that supplements can help have had mixed results. For example, supplements of vitamin E have been shown in one major trial to decrease non-fatal heart attacks and vitamin C supplements have been used successfully in trials too, but other trials have shown negative effects (i.e. increased heart attacks and/or cancer) with vitamin E, beta-carotene and vitamin C.

Although beta-carotene in the diet, as an antioxidant, is often claimed to help protect against cancers and heart disease, experts now say that beta-carotene supplements should NOT be taken for this purpose. Other experts say that it is nearly impossible to get enough vitamin E in a normal diet to offer health protection and so supplementation is indicated. Selenium is another antioxidant which may be in shortfall in many of our diets and some experts recommend supplements. The B vitamin, folate is also linked with heart disease in some and supplementation may be the answer in that case.

Anyone thinking of supplementing their diet to help prevent disease should get professional advice. One problem with supplements is that they may well contain less – or more – of thee 'active ingredient' than is stated on the label, research shows

■ Are there any dangers in taking supplements?

Yes, some are toxic in excess. Too much vitamin A is particularly dangerous for pregnant women, who have also been advised to avoid all herbal remedies as they may contain toxic colchicine, which might harm the foetus. High intakes of iron, zinc and selenium are toxic, and an excess of vitamin C can cause stomach upsets.

Vitamin E supplements shouldn't be taken by those on anti-coagulant drugs nor calcium supplements if you have kidney stones or cancer.

Sometimes supplements are shown to be toxic for other reasons — for instance, fish oil supplements may contain dioxins and other toxins which can be dangerous in moderately high amounts.

Also, some herbal remedies interact with medical drugs and their effect, so if on any medication tell your doctor what supplements you are taking. Almost all vitamins and minerals will have some side-effects if taken in really large doses.

For more on advisable doses, see individual vitamins and minerals in Section One and the recommended maximum doses overleaf.

■ Do supplements create nutritional imbalances?

They certainly can do. This is because vitamins, minerals and other nutrients all work together within the body. Too much of one particular nutrient may have a 'knock-on' effect in various ways. Here are some examples:
* If you take calcium supplements, you should also take magnesium supplements as these work together.
* Iron supplements may reduce zinc absorption.
* High zinc intake may mean copper supplements need to be taken too.
* B vitamin supplements should be taken together rather than just an isolated B vitamin, as the group work together and an excess of one alters the delicate balance.
* High doses of iron can hinder vitamin E absorption.

The best policy when it comes to supplements, if you're not sure what or how much to take, or why you're taking them, is to see a professional nutritionist or doctor for advice. High doses of any one vitamin or mineral are best avoided unless you've been advised to take them. A new EC directive covering supplement doses and labelling may be taken up throughout Europe in the foreseeable future.

■ Can supplements compensate for a poor diet?

Most nutrition experts now agree that there IS no substitute for a healthy diet of real food and that nutrients are best taken as part of that diet. In other words, nutrients extracted from foods (or created synthetically, as many vitamins are), probably don't have the same effect on your body as they do when they come naturally packaged as a part of the food itself. A good example of this is beta-carotene, supplements of which seem to increase the risk of cancer in smokers, one trial has shown.

When nutrients are obtained through

THE MAJOR VITAMIN AND MINERAL SUPPLEMENTS AND THEIR TYPICAL USES

	Typical daily dose	Maximum daily dose**	Typical uses
Vitamin			
A	1-2,000 µg	7,500 µg* women 9,000 µg men	Dry skin, spots, poor night vision
Beta- carotene	6-15 mg	n/k	As vitamin A. Its use as an anti-cancer, anti-CHD supplement is controversial
B group	100% RNI	n/k	Stress and nervous conditions; smokers, drinkers.
B6	10 mg	200 mg	Pre-menstrual syndrome, fluid retention.
B12	100 µg	n/k	Vegans
Folate	400 µg	400 µg	Pre-conception, pregnancy (helps prevent birth defects)
C	250-1,000 mg	2-3,000 mg	Antioxidant; anti bacterial; smokers, drinkers, stress, skin complaints.
D	5-10 µg	10 µg	Elderly and those confined indoors
E	400 i.u. (275 mg)	1,200 i.u. (800 mg)	Antioxidant; wound healing; skin complaints.
Mineral			
Calcium	800-1,000 mg	1,500 mg	Family history of osteoporosis; insomnia
Iron	14 mg	20 mg	Anaemia, heavy periods, pregnancy, fatigue
Magnesium	150 mg	n/k	High calcium intakes, insomnia, stress.
Zinc	7-15 mg	50 mg	High calcium and iron intakes, immune strengthening; poor appetite, wound healing; acne
Selenium	100-200 µg	500 µg	Antioxidant; HIV, cancer, arthritis
Multivitamin/mineral	50-100% RNI	n/k	Slimmers: appetite loss, poor diet

* Avoid in pregnancy ** Adults in normal health, non-pregnant

you are missing out on many nutrients.

Obviously there are cases when it is better to take vitamin and/or mineral pills than nothing at all — for example, anorexia, or loss of appetite through ill health. However, pill popping alongside a poor diet is not a sensible solution.

■ Are vitamins and minerals in supplements easily absorbed by the body?

Not necessarily. Again, the Food Commission found that many were hardly absorbed at all. Fat-soluble vitamins (A, D, E) are less well absorbed when taken without food; iron tablets are notorious for being badly absorbed — help absorption by taking with vitamin-C-rich food, drink or supplement. Don't take mineral supplements with tea or coffee — these hinder absorption.

'Time release' capsules may help vitamin absorption. Mineral supplements are sold with the mineral bound (or 'chelated') to other compounds. Minerals which are chelated to organic compounds, such as amino acid chelates, gluconates, picolinates or citrates, may be more easily absorbed than those bound to inorganic compounds such as sulphates or phosphates (check label).

It is usually agreed that natural vitamin E (d-alpha tocopherol) is absorbed better than synthetic vitamin E (dl-alpha tocopherol),but synthetic vitamin C works as well as the natural extract.

Vitamin and mineral injections are not to be recommended unless administered by a doctor for medical reasons, as there can be potentially dangerous side effects.

■ What else is in supplement apart from 'active ingredients'?

Capsules may be made from gelatine or a vegetarian substitute. Vegetable oils are usually the base for fat-soluble vitamins in capsule form. Tablets may contain binders, fillers and other ingredients, including sugar, artificial sweeteners, yeast, colourings, fat. Check the label.

a varied diet, you cannot overdose. Another important factor is that some researchers say that the 'active ingredients' in the foods that we eat are many compounds other than vitamins — for instance, the phytochemicals in fruit and vegetables. No doubt in time a range of phytos will be packaged alongside the vitamins, but as yet there are few examples of this, although vitamin C is obtainable 'with bioflavonoids'.

A third reason why real food is better than pills is that food contains calories, protein, essential fats, fibre and a whole balance of the things that we need. Take a vitamin C tablet instead of an orange and

Food supplements

A large — and rapidly expanding — supplement market is that of food supplements other than the traditional vitamins and minerals. Often sold in health-food shops or by mail order, but increasingly appearing on the shelves of supermarkets and chemists, these supplements range from thoroughly tested items, such as garlic and evening primrose oil, through to more exotic remedies like kombucha tea and kava kava.

Like vitamin and mineral supplements, their claims vary, but include such things as increased well-being, better health, disease protection, protection against or cure of various ailments, anti-ageing, and so on. Most do not have a medical licence and should therefore not make medical claims. As they aren't medicines, but foods, they also escape medical regulations, which means that they needn't undergo safety tests like drugs do, and scientific proof of their efficacy is therefore scant.

Below we detail some popular supplements and evaluate, where possible, their worth. Benefits are often anecdotal and some products (perhaps in their original herbal form) have been used for centuries or more in their countries of origin. (Fresh herbs and the most common herbal remedies are discussed later.)

Acidophilus, see Pro-biotics

Agnus Castus
This ancient Mediterranean remedy, made from the fruit of the chaste tree, has been shown in properly controlled trials to improve PMS symptoms by 50% in over half of the women who took part in them. The only PMS symptom agnus castus doesn't seem to improve is bloating.

Aloe Vera
Aloe vera has been used medicinally since ancient times. The main active ingredient in the plant is said to be mucopolysaccharide, which may help a range of conditions, including infections, allergies and inflammation. Many skin complaints, including dry itchy skin, rashes, wounds, acne and psoriasis, are said to improve with oral or applied aloe vera preparations.

The plant has also been used for irritable bowel syndrome, candida, ME, arthritis, infections, 'detoxifying', and a variety of other complaints. Another active compound in aloe vera, alloin, is said to help constipation. Fresh aloe vera juice can be taken as a drink (often bitter) or in capsule form. Powdered aloe vera in tablet form is said to be less effective. Aloe vera supplements should not be taken during pregnancy.

Bee Pollen, see Propolis

Bifidus, see Pro-biotics

Black Cohosh
This herb is used to treat menopausal symptoms, like hot flushes, but evidence for its benefits is mostly anecdotal, and regular use may occasionally cause liver damage.

Blue-green Algae
Algae from freshwater lakes in mild climates (or, nowadays, 'farmed' in tanks) are dried and usually offered in tablet form as a food supplement. Spirulina and chlorella are two well-known forms of algae. These supplements contain a wide variety of nutrients, including iron, beta-carotene, selenium and vitamin B12 and also contain EFAs and protein, but the amount of most of these nutrients in a day's supply of tablets or powder (about 1 gram of dried algae) is small, making them an expensive supplement in terms of nutrient returns.

For example, in one brand, a typical day's supply contains just 350 μg (micrograms) iron, which is a very small proportion of a day's average need of 14 mg. Claims are made that algae can boost the immune system, help speed exercise recovery time, detoxify the body and enhance performance. Chlorella has been found to reduce stomach acidity and help repair the gut lining, but research finds that toxins produced by the algae may be linked to brain disease.

Bromelain
An enzyme extracted from pineapples, bromelain is a natural pain reliever, and reduces the swelling of rheumatoid arthritis. In one trial, 73% of patients who took a bromelain supplement reported good pain relief.

Cat's Claw
Derived from a Peruvian vine, cat's claw in capsules or as a tea is used as a healing herb, and is claimed to be anti-viral, anti-bacterial, immune-boosting,

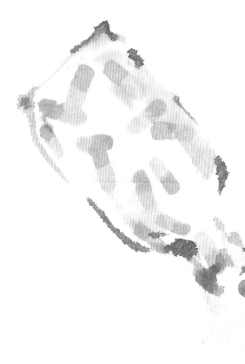

and D can be toxic in excess. A few years ago MAFF found that levels of toxic chemicals in some bottled fish liver oil preparations could be unacceptably high for toddlers. Cod liver oil supplements should not be taken in pregnancy.

Co-enzyme Q10

Co-Q10 is said to help the body convert food into energy, strengthen the heart, increase exercise tolerance, act as an antioxidant, and even help minimize hot flushes. Our bodies can make their own Q10 when young and it occurs naturally in foods, but as we get older or when we're ill, natural levels drop and a supplement may be useful, especially when exercising. Co-enzyme Q10 may even help keep the gums healthy.

Detox Remedies

Several 'detox' remedies are available — sometimes as a single liquid supplement, or as a package containing two or more different remedies, usually to be taken for from three days up to three weeks. These are said to help 'cleanse' the digestive system, purify the blood and help elimination of 'toxic wastes' by improving the action of the liver and sometimes the bladder. (For more on detoxification, see page 156.) They usually contain a range of plant and herbal preparations with these properties and may well come with instructions to follow a semi-fast or a particular diet. In unbiased tests, these products have had mixed results.

Devil's Claw

Another anti-inflammatory, this root from Namibia is said to help arthritic pain though I can't find any scientific trials to prove its efficacy.

Echinacea

The benefits of echinacea as an immune-system supporter are well documented, and a course two or three times in winter

may help shorten the duration of colds, flu and infections, and may help prevent cold sores. However, echinacea's main active compound, echinocosides can react with up to a quarter of prescription drugs (e.g. statins, prozac, asthma treatments) and make them leave the body too quickly.

Evening Primrose Oil

Evening primrose oil is one of the richest sources of the omega-6 (N6) fatty acid gamma linolenic acid, which the body needs for production of prostaglandins which control many vital processes, including fluid balance and the reproductive system. GLA has been shown to help prevent or minimize pre-menstrual syndrome, breast pain and fluid retention, and is also thought to be anti-inflammatory, thus may help sufferers of arthritis and eczema. Some MS sufferers also take GLA-rich supplements, but the benefit is unproven. The body can convert its own GLA from the essential fatty acid linoleic acid, but sometimes this conversion process may not be efficient and evening primrose oil is a convenient way to ensure GLA levels. Therapeutic dose may be up to 3,000 mg a day; maintenance dose 500-1,000 mg (1,000 mg of EPO will yield about 100 mg GLA). There are no known adverse side effects at the recommended doses.

Flax Seed Oil

This is the richest source of the omega-3 (N3) essential fatty acid, alpha linolenic acid, and can be converted in the body to the fatty acids EPA and DHA, which are those present in fish oils. Flax seed oil is useful for vegetarians wanting to increase omega-3 intake. Capsules are the best form in which to take flax seed oil — one 1,000-mg capsule will provide your day's requirement of alpha linolenic acid (about 500 mg) and will also provide some of the other EFA, linoleic acid.

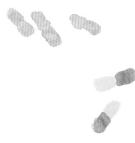

anti-inflammatory, antioxidant, and a cure-all for digestive disorders. Said to have been used by Peruvian tribes for centuries, it is relatively untested in Western trials.

Cod Liver Oil

Rich in vitamins A and D and the essential fatty acids, cod liver oil has been used as a natural source of these for many years. It is also said to relieve joint pain and arthritis, and help the immune system. Recommended doses should not be exceeded, as vitamins A

Garlic

The possible benefits of the garlic plant are well documented in other parts of this book (see particularly Heart Disease, page 119). However, there is some debate about the protective properties of the manufactured forms of garlic — tablets, capsules and so on. Some experts say that the active ingredients in garlic are very volatile and are even deactivated in fresh garlic by cooking. They say that garlic supplements may be far less potent, therefore, and may even be of little use at all.

These theories are being tested, but — until definite answers are found — if you wish to take garlic supplements, avoid those that have been 'deodorized', because it is fairly certain that the active allicin in these products will no longer be potent; avoid those that have been heat-treated, which also destroys the volatile compounds; and go for the purest, least 'treated' capsules that you can find.

Nobody really knows what the optimum daily dose of garlic is — but some experts say that the equivalent of 2 garlic cloves a day is a minimum — for many brands of manufactured garlic capsules this is 2 capsules. Check labels.

Ginkgo Biloba

The leaves of the ginkgo biloba tree are said to be important in helping to maintain brain functions, such as memory, alertness and concentration, by maintaining the supply of blood to the brain and therefore oxygenating it. A few trials have supported this theory. Ginkgo is also said to increase blood supply to the hands and feet. For these reasons it is often promoted as the ideal supplement for older people, and some research indicates that it may help minimize the effects of Alzheimer's disease.

The quality of ginkgo biloba supplements varies — some are just ground-up dried leaf and to be effective you would need at least 1,000 mg of this. Other supplements offer standardized extracts of the leaf, where the active ingredients — flavone glycosides and other compounds — are extracted. A good-quality ginkgo extract tablet will contain about 40 mg extract (of which 24% will be flavone glycosides) and 1-3 tablets a day are normally sufficient. Avoid if pregnant.

Ginseng

The most famous of food supplements from the East, the root of ginseng has been used as a general tonic for at least 7,000 years. There are two main types of 'ginseng' available as supplements — panax ginseng, sometimes called Korean ginseng, and Siberian ginseng. Both are members of the Aralia family of plants, but panax ginseng is a perennial plant while Siberian ginseng (*Eleutherococcus senticosus*) is a shrub. Both are described as 'adaptogens', meaning that they can help the body fight, or adapt to, whatever problems it has.

There are slight differences in the claimed actions of these two ginsengs, summarized as follows. *Panax* ginseng is the 'classic' ginseng containing ginsenoside compounds that are said to be similar to the body's own stress hormones. It is said to help us cope with any kind of physical or emotional stress as well as being a general tonic, and even a sedative. It may also stimulate the immune system and help liver function. Recent trials show that it has marked antibiotic properties.

Panax ginseng is particularly favoured in the East by athletes, by the elderly and by males. A standard dose is 5-600 mg a day in capsule form, but should be taken for periods of a few weeks at a time only. As a stimulant, *panax* ginseng should be taken in the morning and should be avoided during pregnancy or if you have high blood pressure. Panax ginseng seems also to help prevent breast cancer according to one large 2006 USA study.

Siberian ginseng is a stimulant and anti-stress tonic with particular physical benefits — some trials have shown improvement in athletic performance of up to 9%. It also stimulates the immune system and is useful for long-term fatigue. There is also some evidence that it is anti-toxic. A standard dose, which should be taken for a few weeks at a time only, is 1,000 mg in capsule form.

Glucosamine Sulphate

Glucosamine is a 'building block' component of the cartilage and has been shown in scientific trials to help ease the pain and disability of osteoarthritis. Even better, it may actually help regenerate damaged tissue.

Green-lipped Mussel

Green-lipped mussel supplements have been taken for some years by rheumatoid and ostearthritis sufferers and seem to have shown benefits. Research appears to have pinpointed the compound which may provide this effect — lyprinol, which seems to be anti-inflammatory, reducing pain and swelling in joints. Lyprinol is one of the mucopolysaccharides, compounds also found in aloe vera and glucosamine.

Green-lipped mussel can be taken in capsule form and results may show after 4-8 weeks.

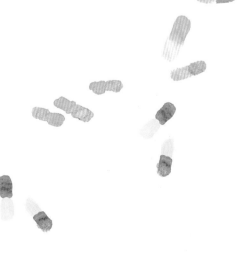

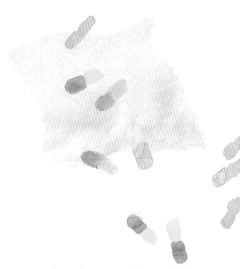

Hypericum, see St John's Wort

Kava Kava
The root of this Pacific island shrub is a well-known relaxant which can relieve anxiety, aid sleep and promote a sense of well-being. The main active ingredient, kawain, is a sedative. Other uses of kava kava are as an antiseptic and analgesic. Capsules are available and recommended dosage shouldn't be exceeded as, in excess, they are intoxicant.

Kelp
Kelp (*Fucus vesiculosus*) is a seaweed also known as bladderwrack, rich in iodine and possibly with immune-system-boosting and thyroid-stimulating properties. Some people believe that kelp will aid weight loss and so it is sometimes sold as a slimming aid, but there appears to be little scientific proof of its effectiveness. Kelp is sold in tablet form and a daily dose of about 150 µg is usually recommended. Excess kelp (and iodine) should be avoided, particularly if you have an over-active thyroid or pregnant.

Kombucha
From Russia and China, kombucha — a fungal brew — has been used for many years there as a tonic and is said to provide a variety of benefits. Apparently it is anti-cancer, anti-bacterial, immune-boosting, a detoxifier, can help arthritis, cataracts, asthma, dandruff, itchy skin, lack of libido ... unfortunately the evidence is, again, anecdotal and not scientific. Kombucha can be brewed yourself in the airing cupboard, or it can be now bought as ready-made tea. Various unwanted side-effects are being reported in long-term users, including jaundice, nausea and allergic reactions.

Lactobaccillus, see Pro-biotics

Linseed Oil, see Flax Seed Oil

Milk Thistle
Milk thistle (*Silybum marianum*) contains the compound silymarin and has been used in Europe for hundreds of years as a treatment for liver disorders. Research seems to back up this claim and modern herbalists use milk thistle to help in cases of jaundice, hepatitis, and to protect the liver in cases of alcohol abuse or other times when it may be under stress. Milk thistle is available in tincture, capsule form as extract of silybum.

Mucopolysaccharides, see Aloe Vera, Green-lipped Mussel

Omega-3 Fish Oils
The benefits of fish oils for a wide range of conditions are well described in other parts of this book. Fish oil capsules are a convenient way to take the 'active ingredients' in oily fish — the omega-3 fatty acids, eicosapentaenoic acid (EPA) and docosahexaenoic acid (DHA).

They are particularly useful for people who have been asked by their physicians to increase EPA and DHA intake but who don't like oily fish. Two to three capsules offering about 400 mg of EPA/DHA per capsule daily should be roughly equivalent to two portions of oily fish a week.

In recent years there have been studies which find high levels of dioxins and other toxic chemicals in fish oil capsules, but some brands are 'cleaner' than others. These contaminants may explain recent findings that fish oil capsule intake actually increased heart attacks in men who already had angina.

Passionflower
Passionflower (*Passiflora*) is an excellent remedy for insomnia and a mild sedative. In tablet form it is a relatively low-cost, non-addictive 'sleeping pill' and, as a supplement, is often combined with other sedative plants, such as hops, camomile and valerian.

Pre-biotics
When we take antibiotics to kill bacterial infections, they not only kill the 'bad' bacteria, but also the 'friendly' bacteria that balance the flora in the body and help to prevent conditions such as thrush, candida and cystitis. If the numbers of 'friendly' bacteria are reduced, they need to be encouraged to re-establish. Pre-biotics are food components called oligosaccharides, a source of soluble fibre which stimulates the growth of the healthy bifido-bacteria by providing a source of food for these bacteria. Particularly beneficial seem to be the fructo-oligosaccharides found in Jerusalem artichokes, onions and chicory, and also in tablet form. Around 5-10 g is a normal dose per day for 1 or 2 weeks after antibiotics have been taken.

Pro-biotics
The work of the pre-biotics can be enhanced by food supplements containing pro-biotics — the 'friendly' gut bacteria, including lactobacillus acidophilus and lactobacillus bifidus. These bacteria can be found in some live yoghurts but taking them in tablet form is a more guaranteed way to get enough of the bacteria to make a difference, as many so-called live yoghurts have been shown to have low levels. Pre- and pro-

biotics should be bought from a retailer who stores them in refrigerated conditions as the bacteria can easily be destroyed by light and heat. Probiotics have been shown to reduce respiratory infection and diarrhoea in children.

Propolis

Propolis — also known as bee propolis or bee pollen —— is made by bees to sterilize their hives and it is said that, taken in supplement form, it provides antibiotic, anti-viral and gut protection for humans. It may also be anti-inflammatory. There is anecdotal evidence that it may offer protection from hay fever, but sufferers should build up over a period of weeks from a micro dose to the equivalent of a teaspoon a day in the run up to the hay fever season.

Royal Jelly

One of the most famous supplements of all in recent years, royal jelly is the sole food fed to the Queen bee by worker bees (who don't eat it themselves). Because the Queen bee lives much longer than the workers, (3-5 years as opposed to 6-8 weeks) it is assumed by fans of royal jelly that this is the reason. However, there is little real evidence to substantiate the claims made for royal jelly in human consumption — increased stamina, fertility, and longevity. The only unusual nutrient to have been found in royal jelly is a fatty acid called trans l hydroxydelta 2 decenoic acid, which is found in no other food — proponents say that this is the 'magic ingredient' but nothing has yet been proved.

Silymarin, see Milk Thistle

Spirulina, see Blue-green Algae

Starflower Oil

Starflower (borage) oil is an even richer source of GLA than evening primrose oil, containing approximately twice as much — i.e., 20%, or 1,000 mg starflower oil will yield 200 mg GLA. Though supplements are more expensive than evening primrose oil, obviously fewer capsules need to be taken to achieve the same GLA intake, which may be of benefit to some people. See Evening Primrose Oil.

St John's Wort

Hypericum perforatum is commonly known as St John's Wort and is a native wild perennial plant of Europe, including the many parts of the UK. The yellow flowers, taken in dried, tincture or supplement form, are an established treatment on the Continent for cases of mild depression and stress, and the plant has gained in reputation and is now used by at least 2 million people .

Conducted trials have shown the efficacy of Hypericum perforatum in treating mild depression, but one recent large US trial found no effect on serious depression. The plant is also thought to be anti-viral, and may help cure menopausal and a variety of other symptoms, though results are mainly anecdotal. Doses to treat depression are usually 1,000 µg (micrograms) daily or 10 drops of tincture in water.

NOTE: St John's Wort interacts with some medical drugs and anyone taking anticoagulants, antidepressants or contraception should always consult their doctor before trying herbal remedies.

Valerian

Another popular supplement for insomnia and often combined with passionflower or hops as such.

Wheat Grass

Sprouted wheat grass is rich in dismutase, which is said to be highly anti-inflammatory. It is said to be antioxidant, immune-boosting, a tonic and detoxifier, containing many nutrients and chlorophyll, said to cleanse the system. In 2006, however, an Australian review of all the research found little evidence for most of these claims.

Herbs for health

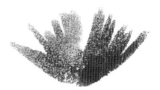

In the west we tend to think of herbs simply as tasty flavourings similar to salt and pepper. We buy them in small jars, ready-dried and -chopped, to be used once or twice, and then they lurk on the shelf for months until we throw them away. However, fresh herbs are not only a wonderful addition to your daily diet but also some of the most potent medicines around.

If you have a windowsill, a tub or two on the patio, or even an area you can turn into a herb garden, it is worth growing at least a few of your own herbs to cook with or to use in other ways to help your health. Others you can pick from the hedgerow, in the meadow — or even from unweeded areas of your garden... for free!

The main 'active' ingredients in herbs are their volatile oils and various phytochemicals, which offer a huge range of therapeutic benefits. Some are sedatives, others digestives, some antibiotics, others stimulant, for example.

Herbs can be used fresh in salads or as a garnish, in cooking, or made into a tea, or they can be dried or frozen and used in cooking, or they can be converted into tinctures which will last a long time. Of course, manufacturers also dry them or extract the oils and convert them into supplement form (see previous pages for more details).

Almost any plant (including its leaves, flowers, buds, seeds, roots and bark) with a medicinal or therapeutic use can be described as a herb, but for our purposes here a herb is an annual, biennial, perennial plant, or small shrub the leaves of which you use, and that you can grow in a small area and/or that would look fine as part of a herb garden — with the exception of the two 'weed' herbs we have included, nettle and dandelion, which may not be so welcome amongst the rosemary and thyme! Both of these are best picked from a 'wild' patch, inside your garden or out.

■ Picking and storing fresh herbs

It is best to pick herbs in the early morning, when they should be at their freshest and most potent. Once picked, they should be taken indoors very quickly, especially if the weather is hot, as they will soon wilt. Leaves can be picked at any time of year if they look green and healthy (some herbs, such as thyme and rosemary, are evergreen and can be picked all year round), especially for cooking purposes. To retain maximum medicinal properties, however, leaves are best gathered before the plant flowers.

If possible, pick enough for immediate use or, if you pick extra to use fresh at another time, pick whole stalks (not just the leaves), immerse these in water as you would a bunch of flowers, and keep them in a cool spot indoors until required, changing the water daily. Herbs which have been de-stalked will also keep well in a plastic bag in the salad compartment of the fridge. Don't chop fresh herbs until the last possible moment before use.

■ Drying fresh herbs

Pick the herbs as above. If you have a dry, warm and airy room, you can simply hang stalked herbs up in bunches to dry. You can, if you like, tie large paper bags around the bunches so that if leaves fall off they fall into the bags.

You can also dry small stalks of herbs on a baking tray in a very cool oven or in an airing cupboard. Turn them once or twice and remove them as soon as they seem completely dry — stalks should break easily if they are dry enough. Once dry, either hang the stalks up in bunches or de-leaf them, storing the dried leaves in airtight containers in a cool dark place.

■ Freezing fresh herbs

Some herbs you can simply destalk, pop into small freezer bags and freeze as they are. Parsley works well this way — when frozen, you can crumble it and save the bother of chopping it when it is defrosted. The softer-leaved herbs, like mint and coriander, can be frozen in ice-cube trays with a little water and used in cooking simply by putting a cube into your cooking pot. Basil doesn't freeze very well; it is better dried.

■ Infusions

For medicinal purposes you can make an infusion of fresh or dried herb leaves, just as you would a pot of ordinary tea. See the recipe on page 255. Infusions will not keep — drink them the same day. NOTE: herbal remedies should not be taken for more than a few weeks at a time.

■ Infused oils

Herbs can also be chopped and covered with a good-quality olive oil, left in an airtight jar in a warm place for two to three weeks, and then the oil strained off and used medicinally or even in cooking or on salads, depending upon which herb has been infused.

For example, infused oils of thyme, rosemary and tarragon make excellent cooking oils.

Some popular herbs for health

Angelica *Angelica archangelica:*
Hardy biennial, up to 2.5 m (8 ft).
Damp soil, needs plenty of space.
Culinary Uses: Stems can be crystallized; leaves chopped and added to salads.
Medicinal Uses: Root and seeds, as well as the stem and leaves, used as a powerful digestive, tonic, expectorant and circulatory stimulant.

Basil, Sweet *Ocimum basilicum:*
Half-hardy annual, up to 50 cm (20 inches).
Dry, sheltered, sunny, good in pots and tubs, window-boxes.
Culinary Uses: Leaves used in salads, good with tomatoes, major constituent of traditional Italian pesto and French pistou, good in most pasta dishes.
Medicinal Uses: Infusion of leaves can aid digestion, flatulence, nausea, stomach-ache, mildly sedative. Oil infusion can be used as insect repellent and sting relief.

Chives *Allium schoenoprasum:*
Hardy perennial, 30 cm (1 ft). Sunny, well-drained bed or tubs, window-sills and -boxes.
Culinary Uses: Chopped into salads, dips, soups, sauces, omelettes, a constituent of bouquet garni or fines herbes, use as onions. Add at end of cooking.
Medicinal Uses: From the same family as garlic and onions, with similar (though less potent) allium compounds. Rich in vitamin C and iron, acts as digestive and help lower blood cholesterol if eaten in quantity.

Dandelion *Taraxacum officinale:*
Hardy perennial, to 30 cm (1 ft). Will grow almost anywhere.
Culinary Uses: Leaves are excellent in salads; root ground as 'coffee'.
Medicinal Uses: Strong diuretic, potassium-rich, blood detoxifier, root is aid to liver action and has also been used to treat arthritis, eczema and constipation.

Lemon Balm *Melissa officinalis:*
Hardy perennial, to 60 cm (2 ft).
Culinary Uses: Excellent tea, leaves can be used in salads.
Medicinal Uses: Calming; anti-viral (infusion good for treating cold sores); may also help over-active thyroid.

Lovage *Levisticum officinale:*
Hardy perennial, to 2 m (6 ft).
Needs plenty of space, sunny, well-drained.
Culinary Uses: Tasty addition to salads, good in soups and casseroles.
Medicinal Uses: Warming tonic which stimulates circulation; digestive; diuretic; and can help cystitis, period pains.

Mint *Mentha spicata, spearmint:*
Hardy perennial, to 90 cm (3 ft). Tub or bed (invasive).
Culinary Uses: Spearmint is the traditional English mint, peppermint (*M. piperita*) and apple mint (*M. rotundifolia*) are similar in use — in sauces, relishes, as vegetable and fruit garnish, as tea and in cold drinks.
Medicinal Uses: Mint contains menthol, used widely for an indigestion remedy, and for clearing congestion in colds and chest infections. It also helps purify the breath, an infusion applied to the skin can help relieve pain, and oil infusion can be used as a massage balm.

Nettle *Urtica dioica:*
Hardy perennial, to 90 cm (3 ft).
Culinary Uses: Young leaves — said to be rich in iron, potassium, vitamin C and carotenoids — can be used as a green vegetable similar to spinach, lightly cooked or made into a soup. Nettle tea is also good.
Medicinal Uses: Diuretic, cleansing and detoxifying herb; proven to help relieve the pain of arthritis, bites and stings, nettle and nappy rash; helps excretion of uric acid in gout; calms hay fever and rhinitis. Nettle root is being used to treat enlarged prostate.

Parsley *Petroselinum crispum:*
Hardy biennial, to 30 cm (1 ft). Most situations, except shade, including window-sills and -boxes.
Culinary Uses: Parsley is rich in iron, carotenoids and vitamin C, and uses are many, including sauces, soups, salads, in herb blends, and with pasta.
Medicinal Uses: Diuretic and stimulating to the liver; breath freshener; can help arthritis and gout.

Rosemary *Rosmarinus officinalis:*
Semi-hardy shrub, to 1.25 m (4 ft). Sheltered, dry, sunny, border or tubs.
Culinary Uses: Pungent herb ideal for cooking with meats, chicken, fish; also good in herb bread.
Medicinal Uses: Tonic and circulation stimulant; said to enhance memory and help mild depression, headaches and migraine.

Sage *Salvia officinalis:*
Shrub, to 60 cm (2 ft) Dry, sunny, borders, tubs.
Culinary Uses: Ideal with duck, goose, pork. Savoury stuffing ingredient and blends well with other herbs, in omelettes, onion and mixed vegetable dishes.
Medicinal Uses: Antiseptic, digestive and stimulant, but is also a calming herb. Said to be tonic for the liver, memory and nerves. Infusion makes a good mouthwash and gargle for sore throats and gum problems. In menopause, has been shown to reduce hot flushes from an average of 10 to 2 a day.

Thyme *Thymus vulgaris:*
Sub-shrub, to 30 cm (1 ft). Dry sunny banks, tubs, window-boxes.
Culinary Uses: Herb widely used in meat cookery, in stuffings, herb blends, omelettes and egg cookery.
Medicinal Uses: A powerful antiseptic, infusion helps bronchitis and respiratory infections, asthma, thrush; anti-flatulence; oil infusion helps bites and stings and fungal skin complaints. Thyme is an antioxidant and tonic.

Demystifying detoxification

Everybody's doing it — detoxing. A 'detox' diet seems to be the millennium's answer to taking the waters or food combining. For anyone who feels run down, tired, or in any other way under par, detoxing appears to be the answer. So what exactly IS a 'detox' diet — and does it really work?

Toxicants can enter your body in or on what you eat (e.g., pesticides, herbicides, hormones, preservatives, etc.) and even a 'healthy' diet may include more of these 'hidden extras' than you would think. Even 'healthy' foods, in the wrong quantities, may become toxins. For example, you can overdose on carrots or cod liver oil. You may also be mildly intolerant to a food without realizing.

Viral and bacterial organisms can enter in or on food, too, or via the skin and lungs, and these are 'toxic' in that the body fights them off. Frequent or recurring minor — and less minor — ailments may be indicative of the immune system's inability to cope. Swollen lymph glands (in the neck or up the arms, for instance) when you aren't exactly ill but feel 'under par' are indicative of too much 'detox' work to do.

Tobacco smoke contains toxins which we breathe in (even if we don't smoke). Alcohol is toxic in large quantities or in moderately large quantities on too regular a basis. Medicines and drugs can be toxic — even over-the-counter painkillers can have a strong effect on the stomach, liver, and so on.

Stress — both physical and emotional — can compound the problems. So, if you feel 'under the weather' and have been subject to more than one or two of these factors, you may possibly feel a lot better for 'detoxing'.

■ How can a detox diet work?

It is the job of the lymphatic system — a network of glands and tubes — to drain excess fluids from all body tissues. At the lymph nodes (glands), foreign material and any unwelcome micro-organisms, such as infections, are filtered out before the lymph fluid joins the blood. A healthy lymph system is therefore important in detoxing the body. Outward signs of a sluggish lymph are swollen or puffy eyes, swollen ankles, dull skin and eyes.

Perhaps the most important of the 'detoxing' jobs are carried out by the liver, probably the most hard-working and versatile organ in the body. One of its jobs is to convert the body's own waste materials — such as ammonia (a poison produced when the body proteins are broken down) and outside toxins such as drugs, alcohol, inhaled toxins and food-borne toxins — into harmless, or less harmful, components, for excretion.

To help this process, a healthy gall bladder and urinary system are also important, and an eating and exercise programme that helps speed up removal of wastes from the body in the urine could also then be regarded as a legitimate part of a 'detox' routine. Unwanted material is also disposed of through the bowels and, therefore, regular bowel movement is important. Waste material is, lastly, excreted in sweat and breath, two processes that can also be enhanced through diet and exercise.

A useful 'detox' diet will, therefore, aim to help by providing dietary items that will encourage the processing and elimination of toxins — and by, as far as possible, avoiding all dietary items likely to be toxic. Lastly, a diet high in antioxidant phytochemicals will help to de-oxidize the body and neutralize harmful free radicals that will be produced during a detox regime. Regular exercise will also help by increasing lymph activity, (lymph flow increases up to 15 times during exercise), by creating urine, by encouraging the bowels to work and by increasing blood circulation, liver activity, sweating and exhalation.

FOODS AND HERBS FOR DETOXING:

To help liver and/or gallbladder function: dandelion root, marigold (flowers and leaves), parsley, burdock (leaves or root), milk thistle (can be taken as a supplement), peppermint, dock root, globe artichoke, apples, olive oil, cucumber, onion.

To help stimulate lymphatic system and circulation: angelica, lovage, marigold, oregano, rosemary, dock root, echinacea, ginger, cayenne.

To help fluid elimination: dandelion, lovage, nettles, parsley, tarragon, apples, cucumber, onion, dock root.

To help purify blood: garlic, onion, leek, dandelion, nettles, echinacea, essential fatty acids.

Laxative effect: olive oil, burdock, dock root, aloe vera juice.

To increase body heat/perspiration: marigold, thyme, garlic, onion, chives, mustard, green tea.

NOTE: Herbal regimes shouldn't be followed for more than 6 weeks without a break of 6 weeks, unless advised by a qualified practitioner.

SAMPLE OF HOW A DAY'S EATING ON A GOOD SHORT-TERM DETOX DIET MAY LOOK:

Glass of pure water 6 times a day

On rising
Water and fresh apple juice; two milk thistle tablets

Breakfast
Fresh fruit salad with live yoghurt and sesame seeds
Dandelion and burdock decoction

Mid-morning
Aloe vera juice

Lunch
Large fresh mixed salad, including marigold petals, cucumber, onion, nettle leaves, with olive oil and lemon juice dressing
Fresh walnuts and almonds
Dandelion and burdock decoction

Mid-afternoon
Green tea

Evening
Globe artichoke dressed with olive oil and lime juice
Selection of crudités with live yoghurt, cayenne and chive dip
Apple and sunflower seeds
Dandelion and burdock decoction

Bedtime
Camomile tea
Small slice of organic whole-grain bread (optional)

NOTE: for detoxes of more than a few days, add starchy vegetables and/or whole grains to at least two meals a day

EXERCISE: Take two 20-minute walks and/or swims a day, concentrating on your breathing

▪ So what kind of diet to follow?

Some detox diets are little more than fasts with water. These may help in avoiding toxin intake, but may also be dangerous if followed for more than a day or two.

A good programme needs to be one you can stay on for more than a day or two — so for most of us, who want to carry on leading a normal active life, it needs to contain a wider range of foods and more calories. Such a diet is more helpful if it contains plenty of the foods, herbs, etc., thought to help the body detoxify itself.

A list appears opposite — choose one or two from each category to eat or drink regularly while on your 'detox' diet.

Several are herbs or roots — see page 255 for how to make infusions and decoctions.

Foods to eat happily are all organically grown fresh fruits, fruit juices, salads and unstarchy vegetables, raw, steamed or, occasionally, very lightly cooked; fresh herbs, olive oils and other uncooked pure vegetable and seed oils, organic live yoghurt, and raw nuts and seeds.

Such a diet can be followed for a few days if you are doing light work and light exercise, and will provide plenty of antioxidants. For longer-term detox, add whole grains and starchy vegetables — e.g. brown rice, quinoa, and a little organic whole-grain bread, potatoes, etc.

Foods to cut right down on — or out completely — include: animal foods, all dairy produce except yoghurt as above, caffeine, alcohol, all processed foods. Also avoid drugs, other than necessary prescription medicines, and smoking.

Drink plenty of pure spring water — 1.75-2.25 litres (3-4 pints) a day — and freshly squeezed fruit and veg juices. You can also drink home-made or organically produced herbal and green tea.

Go to bed early and sleep with a window open or use an ionizer to purify the air, and you should spend at least part of each day outdoors in the clearest air you can find, and learn to breathe deeply.

▪ How long before I feel better?

If you are intolerant to one or more foods and you carry out a detox which eliminates it, you may experience a withdrawal 'headache', or flu-like feeling. Caffeine addicts may experience moderate to severe headache for up to 4 or 5 days on withdrawal. If there are considerable levels of toxins (e.g. pesticides) stored in body fat, a water-only fast may release large amounts at once, causing other symptoms.

This is one good reason not to go headlong into a strict fast without a few days preparation by gradually easing yourself into the regime — say giving up alcohol or smoking. A low-cal, low-carb regime in itself can cause headache. After perhaps feeling worse and tired for a few days, maybe with a bad taste in the mouth, however, most people report an enhanced sense of well-being, feeling much more vital and alert after a week.

▪ When should it end?

Rather than just abruptly stopping a detox it is best to reintroduce a few other foods every day until eating a wide range of healthy foods again. If the detox has benefited you, it is wise to keep to its main principles, using fresh natural organic foods and drink, and avoiding sources of toxins as far as possible.

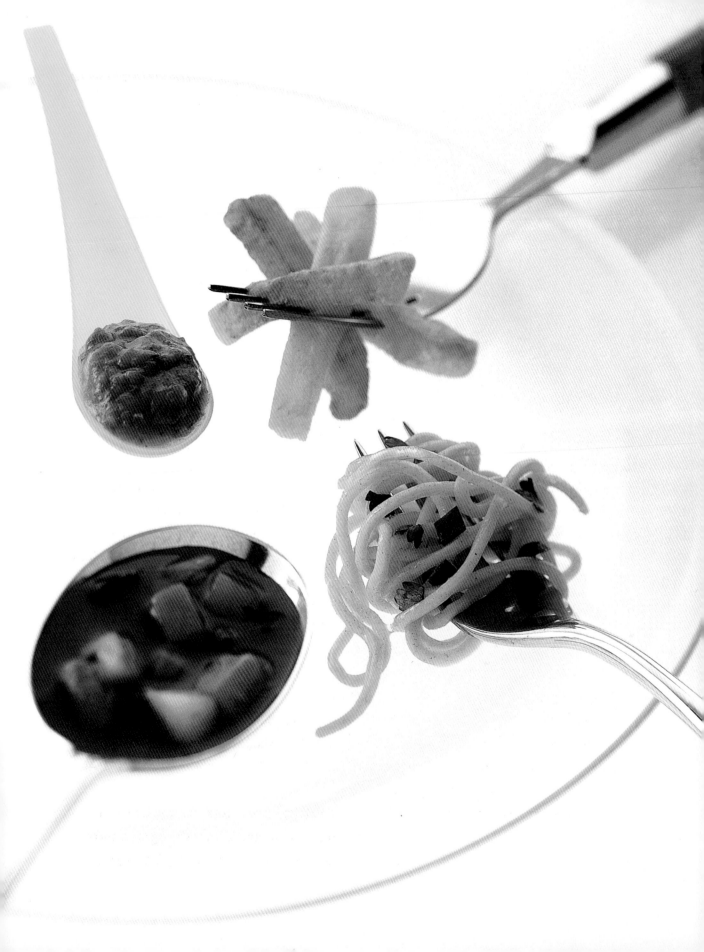

Food for the time of your life

Everyone knows that a baby needs different food from an adult — and that there are special dietary requirements for pregnant women. However, eating right for the time of your life is important at ANY age. Hardly any two decades, from birth to old age, will present the same set of nutritional problems.

What you need now may well not be what is right for your health in several years' time. So here we look at all those different needs. For instance, we examine the many problems that parents face in getting their children to eat well. Then there are the typical teenage food problems — like faddy eating and silly diets.

In their twenties and thirties, many people don't consider nutrition at all, but take their health for granted. Yet, with a little thought, one's 'prime' can be even better — and adults can be better prepared for the years ahead. These may include pregnancy, and getting food right before, during and after the birth is the kindest thing a woman can do for her body — and her baby.

We move on to the middle years and, for women, the menopause. Many of the less wanted symptoms of these years can be reduced or prevented with a suitable diet. For men — well, there is menopause, too. A large number of doctors now believe that it DOES exist and so we look at what men should be doing to help smooth their passage through mid-life.

We also examine the importance of diet in the middle years to help prevent the problems that beset older people. For every 65-plus person who has ever thought, 'It's too late now — it won't make any difference what I eat or drink,' we prove them wrong! It is never too late to begin getting it right.

CHILDHOOD AND TEENAGE YEARS

How much does your child's diet affect his or her health, growth and future well-being? And what IS a healthy diet for most children? The importance of a suitable diet in childhood is recognized by every health professional, and yet a recent Government report says only two out of five children eat properly. In this country, only 30% of mothers breast-feed their babies until three months of age. By the age of $4\frac{1}{2}$, less than 40% of children eat any green vegetables except peas, and only a quarter eat any salad. Yet biscuits, fizzy drinks, crisps and confectionery are eaten by more than 70% of pre-school children. Five- to fourteen-year-olds buy, on average, 57g of confectionery and eat four portions of chips each every week. An alarming proportion of children and teenagers are deficient in major minerals, while eating almost twice as much salt as is recommended.

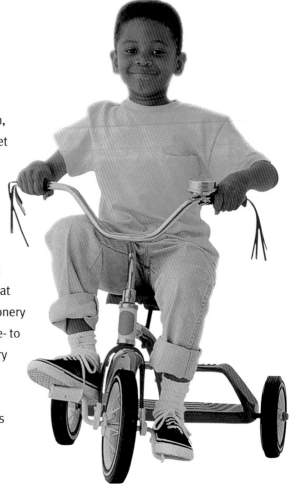

Birth to six months

Up to six months (according to a WHO report), most babies need nothing other than breast milk, apart from vitamin K, which is routinely given at birth by injection.

Few will need vitamin supplements or any other food (there are always exceptions, particularly if nutrition during pregnancy was inadequate). Breast feeding is beneficial to the baby's health in many ways:

* Breast milk contains the antibacterial compounds lactoferrin, IgA and lyso-zome, which reduce risk of gastro-enteritis, and ear and respiratory infections.
* It provides protection against asthma, eczema and jaundice.
* Breast feeding builds up immunity in the baby. It may offer protection against diabetes, coeliac disease and food allergies.
* Breastfeeding helps reduce the risk of obesity in childhood, as well as of strokes, CHD and high blood pressure later in life.
* Breast milk is high in the long-chain omega-3 polyunsaturated acids e.g. DHA (contained in fish oils) and also high in oligosaccharides, both of which may have an effect on 'cognitive' (brain) development. Breast-fed children appear to have a higher IQ than bottle-fed children.
* Breast milk is natural, free, convenient and easily digested, with a perfect balance of nutrients in a highly available form. For instance, the iron in breast milk is 70% absorbed, while that in formula milk is only 10% absorbed.

Bottle feeding, however, is necessary for some and adequate without further nutrition again, normally until the baby is around 6 months old, although one report has suggested that babies fed exclusively on formula milk may be at risk of selenium deficiency. An approved infant formula should be used (NOT ordinary cows'-, sheep's- or goats'-milk). About 2% of babies develop an allergy to the protein in cows' milk, which can cause vomiting, diarrhoea, skin and respiratory problems. Some also are intolerant of the lactose in cows' milk, which will also result in intestinal upsets (see Allergies, page 88).

Alternatives in these cases are infant formulas based on goats' milk (to which some are also intolerant or allergic) or soya milk, to which up to 10% of cows'-milk-intolerant infants are also intolerant. Soya milk is also high in natural oestrogens which may affect sex hormones and should only be given to babies on medical advice. Cows'-milk intolerance may be only temporary in infants, and medical advice should be taken.

Weaning

Weaning by 6 months is recommended by the DoH. Earlier weaning has been linked with the development of coeliac disease, food sensitivity, infection and possibly with obesity in infants, and there is no advantage for most babies in introducing solids at an earlier age. However, by the time a baby has doubled his or her birth-weight, breast milk supplies of iron, zinc, copper and vitamin D and A, protein and energy supplied may not be adequate for the growing infant, and by six months all babies will need some solid foods.

Research indicates a link between poor growth rate in infancy and disease in adult life. Low-weight infants at one year old have an increased risk of CHD in later life, for example. Breast feeding may continue to advantage until 1 year old or even longer, but if breast feeding is discontinued at weaning, the baby

COMMERCIAL BABY FOODS

It is possible for a weaned infant to get all his nutritional requirements from a diet based on commercial, ready-made (or dried) baby foods and formula milk. Artificial flavourings and other additives are normally not allowed, and sugar content should be stated on the label. Organic baby foods are available.

However, the EC recognizes the importance of home-prepared food for the infant and suggests that it is ideal if home cooking is introduced to the diet early. There is evidence that infants fed only, or mostly, on commercial baby foods may be reluctant to change to home cooking as they grow older. It is also likely that the range of phytochemicals present in fresh foods, which we now know are so important to health, are just as important whatever one's age.

should receive infant formula to 6 months, then a 'follow on' milk formula can be used. Cows' milk should not be given as a main drink until one year old, although it can be introduced in small quantities as part of the baby's food.

First weaning foods are usually bland, puréed gluten-free cereals, such as rice, potatoes and some vegetables. These can be home-cooked or commercial, and a wider variety of items can be introduced from day to day -– yoghurt, custard, fruit, pulses and other vegetables, cereals and meat can be offered, all still puréed. Water or milk should be the main drink; fruit juices (although most contain good amounts of vitamin C) also contain extrinsic sugars and should be limited, diluted and offered only with a meal (when the vitamin C will help iron absorption in the food), unless no fresh fruit is eaten. Fruit squashes, cordials and fizzy drinks, tea or coffee should not be offered, and neither should 'diet' drinks containing artificial sweeteners. Sweet drinks should not be given in a bottle -– infants can drink out of a cup after 6 months to avoid tooth decay. Bottles containing sweet drinks should never be given at bed- or nap-time.

Second-stage weaning foods (from the age of 6 to 9 months) can include finger foods and foods with

more texture, to encourage chewing, and wheat-containing foods and bread can also be introduced.

Third-stage (9 to 12 months plus) infants can begin to eat a diet similar to that of the rest of the family, with three meals a day plus snacks, and infants should be encouraged to feed themselves as much as possible. However, an infant diet shouldn't mimic the diet of a healthy adult exactly -– a high-fibre, low-fat diet should be postponed. Salt should not be added to weaning foods at all.

Pre-school children

From weaning to the age of five, children need more of some nutrients than adults and less of others. They need:

✱ More fat. Breast milk is over 50% fat; follow-on milks about 42% fat. Children should only gradually reduce the amount of fat in their diets, down to the recommended adult level of 30-35%. From 1 to 2 years old, whole milk should be given, and from 2 to 5, semi-skimmed can be given, but skimmed milk not used until after 5.

Whole-milk yoghurts and cheeses are also preferable. The higher fat levels are important because of the high energy needs of young children (fat is the most calorie-dense food), and fats provide the fat-soluble vitamins A, D, E and K. Children up to two can also cope only with moderate amounts of starchy foods.

✱ Less fibre. Young digestive systems are not equipped to deal with large amounts of high-fibre foods. High-fibre diets may hinder absorption of vital minerals, such as iron and calcium, and because high-fibre foods tend to need more chewing and appear to satisfy appetite more quickly than low-fibre foods, may also mean that a child may have trouble consuming enough food at each meal to take in adequate calories.

✱ Small children should not be given nuts until age 5. They can choke on them — and nut allergy, particularly to peanuts, is a growing problem in children.

Most of all, small children need to enjoy their food and be encouraged to eat as wide a variety of new foods as possible. Young children are sometimes more willing to do this than school-age children. Almost any child dislikes some foods, but using Section One you can easily find replacement foods for all the nutrients. Often, a few weeks or months later, the refused food will become acceptable. It is important not to make an issue of food refused or the odd meal where a child doesn't seem hungry. Negative associations with food can begin through a child being made to feel 'naughty' or guilty through refusal.

How do you tell if a young child is getting all the nutrients he or she needs? If the child is growing well, has a good appetite, seems strong and active, and is neither fat nor thin, then all is well. A child who doesn't appear to be thriving, eats only a few foods, has an under- or overweight problem, is ill a lot, or suffers problems which may be linked to food intolerance, should see a physician and perhaps be referred to a dietician. Poor growth-rate in young children has been linked with heart disease, stroke and diabetes in later life. A survey of British pre-school children revealed that 8% have lower-than-recommended levels of vitamin A intake, 20% have low iron intake (with one in 12 of all under-five-year-olds anaemic) and 14% of under-four-year-olds are deficient in zinc.

Ages 5 to 11

When a child reaches school age, good groundwork in previous years pays off. By this time, he or she should be enjoying a wide variety of meals, including plenty of fruits and vegetables. Normal healthy children of this age usually have very healthy appetites and, if plenty of activity is undertaken, may eat as much as an adult in order to gain enough weight and growth. The chart below lists nutrient requirements of children aged 1 to 11.

■ Packed lunches vs school meals

Since compulsory nutritional standards were abolished in the UK in 1980, the nutritional content and value of school meals has varied tremendously. In 2001, new school lunch guidelines came into force — limiting chips, for example, and ensuring that fruit and veg are on the menu. However, a large element of choice is still left to the child. To be sure of what your child is getting at lunchtime, a packed lunch is a sensible answer.

A packed lunch should be similar in style to those recommended for adults on page 46, containing at least one high-carbohydrate item (e.g. sandwich, pasta), some protein (e.g. cheese, tuna), some fruit, something sweet but nutritious (e.g. malt loaf, a slice of fruit cake), and a drink of milk or pure juice. To that you can add what your child will need to satisfy his or her appetite (e.g. dried fruit, a hard-boiled egg). In winter, a small flask of soup is good. It is also important to vary contents as much as possible from day to day — otherwise the child gets bored and may not get a complete range of nutrients.

Remember that young children don't need a very low-fat diet, so don't feel guilty about contributing to the calorie content with fat — for instance, spreading bread with real butter, adding mayonnaise to a sandwich, giving whole milk, even a chocolate biscuit bar if the school allow it. What you need to do is pack a lunch containing plenty of fresh items and not too many highly refined, coloured, additive-heavy items. Just make sure things are colourful and tasty.

SELECTED NUTRITIONAL NEEDS OF CHILDREN (girls/boys)

Age	Calories	Protein g	Folate μg	C mg	A μg	D μg	Calcium mg	Iron mg	Zinc mg
1-3	1,165/1,230	14.5	70	30	400	7	350	6.9	5.0
4-6	1,545/1,715	19.7	100	30	500	*	450	6.1	6.5
7-10	1,740/1,970	28.3	150	30	500	*	550	8.7	7.0
11	1,845/2,220	42	200	35	600	*	800/1000	14.8/11.3	9

Weight control

Parents are often worried about their children getting overweight, and overweight and obesity rates for children in the UK are still rising – now a quarter of all children under the age of 11 are either overweight or obese. Mainly because of this increase in weight – and in the size of children's waists – illnesses such as type-2 diabetes and heart disease are increasing in the young, year on year. However, around 5% of children still suffer from malnutrition – either underweight or lacking in vital nutrients.

If your child looks fat (compare with the other children in the class to get a sensible comparison), however, the best course of action is to reduce portion sizes slightly, cut back a little on the very-high-fat and sugar items, like puddings, cakes, biscuits, chocolate and sweets, and offer slightly more lower-calorie items like yoghurts, fresh fruit, and so on. Don't mention the word 'diet' to your child; there's no need. Over the months, most children will grow taller, while staying the same weight or losing a little — and so look much slimmer.

Without appearing over-anxious about childhood overweight, it is more sensible to do something about it early on, in as relaxed a way as possible, rather than leaving it and hoping the child will 'grow out of it'.

Children's high energy needs in comparison with their age should not become an excuse to feed them exclusively on a high-saturated-fat, high-sugar, low-fresh-food diet.

More importantly, exercise and good nutrition will help to prevent heart disease and other health problems in adulthood. Although low birth-weight and low infancy-weight can increase risk of CHD, research shows that a child who is overweight at 6 to 9 has a ten times greater chance of being obese in adulthood and a child overweight at 10 to 14 has a 28 times greater chance.

The height/weight charts for children given here are only a guide — there is much individual variation. Weight for height is a better guide than weight for age. Use common sense in interpreting this chart: if your child is in the centre of the lower and upper figures there is no problem; if right at the maximum average, there may be a weight problem in the making. If he or she is right at the minimum weight, care should be taken that weight does not fall further.

AVERAGE WEIGHTS AND HEIGHTS OF CHILDREN

Age	Weight			Height		
	Bottom	Average	Top of range	Bottom	Average	Top of range
Girls						
5	13.05 kg	18.00 kg	27.00 kg	0.94 m	1.06 m	1.18 m
	(2 st 1 lb)	(2 st 12 lb)	(4 st 4 lb)	(3 ft 1¾ in)	(3 ft 6½ in)	(3 ft 11¼ in)
6	14.40 kg	19.80 kg	31.05 kg	1.01 m	1.13 m	1.26 m
	(2 st 4 lb)	(3 st 2 lb)	(4 st 13 lb)	(3 ft 4¼ in)	(3 ft 9¼ in)	(4 ft 2¼ in)
7	15.75 kg	22.95 kg	36.90 kg	1.05 m	1.19 m	1.33 m
	(2 st 7 lb)	(3 st 9 lb)	(5 st 12 lb)	(3 ft 6 in)	(3 ft 11½ in)	(4 ft 5 in)
8	17.55 kg	25.20 kg	43.65 kg	1.10 m	1.25 m	1.39 m
	(2 st 11 lb)	(4 st)	(6 st 13 lb)	(3 ft 8 in)	(4 ft 2 in)	(4 ft 7½ in)
9	18.90 kg	28.35 kg	50.40 kg	1.15 m	1.30 m	1.46 m
	(3 st)	(4 st 7 lb)	(8 st)	(3 ft 10 in)	(4 ft 4 in)	(4 ft 10¼ in)
10	20.70 kg	31.95 kg	57.60 kg	1.19 m	1.36 m	1.53 m
	(3 st 4 lb)	(5 st 1 lb)	(9 st 2 lb)	(3 ft 11½ in)	(4 ft 6¼ in)	(5 ft 1 in)
11	22.95 kg	35.55 kg	64.35 kg	1.23 m	1.42 m	1.60 m
	(3 st 9 lb)	(5 st 9 lb)	(10 st 3 lb)	(4 ft 1 in)	(4 ft 8¾ in)	(5 ft 3¾ in)
Boys						
5	13.95 kg	18.45 kg	26.10 kg	0.95 m	1.08 m	1.19 m
	(2 st 3 lb)	(2 st 13 lb)	(4 st 4 lb)	(3 ft 2 in)	(3 ft 7 in)	(3 ft 11¾ in)
6	14.85 kg	20.70 kg	30.60 kg	1.00 m	1.08 m	1.27 m
	(2 st 5 lb)	(3 st 4 lb)	(4 st 13 lb)	(3 ft 4 in)	(3 ft 7 in)	(4 ft 2¾ in)
7	17.10 kg	22.95 kg	35.55 kg	1.06 m	1.20 m	1.33 m
	(2 st 10 lb)	(3 st 9 lb)	(5 st 12 lb)	(3 ft 6½ in)	(4 ft)	(4 ft 5 in)
8	18.45 kg	25.20 kg	41.40 kg	1.11 m	1.26 m	1.40 m
	(2 st 13 lb)	(4 st)	(6 st 13 lb)	(3 ft 8½ in)	(4 ft 2¼ in)	(4 ft 8 in)
9	19.80 kg	27.90 kg	48.60 kg	1.16 m	1.31 m	1.46 m
	(3 st 2 lb)	(4 st 6 lb)	(8 st)	(3 ft 10¼ in)	(4 ft 4¼ in)	(4 ft 10½ in)
10	22.05 kg	30.60 kg	56.70 kg	1.20 m	1.36 m	1.53 m
	(3 st 7 lb)	(4 st 12 lb)	(9 st)	(4 ft)	(4 ft 6¼ in)	(5 ft 1 in)
11	23.85 kg	34.65 kg	63.45 kg	1.23 m	1.41 m	1.58 m
	(3 st 11 lb)	(5 st 7 lb)	(10 st 3 lb)	(4 ft 1¼ in)	(4 ft 8¼ in)	(5 ft 3¼ in)

Data from Child Growth Foundation, 1995

Childhood eating problems

The nutritional needs of children, as outlined on the previous page, are fairly straightforward. For many parents, however, putting those needs into practice — in the form of an everyday diet that their children will actually eat — is far from straightforward.

From toddler to twelve-year-old, how do you persuade your child to eat what you want him or her to eat, rather than the 'junk' he or she seems to want? And what can you do with a child who will eat only one or two types of food for weeks at a time, or the child who will hardly eat at all?

Persuading children to eat a healthy diet is rarely easy, but recent research has confirmed that a love of healthy foods – such as vegetables, fruit, wholegrains and fish – can be instilled in children by parental example. If you enjoy healthy food, they will too. It has also been shown that it takes up to 10 tries to persuade a young child to eat a new food item. Thus, children all need showing by example and encouraging to eat a healthy diet from weaning on.

◾ The junk food dilemma

You want your child to eat fresh fish, green vegetables, citrus fruits and wholewheat pasta, but he or she hates all that and only wants commercial burgers, pizza, chips, baked beans, ice-cream, chocolate and sweets. In truth, your ideas on good food are so far apart that you can't see how you're ever going to reach a compromise... but you will. You simply need to understand why children like 'junk' food and then apply the same criteria to the kinds of food they should eat for good health — if that proves to be necessary. For the fact is that much of what we dismiss as 'junk' is a perfectly acceptable part of your child's diet (see the panel opposite).

First, let's look at the reasons why most children like 'junk' food and how you can deal with that:

∗ They are familiar with it. Children like to experiment with new foods to a certain degree, while wanting to find something familiar on their plate at each meal. Children who have been raised on burgers and chips can't be expected to forsake them overnight and turn to lentils and brown rice.

Solution: 'Starting as you mean to go on' is a sensible idea when it comes to feeding your family. Children who are weaned on to a healthy varied diet, with plenty of fresh fruit, vegetables and salads, will tend to carry on being happy to eat this way even if in later years they crave the odd 'junk' item.

If, in your child's case, it is too late for that, you need to introduce the healthier foods into the diet very slowly and in small amounts, disguised, as necessary (see the next point).

∗ It is easy to eat with minimal chewing. Many children hate anything at all difficult to chew or swallow — lumps of meat, fibrous vegetables or fruits, even bread crusts. This is understandable because, of course, children are one stage on from babies whose diet is mainly liquid.

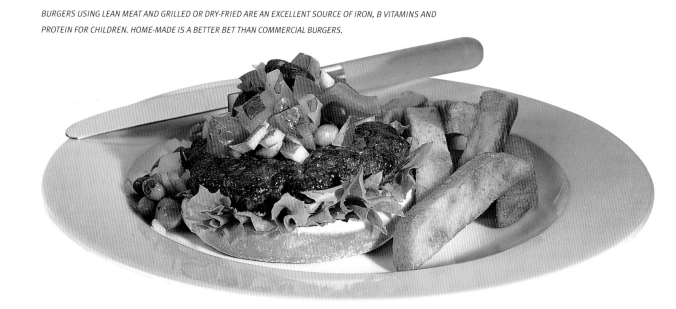

BURGERS USING LEAN MEAT AND GRILLED OR DRY-FRIED ARE AN EXCELLENT SOURCE OF IRON, B VITAMINS AND PROTEIN FOR CHILDREN. HOME-MADE IS A BETTER BET THAN COMMERCIAL BURGERS.

Solution: all 'healthy' foods can be served in child-palatable form without much trouble. If you want your child to eat meat, offer it in minced form as home-made burgers, cottage pies, lasagnes, soups, pasta sauce and so on. Most vegetables and fruits can be puréed or mashed, or the tougher bits of stalk, etc., removed — children don't need to eat them to get their fibre. You can get most children to eat fresh fruit by converting it into fruit juices and squashes, fruity milk shakes, ice-lollies, ice-creams and fruit fools. You can also cut crusts off bread and feed the birds or grind them into crumbs and freeze them for savoury toppings, gratins, etc.

∗ Children like attractive colourful food — junk food isn't always, but it often is, with golden chips, crimson tomato ketchup, golden crumbed fish fingers, and brightly coloured drinks and desserts.

Solution: try to present all food attractively and use plenty of the more colourful fruits and vegetables, cut into small pieces. Don't serve over-boiled soggy vegetables — besides looking and tasting totally unattractive, they have hardly any of their inherent nutrients left.

∗ Children like tasty food... things that really hit the palate, and quickly learn to mistake the high salt content of most savoury junk foods, and high sugar content of most sweet junk foods, for 'taste'.

Solution: make your own healthy offering as tasty as you can by using natural flavours and healthier items. Make full use of the sweeter fruits, dried fruits, raw cane sugar, Greek-style or bio yoghurt and honey for home-made desserts. Cut down on salty and sweet items slowly, a little at a time. An average child's palate can be re-educated to accept less salt and sugar in a few weeks.

■ Junk food — the truth

The fact is that a lot of the foods that you may consider to be complete junk actually contain a lot of valuable nutrients for growing children. Children need plenty of energy (calories), protein and calcium, as discussed. In fact, when 'health food' eating became widely popular in the l980s, the children of many 'health food' converts became nutritionally and calorifically deficient because the parents' so-called healthy diet was depriving them of all three.

There have also been many documented cases of children who have existed for months on only two or three different types of food — e.g., jam sandwiches and milk, or bananas and orange juice — and on later examination have proved to be in perfectly good health and making normal good growth.

So, instead of fighting with a child over yet another request for burger and chips for tea, perhaps the answer is to find ways of making that burger and chips more acceptable to you both, by, say, making the burger out of extra-lean meat, and using large chips that are brushed with oil and baked.

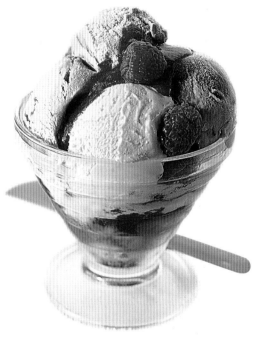

ICE-CREAM IS A GOOD SOURCE OF CALCIUM AND PROTEIN. TOP WITH A HOME-MADE FRUIT PURÉE FOR A HEALTHY TREAT.

JUNK FOOD-OR IS IT?

Chips: can be a good source of vitamin C, calories and some fibre and, if cooked well in fresh oil (or brushed in oil and oven-baked), have no negatives unless your child tends to be overweight, in which case deep-fried chips should be limited as they are high in calories.

Burgers: made with lean meat and grilled or dry-fried are an excellent source of iron, B vitamins and protein for children. Home-made is a better bet than commercial burgers, which are usually higher in fat. If choosing beef you may prefer to use organic.

Baked Beans: high in protein and fibre and low in fat.

White Bread: good source of calcium and ideal for children who generally don't need as much dietary fibre as adults. Try to buy good-quality bread made from hard wheats.

Chocolate: contains iron and calcium and, if a child isn't overweight, is a better occasional snack than sweets.

Pizza: good food for children, containing calcium, vitamin C and fibre. Go for vegetable-topped pizza rather than the high-fat meat and salami versions.

Ice-cream: good source of calcium and protein. Top with a home-made fruit purée for a healthy dessert for children.

White pasta: fine for children, who don't necessarily need the extra fibre that wholewheat pasta provides.

The truth is that there are few genuine completely 'junk' foods. The exceptions are the sweet and sugary products that offer little if any nutritional benefit, but too many E numbers for comfort — the coloured fizzy drinks and squashes, bags of brightly coloured sweets, commercial ice-lollies and packet dessert mixes that line our supermarket shelves. Don't buy them, and don't give your child the impression that these are 'treats' for special occasions — explain in the simplest terms that they are poor food lacking in real substance.

It's also wise to limit the amount of commercial pies, pastries, biscuits, cakes and bakery items that you let your child eat, especially the cheaper ones. They are often extremely high in saturated fat and/or hardened margarines (trans fats) and (in the case of sweet items) sugar, but little else in the way of good nutrients, and are also often high in salt (both the savoury and the sweet ones). Active children may be able to eat these foods and stay slim and apparently healthy, but a diet high in saturated fat is linked with heart disease and obesity in adult years. Tests have also shown that children as young as 10 who eat such a diet already show signs of atherosclerosis (the 'furring' of the arteries that is an early sign of possible heart disease). It is, therefore, best to keep an eye on saturated fats in your child's diet right from the early years.

Those items apart, most other foods can be eaten and enjoyed by your child as part of a varied diet without you having to feel guilty in any way, as long as you always remember to add some fresh fruit and fresh or frozen vegetables to every meal of the day in one form or another.

Think of your child's diet as something you are constantly trying to improve. It may not be perfect now — but children's tastes evolve and can be manipulated with patience and a 'softly softly' approach.

The teenage years

Teenagers (especially those aged between 14 and 18) have greater nutritional needs than any other age-group in terms of calorie, protein, vitamin and mineral requirements. This is the crucial time for making height and muscle, for building bone-mass and for sexual development. Health problems later in life, including osteoporosis and heart disease, may be influenced by what people eat in their teens. Yet, sadly, many teenagers get a poorer diet than most other social groups. Here we discuss the main areas of concern in the teenage diet and offer solutions.

■ Girls and iron intake

The iron RNI for female teenagers is higher than that for boys of the same age (see the chart on the right) because iron is lost each month in the blood during menstruation, and young teenage girls tend to have heavier periods than women in their 20s and 30s. However, research suggests that optimum iron intake is actually being met by few girls. On average, female teenagers get only 60% of the RNI and one in four of girls aged 11 to 15 is anaemic.

All the general notes on the importance of iron in the diet (see page 30) also apply to teenagers, but the shortfall is of particular importance because it has been shown in more than one scientifically controlled trial that iron deficiency in the teens can affect academic performance.

One 1989 trial showed that in schoolchildren with moderate iron-deficiency anaemia, a three-month course of supplements improved both physical and academic performance in measurable quantity. Another 1997 trial showed that iron-deficient teenage girls have IQ scores almost ten points lower than others (equivalent to one grade in GCSE), and that a ten-week course of

---

SPECIAL POINTERS TO CHILD HEALTH THROUGH FOOD

Sweet tooth: children have a naturally sweet tooth, probably because breast milk and formula milk is sweet. Try to satisfy this throughout childhood with fruits first. Sweet drinks consumption in kids is linked to obesity, a US survey found, and tooth decay.

Asthma: childhood asthma, coughing and wheezing has been shown to be reduced in children who eat enough fresh fruits, vegetables and essential omega-3 acids. There is also evidence that a diet low in vitamins E and A may increase risk of asthma-type illnesses. For foods high in these vitamins, see the lists on pages 24 and 22.

Breakfast: is an important meal for children, tests show. Energy, concentration and brain power are all better in children who get a good breakfast. They are also more creative and have more physical endurance. If a child is having a packed lunch, a hot breakfast such as beans on toast, porridge or a boiled egg and toast is a good idea. A small bowl of highly refined sugary cereal does not really provide enough calories.

Nutrients: most likely to be in shortfall in schoolchildren up to age 11 are folate and zinc. At age 11, calcium and iron deficiencies are fairly common.

Oily fish: trials have concluded that regular intake of omega-3s in oily fish can help improve children's brainpower, concentration, memory and performance, and improve anti-social behaviour, but few eat the necessary 1–2 portions of oily fish weekly.

DAILY ENERGY REQUIREMENTS AND RNIS FOR SELECTED NUTRIENTS FOR TEENAGERS

Age	Calories g	Protein g	Calcium mg	Iron mg	Zinc µg	A µg	Folate mg	C
Boys								
12-14	2,220	42.1	1,000	11.3	9.0	600	200	35
15-18	2,755	55.2	1,000	11.3	9.5	700	200	40
(19 plus as adult)								
Girls								
12-14	1,845	41.2	800	14.8*	9.0	600	200	35
15-18	2,110	45.0	800	14.8*	7.0	600	200	40
(19 plus as adult)								

* 10% of girls may need more than this.

(Based on information from the Department of Health)

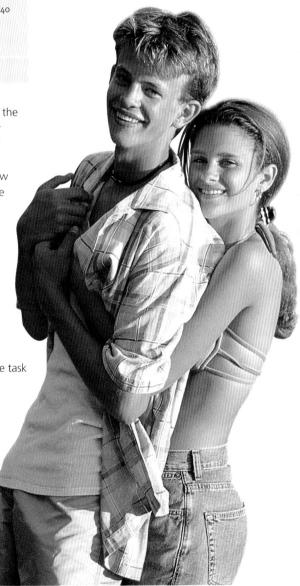

in winter, both of which are vital to help build bone mass during the enormous growth spurt (12–16 for girls and 13–18 for boys). Vitamin D intake in adolescence is also linked to protection from breast cancer later in life. Folic acid intake may be low in both sexes in the teens. Recent research reveals low intakes of zinc, potassium and magnesium in 15–18-year-olds, and of iodine in 15–18-year-old girls.

supplements levelled out the difference.

Why do so many teenage girls not get enough iron from their diets? There seem to be four reasons: one, many follow faddy low-calorie diets so they don't eat enough food to provide the iron; two, many are vegetarian or semi-vegetarian, and some of the richest and most easily absorbed sources of iron are meats and meat products; three, many others eat a 'junk' diet low on variety and particularly low on green vegetables (another good source of iron). Such a 'junk' diet also affects iron absorption — tea, coffee, caffeine drinks and lack of vitamin C in the diet all lower the amount of iron that can be absorbed.

Finally, in one analysis, school meals were found to contain only 60% of the recommended iron content and, for many teenagers, a school meal may be the main meal of the day.

Iron-rich foods (see the box below and the chart on page 30) should be introduced at each meal to help prevent teenage anaemia and, if you suspect that your daughter is already anaemic, a physician can do a blood test and prescribe iron tablets as necessary, which should be taken with food including items rich in vitamin C, such as fruit or fruit juice.

Of course, however, the four problems listed above may mean the task is difficult.

IRON-RICH FOODS:

offal, red meat, liver pâté, dark green leafy vegetables, wholemeal bread, seeds, fortified breakfast cereals, seaweed, cocoa powder, soya mince, vegeburger mix, quinoa, lentils, pulses, cashew nuts, pot barley, dried apricots and peaches, whole grains, eggs, baked beans in tomato sauce, curry powder.

■ Other teenage nutritional deficiencies

Teenagers with poor or insufficient eating habits are likely to be deficient in a range of important nutrients but, importantly, research shows that many teenagers (both boys and girls) are significantly deficient in calcium and vitamin D

AVERAGE WEIGHTS OF TEENAGERS

Boys

Age	Average Weight
12½	39 kg (6 st 3 lb)
13½	45.5 kg (7 st 3 lb)
14½	52 kg (8 st 5 lb)
15½	56.5 kg (9 st)
16-19	64.5 kg (10 st 3 lb)

Girls

Age	Average Weight
12½	41 kg (6 st 7 lb)
13½	47 (7 st 6 lb)
14½	50.5 (8 st)
15½	52.5 (8 st 5 lb)
16-19	55.5 (8 st 11 lb)

(Based on information from the Department of Health)

■ Weight problems

Calorie intake is also too low in many teenage diets. In one survey, 25% of older teenagers and young women had a BMI (Body Mass Index, see page 188) lower than 20, meaning that they were clinically underweight, whereas throughout all adult age groups of women only 12% were lower than 20.

However, about 25% of UK teenagers are now overweight or obese, according to the International Obesity Task Force. This is partly due to lack of exercise and partly to overconsumption of high fat/sugar foods and drinks. Overweight teenagers will be unlikely to develop into slim and fit adults unless encouraged to take more exercise and eat a healthy diet. For more information, see Section Four.

■ Vegetarianism

According to one national survey, 19% of teenagers are vegetarian and those between 16 and 24 have a higher concentration of vegetarians than any other age group. The guidelines on a safe and enjoyable vegetarian diet which appear on pages 60-63 also apply to teenagers. Special points to watch if your child decides to give up meat are:

✱ Make sure that the protein content of the diet remains reasonable by replacing meat with dairy produce (sometimes the lower-fat versions, especially if the teenager inclines towards overweight), pulses, and other acceptable sources (see lists of protein sources on page 21).

✱ If your teenager is female, pay special attention to ensuring that she eats plenty of iron-rich foods and folate-rich foods.

✱ Find out what provision is made at school/college for vegetarian meals. If these meals are not adequate, the teenager should take a packed lunch.

✱ Make sure that your child is aware of what constitutes a healthy diet for vege-tarians and knows how to prepare simple nutritious meat-free meals.

AN IDEAL VEGETARIAN LUNCH-BOX FOR TEENAGERS — SLICED WHOLEWHEAT PITTA, HUMMUS, CRUDITÉS, FRUIT CAKE, SMALL PACK OF SUNFLOWER SEEDS, DRIED APRICOTS, BANANA, MILK SHAKE, SATSUMA.

■ Anorexia and eating problems

The incidence of anorexia, bulimia and over-strict dieting is high amongst teenagers, particularly teenage girls. There is a large article on these problems in Section Two (see page 107). If you feel that your teenager may have an eating problem, it is always best to attempt to sort it out at the earliest opportunity first by discussing what you perceive to be the problem with the child, and secondly by taking medical advice or other appropriate action (e.g. counselling or nutritional advice) and by contacting the Eating Disorders Association, who can give plenty of help. (For their address, see the Appendix.) The following danger signals will help you decide if your child does have, or may soon have, an eating problem:

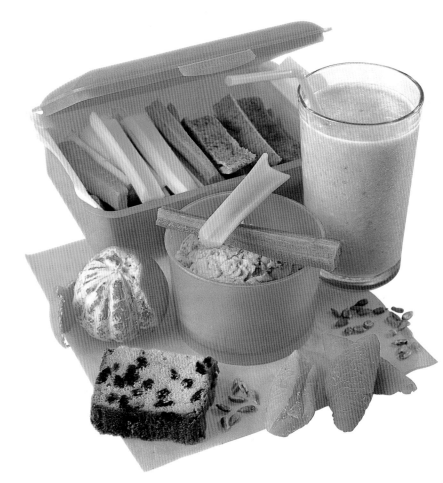

* Wanting to diet although not over-weight.
* Preoccupation with calories and food.
* Eating too little and making excuses for not eating.
* Fluctuating body weight.
* Over-activity.
* Disappearing after meals (may have bulimia).
* Secretiveness, moodiness.
* Wants to hide their body from you.

◼ Refusal to eat a varied healthy diet

For every teenager who is faddy about her or his diet in one way — wanting, for instance, no red meat and lots of healthy salads — there is another who tends to want nothing but foods like crisps, chips, fried foods, pies, pastries, sweet things and fizzy drinks, and will balk at having to eat anything like fresh vegetables, salad and fruit.

Much of what has been said on page 164 about the 'junk food dilemma' also applies to teenagers. They are, however, less likely to be compliant to your solutions than younger children! Teenagers also spend more time outside the home and outside the control of parents, and have more money to spend on the kind of food and snacks they wish to buy.

Appeals to vanity may work ('Your teeth will decay if you carry on eating so much sweet food!') or the official approach may do the trick — getting leaflets from school or The Health Education Authority (for their address, see the Appendix) on the importance of a healthy diet in the teenage years, for instance, or getting the area dietician to outline to him or her the dangers of a poor diet.

The key is, perhaps, to build on any areas — even if only one or two — of common ground. If possible, cook the things the teenager enjoys most yourself — e.g., he loves pies and chips, well your homemade pies and chips are likely to be

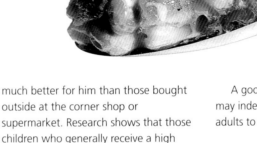

THIS MACARONI CHEESE, MADE WITH SEMI-SKIMMED MILK AND INCLUDING PARBOILED BROCCOLI, PEAS AND SLICED TOMATO, FORMS THE HEART OF AN EVENING MEAL WHICH ALMOST ANY VEGETARIAN TEENAGER WILL ENJOY — SERVED WITH A CRISP SIDE SALAD AND FOLLOWED BY ICE-CREAM AND FRESH FRUIT SALAD.

much better for him than those bought outside at the corner shop or supermarket. Research shows that those children who generally receive a high proportion of home-cooked food tend to choose a better diet for themselves in later life.

Lastly, if all else fails make sure the teenager gets a daily multi-vitamin and -mineral tablet.

◼ Acne

Teenage acne is very common indeed; few boys are likely to escape completely. The subject is covered in Section Two on page 86.

◼ Behaviour and co-ordination

There is new evidence emerging from a long-term UK-Government-sponsored study into violence and anti-social behaviour in young people, that diet has a part to play, particularly vitamins, minerals and essential fatty acids. A deficiency of omega-3s and omega-6s has been linked to dyspraxia — 'clumsy child' syndrome.

A good general varied healthy diet may indeed help your children and young adults to behave and function better.

◼ Academic performance

As we've already seen, lack of iron in teenage girls can cause lowered mental ability and performance. Other trials have shown that there may be a link between lack of a wider range of vitamins and minerals and poor academic performance, but the evidence on this does vary quite considerably. However, there is strong evidence that intake of omega-3 fats is linked to brain power and dyslexia.

The most likely conclusion is that if children and teenagers are falling short on nutrients then their performance may be impaired, but that if they already have a healthy diet and get their RNI of all the nutrients, then giving them more won't make any difference to their intelligence. As with any age group, it is better for them to get vitamins and minerals within a healthy diet rather than as supplements.

ADULTHOOD

That period between the teens and the start of 'middle age' in the mid-forties is a time when many people ignore, or even abuse, their health — eating poorly, drinking too much alcohol, coping with stress, lack of sleep, an over-busy lifestyle, and so on. Yet how you treat your body in this period has a very important bearing upon health later in life. This is the ideal time to look after yourself and your diet, so that middle- and old-age can be enjoyed in robust, optimum health, with as few illnesses and physical problems as possible.

Ages 20-35

These are the years when people tend to take fitness and good health for granted, and yet it is wise to use this time sensibly to build up a healthy body, fit for anything you care to do, including, for women, the stresses of pregnancy and child-care.

The Basic Healthy Diet and healthy eating guidelines described in Section One will ensure that such needs are met, but it is worth emphasizing here some of the most important nutritional points for young adults:

Bone building: at this age you are still building bone until peak bone-mass is reached around the age of 35. Optimum peak bone-mass means that the effects of osteoporosis in later life will be minimized. It is therefore vital to get enough calcium in the diet and to absorb enough calcium from that diet so that adequate bone is made. You won't get another chance to do this! Regular weight-bearing exercise, such as walking, will also help build bone. Follow all the guidelines on pages 28-9, eating plenty of lower-fat dairy produce, tofu, pulses, leafy greens, nuts and seeds.

Weight control: many previously slim people tend to begin putting on weight, especially around the midriff, as they reach the mid- to late-twenties. This is usually because activity levels have slowed (e.g. many men give up playing regular sport at this time) and with, perhaps, marriage and more home cooking, and more money to be able to afford to eat out often, calorie intake increases.

A very gradual and small weight gain from the 20s to middle-age is acceptable (up to 6.5 kg/1 stone), but it is sensible to watch diet and exercise if weight seems to be escalating more quickly than this as maintaining a reasonable weight is one simple way to help prevent many ills, including CHD, arthritis, mid-life onset diabetes, breast cancer in women, and others. It is also easier to keep weight off for most people than it is to lose stones which have been in place for years.

Up until the age of 30 or so, your metabolic rate remains constant (all other factors being equal), but after that age it begins to slow down. It has been estimated that you need 50 calories a day less for every five years you are over 30. For example, at 40 you will need 100 calories a day less than you did at 30, and by 50 you will need 200 less. See Section Four for more information on weight control and slimming.

Family planning: in their 20s or 30s many people plan a family. For women, this means following a healthy diet and maintaining a reasonable body weight, as a low BMI may increase the risk of periods ceasing and therefore will reduce fertility. Before actively trying to conceive, women should consider pre-conceptual care for optimum health for mother and baby during pregnancy and afterwards — a subject discussed overleaf. For men, a healthy diet high in zinc, selenium, and vitamins E and C has been shown to help fertility. There have been studies linking high coffee intake to lowered fertility levels and the Royal College of Obstetricians and Gynaecologists reports that alcohol intake affects female fertility too, and that more than 5 drinks a week can raise the risk of early miscarriage.

Women's needs: menstrual losses mean that throughout the reproductive years, women will always need more iron intake than men (for a list of good sources, see page 30) to prevent iron deficiency diseases, including anaemia. They may also have to cope with problems such as PMS, menstrual problems and fluid

retention. All these topics are discussed in detail in Section Two. Here are a few more pointers for women in adulthood:

* Diet should be adequate in calories and all nutrients. It is not wise to follow a diet too low in fats as the role of the essential fatty acids, found in a variety of plant foods, is important not only for health but also to keep skin soft and supple and hair in good condition.

* Women on the contraceptive pill may find they gain up to 3 kg (half a stone) in weight. This is partly due to fluid retention; the PMS and Diuretic Diet on page 145 will help minimize this, as will exercise.

* Drinking more than one alcoholic drink a day may increase the risk of breast cancer in young women.

Ages 35-45

As the metabolic rate begins to slow, it is important to keep a watch on the intake of high-density low-nutrient foods, such as many desserts, pastries, sweets and animal fats, and to take adequate exercise. A weight gain of 3-6.5 kg (half a stone to 1 stone) over your weight at 20-25 is acceptable.

The basic healthy diet should still be followed, paying particular attention to the 'superfoods' highlighted in the Food Charts at the back of the book. These are the foods that seem to offer most protection against the major diseases of middle- and old-age, and against the ageing process. Plenty of fresh fruits and vegetables is vital, not only for the well-known antioxidants, vitamins C, E, beta-carotene and selenium that they contain, but also for the other phytochemicals which are protective too (see page 34).

A healthy diet at this time can also give a perhaps much-needed boost to brain power. Research has shown that various dietary factors

can influence how well our brains work. A diet low in saturated fat encourages circulation of blood through the brain, and eating a diet slightly lower than average in calorie content has been shown to help prevent the brain from deteriorating as we get older, as well as helping to improve mood, memory and other factors.

Brain power can also be adversely affected by eating a big meal OR by crash dieting, so that blood sugar levels fall too low. As Section One explains in detail, mental powers can also be improved by eating a breakfast high in protein and not too much carbohydrate at lunch-time. Lastly, 'eat little and often' is the best way to benefit your brain and keep one step ahead.

A good night's sleep also becomes very important in the 30s and 40s, both to help the body rest and repair itself and to keep the brain alert. If having trouble sleeping, see Insomnia on page 123.

See also: Eating Out (page 64), Fast Food (page 55), and Alcohol Abuse (page 86).

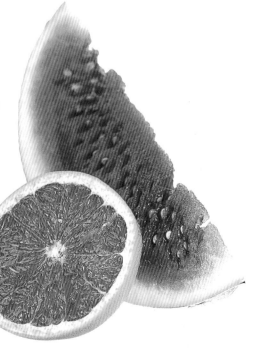

Pregnancy and pre-conceptual care

We now know that your health and nutritional status both before and during pregnancy may have a bearing not only on your baby's health in infancy but on his or her health right through to adulthood, and even on the length of his or her life.

■ Pre-conceptual care

If a pregnancy is planned, it is now accepted that it is sensible for the prospective mother to prepare herself for the pregnancy with suitable diet, folate supplements, exercise and weight control. She should also give up, if

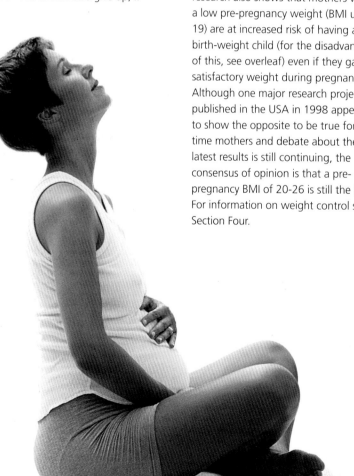

necessary, smoking and cut back on alcohol. The reason for the importance of pre-conceptual care is that this will reduce the risk of birth defects and of giving birth to a low-weight infant, which is a proven risk factor in various lifelong health problems. Here we look at the various pre-conceptual factors that can influence ease of conception, a healthy pregnancy and baby.

Weight: if you have a BMI (Body Mass Index, see page 188) within the accepted normal range of 20-25 you have a greater chance of becoming pregnant. With BMIs under 20 and over 30, the rate of conception is lower. Most research also shows that mothers with a low pre-pregnancy weight (BMI under 19) are at increased risk of having a low-birth-weight child (for the disadvantages of this, see overleaf) even if they gain satisfactory weight during pregnancy. Although one major research project published in the USA in 1998 appeared to show the opposite to be true for first-time mothers and debate about these latest results is still continuing, the consensus of opinion is that a pre-pregnancy BMI of 20-26 is still the ideal. For information on weight control see Section Four.

Diet: The mother's diet both before conception and during the first few weeks after conception (when many women still don't realize that they are pregnant) is important for the growth and proper development of the embryo, as from conception for the first few weeks it grows more rapidly than at any other time. Any abnormal cell development also seems to happen at this early stage.

To help prevent neural tube defects, such as spina bifida, adequate amounts of the B vitamin, folate should be taken. The normal RNI for non-pregnant adult women is 200µg a day, but pre-conceptually and for the first three months of pregnancy it is recommended that a supplement of 400µg is taken and that an extra 100µg is taken in the diet. (More than this will be prescribed for women who have already given birth to a baby with a neural tube defect.)

This means eating a basic healthy diet containing plenty of naturally folate-rich foods, such as green vegetables, yeast extract, pulses, nuts, fruits and potatoes, and fortified breakfast cereals. For a more detailed list of rich sources of folate, see page 28. Even with a healthy diet the supplement is important, though. There is some evidence also emerging that supplements of the compound inositol can also help to reduce possible neural tube defects.

It may also be a good idea to take in extra calcium and iron during the pre-conception period, as women with low iron stores at the start of pregnancy may become anaemic and there is evidence that the foetus will deplete maternal bone if calcium runs short during the pregnancy.

Fitness: the mother-to-be should aim to get fit for pregnancy, taking regular walks or similar, and cutting out smoking (one of the major causes of low-birth-weight babies).

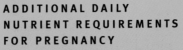

Alcohol: According to the DoH, while the safest approach may be to avoid any alcohol during pregnancy, there is no evidence of harm from low levels of intake, defined as no more than 1–2 units of alcohol once or twice a week. But in the USA since 1981, the advice has been to avoid all alcohol during pregnancy, and the UK Medical Council on Alcohol advises women to avoid it during the first trimester.

The latest research on alcohol and pregnancy finds that drinking is linked to major structural malformations in the foetus, increase in pre-term birth, disturbance to foetal growth and later cognitive and behaviour problems in children. For more see page 36.

■ Pregnancy

Once a pregnancy is confirmed, it is important to continue to live healthily, eating a balanced, healthy and adequate diet. This is not only for the sake of the growing foetus (research even shows that what you eat also affects the baby's tastebuds and food preferences after birth and henceforth!), but also in the interests of the mother's own health and wellbeing, — avoiding excessive tiredness, constipation, nausea, and so on.

ADDITIONAL DAILY NUTRIENT REQUIREMENTS FOR PREGNANCY

(For nutrients not listed here, requirement is the same as for non-pregnant adult females.)

Calories	+200*
Protein	+6g
Vitamin A	+100µg
Vitamin B1	+0.1mg*
B2	+0.3mg
Folate	+400µg**
Vitamin C	+10mg
Vitamin D	+10µg

* For last three months only
** Preconceptually and until 12th week of pregnancy.

ADDITIONAL DAILY NUTRIENT REQUIREMENTS FOR LACTATION

(For nutrients not listed here, requirement is the same as for non-pregnant adult females.)

Calories:	
up to 1 month	+450
1-2 months	+530
2 to 3 months	+570
4-6 months	+480-570*
over 6 months	+240**
Protein	+11g***
Vitamin B1	+0.2mg
Vitamin B2	+0.5mg
Vitamin B3	+2mg
Vitamin B12	+0.5µg
Folate	+60µg
Vitamin C	+30mg
Vitamin A	+350µg
Vitamin D	+10µg
Calcium	+550mg
Phosphorus	+440mg
Magnesium	+50mg
Zinc	+6mg****
Copper	+0.3mg
Selenium	+15µg

* Depending upon amount of weaning foods given; if primarily breast milk is fed, upper limit may be used.
** Assuming non-breast milk foods form majority of baby's diet.
*** 4 months plus, reduces to +8g (due to weaning)
**** 4 months plus, reduces to +2.5mg

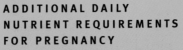

Surprisingly, the need for most nutrients doesn't increase during pregnancy, but there is a need for more of some of them. The chart above lists the recommended nutrient intake for all major nutrients in pregnancy and when lactating.

The lists on pages 22–33 show rich sources of all the extra nutrients needed in the charts above. Some omissions may seem surprising; for example, there is no extra requirement for iron or calcium in pregnancy. This is because absorption of both iron and calcium rises during pregnancy. In addition, loss of iron through the process of menstruation ceases but, if iron stores are low at the start of pregnancy, supplements may indeed be prescribed.

Less calcium is also excreted in the urine during the period of pregnancy, thus conserving supplies, and if more calcium is needed the mother's bone mass will supply this. However, extra calcium intake is, in fact, recommended in the case of teenage pregnancies.

'Eating for two' during most of the course of pregnancy is also not necessary. A mere 200 calories extra a day for the last three months will be enough for most women's needs — representing a small baked potato or 300 ml (1/2 pint) of skimmed milk and a small piece of cheese.

It is thought that part of the reason why pregnant women don't need to eat a lot extra is that the metabolic rate slows down during pregnancy, and also that they naturally become less active. However, women who are significantly underweight at the start of their pregnancy may need to consider eating more than this.

OILY FISH, SUCH AS SARDINES, ARE A GOOD SOURCE OF VITAMIN D AND ESSENTIAL FATTY ACIDS – AS WELL AS MANY OTHER NUTRIENTS – FOR THE PREGNANT WOMAN.

Although vitamin A need is increased during pregnancy (especially in the last 3 months), most women generally get plenty in their diets; and, in excess (above 3,300µg a day), vitamin A (in the form of retinol, not pro-vitamin A beta-carotene) is toxic in pregnancy and can cause birth defects.

For this reason, pregnant women are warned not to eat liver or liver products, as liver contains potentially toxic amounts of vitamin A. They should also not take supplements containing retinol (e.g. cod liver oil) unless prescribed by their physician.

Extra vitamin C is needed in pregnancy, especially in the last three months, and 10µg vitamin D should be given as a supplement as it is hard to get this amount from the diet unless quite a high-fat diet is followed.

There are no additional requirements for total fat or carbohydrate during pregnancy (except as a means of increasing calorie intake in the last 3 months), but the essential fatty acids and their derivatives such as GLA, EPA and DHA, found in plant and fish oils, may be very important to a healthy pregnancy and baby. Research has linked a diet rich in EFAs with longer pregnancies (and therefore higher birth-weight, see

below), a reduced risk of high blood pressure in the mother, and optimum brain and eye development in the baby — and therefore intelligence. EFA intake in the last three months of pregnancy, when the brain of the foetus increases in weight by four or five times, is believed to be the most crucial.

There is no official recommendation for fibre increase in the diet for pregnancy, but many pregnant women experience constipation; increasing fibre intake (see list of rich sources on page 14) as well as water will help prevent this, as will regular gentle exercise.

■ Foetal health

Almost all research to date shows that a baby's weight at birth has great relevance to its future health, both in the immediate- and long-term. Low-birth-weight babies are more at risk of CHD, high blood pressure, stroke and diabetes in later life. They also appear to suffer poorer cognitive (brain) function in childhood. Low birth-weight is 2.5 kg (5½ lb) or less. Nutritional factors that may produce a low-birth-weight baby include:

✴ Excess alcohol intake during pregnancy. Alcohol is best avoided.

✴ Smoking — this should be stopped.

✴ Inadequate calorie intake. Most researchers agree that thin mothers and mothers who fail to put on adequate weight and/or fail to eat adequate calories during the pregnancy may run greater risk of having a low-birth-weight baby. A child's potential adult bone density (and risk of osteoporosis) is linked to magnesium, phosphorus and potassium levels in the mother's diet during pregnancy, and to a high saturated fat diet.

✴ Poor diet. Shortages of B vitamins, magnesium, iron, phosphorous, potassium and zinc in the first three months of pregnancy have been associated with low birth-weight. Shortage of vitamin D in the womb can cause reduced bone mass in children as they get older.

WEIGHT GAIN GUIDELINES FOR PREGNANCY

BMI at Start of Pregnancy	Total Optimum Amount of Weight to Gain
under 20	12.5-18 kg (27-38 lb)
20-26	11.5-16 kg (25-34 lb)
26-30	7-11.5 kg (15-25 lb)
over 30	minimum of 6 kg (13 lb)
	maximum to be decided in individual consultation.

Gaining too much weight is not a good idea — gains over those listed are associated with several complications in pregnancy, such as high blood pressure and prolonged labour, as well as overweight after the pregnancy.

DIET TIPS FOR A TROUBLE-FREE PREGNANCY

The three most common complaints mentioned by pregnant women and how to deal with them:

Morning sickness: this can occur at any time of day but is usually worse in the morning. Probably caused by low blood-sugar levels and so eating several small high-carbohydrate snacks throughout the day will probably effect a cure, or at least minimize the nausea. Sickness on waking may be helped by eating such a snack as soon as you wake (have it ready by your bed). Ideal snacks: a banana; a slice of wholemeal bread and jam; ginger biscuit; oatcake. See also the ideas on curing nausea on page 129.

Tiredness: especially common in the first three months of pregnancy and is often the first sign that a woman is pregnant. Good pre-conceptual care will help, including a healthy energy-giving diet and an exercise programme to increase heart/lung capacity. Follow this on with a healthy diet for pregnancy (Basic Healthy Diet, page 53, plus supplements as necessary) and make sure to get enough calories. Dieting is out. Alcohol and caffeine will increase fatigue. Adequate rest is essential. Check with a doctor that you aren't iron-deficient. For more information see Fatigue, page 111.

Food cravings: many women do find themselves craving foods that they possibly wouldn't even usually consider. These cravings can be for almost any food, from pickled onions to oranges, and some women want strange combinations of foods. There is little scientific basis for the idea that the cause of such a craving is the need for a food high in a particular nutrient that the mother is lacking; e.g. if she craves oranges she must be lacking vitamin C.

If such cravings are for reasonably nutritious food then there is no great problem, unless the craved food is eaten regularly and to such an extent other types of foods are avoided, which will create nutritional shortages, or to such an extent that too much weight is gained, in the case of the higher-calorie foods.

If cravings are for the less nutrient-dense foods and/or 'junk' foods, the pre-natal dietician should be told and she or he can then work out a suitable strategy, which may include supplements.

■ Foods to Avoid

When pregnant, it is even more important than usual to avoid getting food poisoning; such bacteria as salmonella and listeria can seriously affect the unborn baby.

* Avoid soft mould-ripened cheeses, like Brie and Camembert, and unpasteurized cheeses, such as most Parmesan, and blue-veined cheeses like Stilton and Danish Blue, which may harbour listeria. Cheddar and cottage cheese are fine.
* Avoid pre-packed salads, deli salads in dressings, and other items sold loose from chill cabinets in shops and restaurants.
* Avoid raw or lightly cooked eggs and anything containing them, e.g. real mayonnaise, tiramisu, in case of salmonella.
* Avoid pâté, unless pasteurized, in case of listeria, and all liver products because of high levels of vitamin A.
* Avoid raw or partly cooked meat, unpasteurized milk, soil-dirty fruits and vegetables, to avoid toxoplasmosis.

* Avoid shark, swordfish and mackerel which may contain harmful levels of mercury, according to the USFDA.
* Avoid herbal supplements and chinese herbs and herbal medicines which may contain toxins.
* Avoid more than 5 cups of coffee a day — higher levels may increase risk of miscarriage.
* Avoid alcohol — DoH guidelines are maximum four units a week but research indicates even as little as this may affect a baby's nervous system and brain.

BANANAS AND WHOLEMEAL BREAD MAKE IDEAL FIRST-THING-IN-THE-MORNING SNACKS TO HELP ALLEVIATE MORNING SICKNESS.

THE MIDDLE YEARS

For most people between the ages of 45 and 65 the good health of youth is eroded, and problems like arthritis, atherosclerosis, obesity, diabetes and general physical deterioration take its place. With dietary and lifestyle intervention, however, it really is never too late to make significant improvements to long- and short-term health and to keep many of the typical signs of ageing at bay. Experts are also unlocking the secrets of increasing life-span through diet!

In the middle years, some changes — such as the menopause in women — are natural and inevitable, while others which many people regard as natural may, in fact, be undesirable and possibly preventable. Our health in so-called 'middle age' is, in part, dependent upon what has gone before, and obviously good diet, enough exercise and a healthy lifestyle throughout youth are important factors. However, many people don't, in fact, 'look after themselves' until their youth is gone. It isn't until they hit 40 or 50 that they begin to realize that perhaps their own body deserves a regular service as much as their car does! Even if you do leave it this late to begin paying attention to what you put in your body for fuel and other lifestyle factors, however, you can still see great benefits.

One recent twenty-year international study published in the British Medical Journal, which examined the link between the diet of men aged 50 to 70 and their death rates, found that a healthy diet (as laid down by the WHO) is associated with a reduction of 13% in all causes of death in men of those ages.

Other important US and UK studies on mice, rats, fruit flies and monkeys have found that life-span can be increased by up to 50% on a calorie-restricted but highly nutritious diet and that such a diet also reduces the risk of CHD, cancer, stroke and diabetes, and increases the functioning of the immune system (see Anti-ageing, opposite).

On a more mundane level, we now know that all kinds of health problems and signs of 'getting older' — from Alzheimer's and osteoporosis to hair-loss and lack of libido — can be minimized, or even prevented, by particular diets or foods. Middle-age really is the time to pay attention to your diet.

■ Your Starting Point

If you don't know where to begin, the best place is the Basic Healthy Diet on page 53. A complete health check-up by a physician is a good idea — this should reveal any health problems you may have; or perhaps you already know what they are. In that case you should follow the particular type of diet that suits your ailment. You will find all the information and special diets for major ailments in Section Two.

Many more people will be in reasonable health now, but perhaps have higher than average risk factors for a particular disease or ailment. Here are the major risk factors for the most prevalent ailments of middle- and old-age:

Arthritis: family history; obesity; lack of exercise.

CHD and stroke: smoking; heavy drinking; obesity; family history of CHD; diet high in saturated fat and low in fresh fruits and vegetables; stress; lack of exercise.

Cancer: smoking; heavy drinking; diet low in fresh fruits and vegetables; family history of some cancers; possibly high-meat or -animal-fat diet; possibly obesity (link between breast cancer and obesity in post-menopausal women established).

Diabetes: obesity.

Alzheimer's: smoking; heavy drinking; poor diet.

Osteoporosis: low BMI throughout life; family history; insufficient calcium/magnesium/vitamin D in diet; lack of exercise; female.

A: If you have one or more risk factors, apart from obesity, for any particular ailment the corresponding diet in Section Two may be right for you, though you should see your GP and discuss those risk factors.

B: If you are obese, with no other risk factors, then you should lose weight by following a sensible diet plan. Obesity, even moderate overweight, is a risk

ANTI-AGEING AND CALORIE RESTRICTION

If you want to live to be 120 — or more — there is fascinating evidence emerging that the way to do it is to restrict your calorie intake on a permanent basis. Several different research trials in the USA and UK have discovered that restricting calorie intake to 30–70% of normal extends lifespan in monkeys and other animals by up to 50%. Now one human study in the USA (2006) finds evidence to back this up – humans on a calorie-restriction plan for 6 months showed reduced fasting insulin levels and average core body temperature – both linked to longer lifespan.

It seems that a calorie-restricted diet can have many beneficial effects on health, including much reduced risk of certain cancers, heart disease and stroke, as well as increased energy levels and improved efficiency of the immune system. The US Government is so impressed with the research that it is funding an official trial for 120 volunteers who will aim to restrict their calories to about 1,800 a day on average (for men) and reduce their body weight by 10-20%.

The concept of calorie restriction is not without its risks, however, and shouldn't be undertaken by people of normal weight until the results of the trials come through and are evaluated, a task that will take some years. The risks include malnutrition (although the humans in the experiment will be fed carefully to ensure this doesn't happen), increased risk of osteoporosis, and lack of menstruation and fertility in younger women.

Perhaps some time in the future, calorie-restriction will prove to be a safe method of extending healthy life for all — meanwhile, the message for most people in mid-life is to think slim, but not too slim!

factor for so many illnesses and problems in later life that it really is worth getting a grip on your size as soon as possible. All the information you need about weight and health, your optimum weight and slimming information is in Section Four. (See also Anti-ageing above.)

C: If you are obese, with other risk factors, you should lose weight as in B. After you have lost weight, you should revert to plan A.

D: If you have no risk factors, follow the Basic Healthy Diet, taking into consideration any further information in this article that applies to you; or, if in the menopause, try the diet overleaf.

■ The menopause

For every woman the menopausal years — when hormonal changes in the body bring about the gradual decline in her fertility and an end to her ability to bear children naturally — are an inevitability. For many, the menopause brings a variety

of symptoms, ranging from the mildly upsetting to those severe enough to disrupt their lives.

The majority of these symptoms — such as hot flushes, tiredness, mood swings and depression, libido problems and insomnia — can be alleviated by correct diet or, on the other hand, made worse by a poor diet. We look at the dietary options here and consider also the long-term effects on your health in old age of what you eat at this time. We also provide solutions to the 'male menopause' dilemma.

As 50% of the human population will one day face the menopause, it is difficult to understand why so little information is available on the prevention of the symptoms and consequences of the female menopause by natural methods. Medical intervention through hormone replacement therapy — and often through prescription of anti-depressants and tranquillisers — may provide relief for quite a lot of women, but the side-effects of HRT are, for many, almost as unpleasant as the symptoms of the menopause themselves, and the long-term effects are still uncertain, though it is now generally agreed that HRT does increase the likelihood of breast cancer.

One of the major benefits of HRT is that it helps to prevent the loss of bone density which accelerates greatly in menopausal and post-menopausal women, causing osteoporosis. HRT works mainly by replacing the female hormone oestrogen, which allows calcium to be absorbed more effectively. There are, however, various dietary means by which bone-loss can be slowed in susceptible women. A diet high in soya and soya products has been shown in studies to mimic the effects of oestrogen in maintaining bone density. Other foods which may have an oestrogen-like effect include nuts, yams, linseeds, pulses and grains, and most fresh fruits and vegetables.

Adequate calcium intakes during menopause and beyond are essential — 1,500mg per day is ideal. Good sources of calcium are dairy products (which should be low-fat versions, rather than full-fat, because there is evidence that saturated fat 'binds up' calcium and inhibits its absorption), calcium-enriched soya milk and yoghurt, tofu, seaweed and other dark green leafy vegetables, nuts, sunflower seeds, white flour, soya flour, pulses, sardines, whitebait and shellfish.

Even if calcium intake is adequate, absorption is affected by various factors. It is hindered by eating raw bran at the same meal; by oxalic acid in spinach and rhubarb; by high alcohol intake; by caffeine found in tea, coffee, cola, cocoa, chocolate and some herbal supplements; by smoking; by saturated fat, and possibly by a diet high in highly processed junk foods.

It also appears that calcium is leached from the bones by a high intake of protein — particularly animal protein — so it makes sense to choose more plant proteins in your diet and not to eat more protein than your body needs for good health and maintenance (see page 20 for more detail).

Absorption is helped by adequate vitamin D. Zinc — found in shellfish, nuts, wheatgerm, seeds, soya, whole grains, pulses and cheese — and magnesium — found in nuts, whole grains, soya and other pulses, seeds, wheatgerm and fruits and vegetables — are important for bone status. Absorption of all the minerals, including calcium and zinc, is helped considerably by eating vitamin C-rich foods at the same time.

Calcium is also important in the diet for menopausal women as it helps to maintain a healthy nervous system and a healthy heart and blood pressure.

Osteoporosis, and its prevention and management from childhood through to old age, is dealt with in more detail on pages 130–32.

■ Hot flushes and other menopausal symptoms

In the West, approximately half of menopausal women suffer from severe or prolonged 'hot flushes', with flushing of the face and neck, a feeling of suffocating heat and sweating, often followed by chilling. Some experts believe that these can be alleviated by soya-based foods such as tofu, which contain powerful phyto-oestrogens, and other oestrogenic foods, like other pulses, linseeds, beansprouts and other fresh vegetables. But the recent COT report on phytoestrogens found the evidence inconclusive and that there was a strong placebo effect. Eating plenty of foods rich in the amino acid tryptophan, is also known to help the brain produce serotonin, the 'mood-calming' chemical.

Vitamins E and C are said to help minimize hot flushes. Yams are rich in natural progesterone which may also help symptoms. Zinc helps regulate hormones.

Weight gain is not an inevitable consequence of the menopause, but a change in body shape happens to many women — the waist may thicken and mid-body fat increase, due to altered levels of hormones. It is important not to attempt to maintain a very low body-weight as thinness will have a detrimental effect on bone-loss and calorie intake needs to be sufficient to give your body all the nutrients it needs. Yet it is also important not to put on too much body fat during and after menopause, as obesity in post-menopausal women is linked with an increased risk of breast cancer as well as increased risk of heart disease (THE biggest killer of women aged 50-plus in the UK), high blood pressure, diabetes and arthritis of the weight-bearing joints. Most women who were slim in their teens and 20s should aim for a weight approximately/no more than 6.5-9.5 kg (1-1½ st) heavier in their late 40s and 50s. The best diet in and after menopause may be one that includes plenty of low Glycaemic Index foods (see page 195) – this will also help prevent breast cancer.

Lack of libido may improve if your overall diet and lifestyle improve and your menopausal symptoms diminish — tiredness and depression are passion-killers at any age. A diet rich in zinc is

MENOPAUSE MANAGERS

Moderate alcohol consumption can delay the menopause by up to 18 months, and in post-menopausal women a little alcohol can protect against CHD.
Smoking induces an earlier menopause.

said to help libido. The 'anti-ageing' mineral, selenium, may also help, and adequate essential fatty acids and vitamin E may help minimize vaginal dryness.

Mood swings, depression and insomnia can be helped by adequate intake of B vitamins, zinc, magnesium and tryptophan. A calcium-rich snack before bed can induce sleep.

Headaches can be minimized by regular meals and snacks, including complex carbohydrates, such as whole grains, and foods rich in vitamin B group.

Fluid retention can be largely avoided by a diet low in sodium, junk foods and highly refined foods, and high in natural diuretics like parsley, celery and asparagus.

Dry skin and poor hair condition is improved by eating plenty of the antioxidants selenium (found in shellfish, dairy products especially butter, avocado, whole grains, pulses and leafy greens) and vitamin E (found in plant oils, seeds, nuts, wheatgerm, cabbage, tuna in oil and asparagus) as well as omega-3 fats found in fish oils and flax seed (linseed) oil, and GLA oils found in evening primrose and starflower oil.

■ The male menopause and other problems

Up to 40% of doctors believe that, yes, there really IS a male menopause. Many more middle-aged males know that there is. It may not carry clinical symptoms, as the female menopause does, but there are indeed symptoms. Here are those most frequently mentioned:

* Diminished sex drive (libido).
* Depression and/or negative mood or mood swings.
* Lethargy/fatigue.
* Weight gain.
* Loss of hair and skin-tone.
* Problems getting or maintaining an erection even when aroused.
* Loss of muscle-tone/strength.

Many of these problems can be helped by the Basic Healthy Diet (see

SUPPLEMENTS FOR THE MENOPAUSE

If one or more of your own menopausal symptoms is severe, it may be worth considering a food supplement, along with the menopause diet overleaf. Actual scientific evidence for their worth is fairly scant, but anecdotal evidence for all is quite strong.

Hot flushes: vitamin E supplements (look for d-alpha tocopherol on the label, which is the natural vitamin E, rather than the synthetic, which is less effective) — minimum 200mg a day. Herbs — try black cohosh (but see page 149), sage, agnus castus and red clover. (For stockists of herbs and herbalists, see the Appendix.)

Depression, mood swings: Korean ginseng, trytophan (available from health food shops), St John's Wort (*Hypericum perforatum*).

Nerves: motherwort, calcium, B complex.

Insomnia: kava kava root (from health food shops), melatonin (on prescription only in UK, available by mail order from USA), camomile. See also Ailments and Solutions section, page 123.

Fluid retention: hawthorn, motherwort, dandelion. (For stockists of herbs and herbalists, see the Appendix.)

Libido: St John's Wort (*Hypericum perforatum*). (For stockists of herbs and herbalists, see the Appendix.)

page 53). Extra help can be found in the relevant entries in the Ailments and Solutions section (e.g. fatigue is discussed on page 111, depression on page 103, skin problems on page 134 and libido on page 122). Surplus weight can be lost by using the advice in Section Four, and muscle- and skin-tone can be improved and/or maintained by regular weight-bearing exercise. Skin-tone can be improved further with good diet, including plenty of fresh fruits, vegetables, essential fatty acids and water. With improvement in general wellbeing, appearance and mood, the sex drive generally tends to improve as well. Dopamine-rich foods, like yoghurt, fish and lean steak, may help. Stress levels can be helped with the right

diet — if this is a major part of your life, try the anti-stress diet hints on page 138.

A high proportion of middle-aged men begin to have prostate troubles — an enlarged prostate gland can be uncomfortable and tests show a diet high in zinc and vitamin E can help (for rich sources, see pages 31 and 24). To help prevent prostate cancer, avoid heavy drinking and saturated fats, and eat a diet rich in brightly coloured vegetables (e.g. tomatoes).

One area often forgotten in mid-life is oral care. Regular dental checks, thorough cleaning twice daily and a diet low in sugar and refined produce and high in natural, crunchy, fruits and veg will help avoid problems. Nothing ages you more than a set of teeth that aren't your own.

■ The menopause diet plan

This plan is a sample of the kind of eating that should help reduce menopause symptoms as well as minimizing bone-loss. After the menopause is over it is acceptable to continue with a similar diet.

Instructions:

✳ Choose plenty of foods low or medium low on the Glycaemic Index (see page 195).

✳ Choose skimmed milk and lower-fat dairy produce rather than full-fat, most of the time.

✳ Drink only decaffeinated tea and coffee and avoid all cola drinks and cocoa. Keep all types of chocolate for only a very occasional treat.

✳ Drink a maximum of 1 or 2 glasses of wine a day.

✳ Drink plenty of water, freshly squeezed fruit/vegetable juices and soya milk.

✳ Eat as much fresh fruit and vegetables as you can, getting a wide variety.

✳ Avoid junk food — any processed foods high in saturated fat/sugar/phosphates (read labels).

✳ Keep salt to a minimum — use sea salt when you do.

Unlimiteds:

Drinks as left; fruits and vegetables as above (plainly cooked or with pure vegetable oils); fresh and dried herbs and spices.

Breakfast every day:

Have either fortified soya milk OR yoghurt with a portion of whole-grain low-salt cereal — e.g. muesli, Weetabix, Shredded Wheat, porridge.

Add one orange, a few chopped nuts, preferably Brazil nuts, a dessertspoon of sesame and/or sunflower seeds, and a good dessertspoon of wheatgerm.

For a change, have a pink grapefruit or 1 or 2 satsumas or other citrus fruits instead of the orange.

If still hungry, have a slice of whole-grain bread with a small amount of butter and honey or Marmite.

Snacks every day:

Twice a day between meals have a small snack of any of the following:

Fresh nuts; seeds; fresh fruit; dried fruit; fortified soya milk; low-salt rye crispbread with a little low-salt peanut butter or hummus.

NOTE: Recipes for dishes that are capitalized are to be found in Section 5.

SPINACH, BROCCOLI AND WALNUT STIR-FRY (SEE PAGE 244)

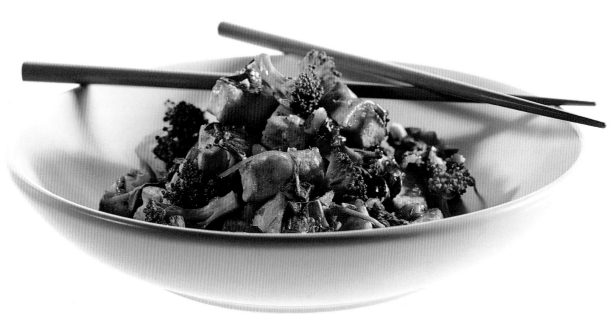

THE MENOPAUSE DIET

DAY ONE
Lunch

salad of mixed green leaves (some dark green, e.g. rocket, lamb's lettuce, watercress) with celery, cucumber, tomato, one hard-boiled egg and two anchovies, dressed in olive oil and vinegar dressing
wholemeal, rye or white bread
1 banana

Evening

Chicken Cacciatore
brown rice
Brussels sprouts or spring greens
fruit and soya yoghurt

DAY TWO
Lunch

salad of drained tuna in oil mixed with cooked butter beans, sliced ripe tomatoes, red onion and lightly cooked asparagus tips, garnished with chopped parsley and olive oil and red wine vinegar.
French bread

Evening

stir-fried tofu
Spinach, Broccoli and Walnut Stir Fry
brown rice
berry fruits with yoghurt

DAY THREE
Lunch

lentil and spring green soup
rye bread
dried apricots

Evening

omelette
pepper and onion salad
1 banana

DAY FOUR
Lunch

Smoked Mackerel Pâté Salad
rye bread
coleslaw made with white cabbage, carrot, onion, dried apricots, and mixed nuts, dressed with low-fat bio yoghurt mixed with lemon juice and a little honey and black pepper

Evening

Pasta with Broccoli and Anchovies
mixed salad with balsamic vinegar dressing
1 orange

DAY FIVE
Lunch

Hummus
pitta bread
salad of cucumber, olives, tomatoes, onion, dark green lettuce leaves

Evening

grilled sardines or herring fillets dressed with ginger and coriander
peas
new potatoes
fresh fruit of choice

DAY SIX
Lunch

salad of slices of ripe avocado, tomato and halumi cheese dressed with olive oil and red wine vinegar, seasoned and flashed under grill for a minute
ciabatta bread
selection of seeds and dried fruits — e.g. pine nuts, sunflower seeds, dried figs, dried peaches

Evening

salmon fillet with a herb and ginger crust
brown rice
mange-tout peas
Green Lentils with Herbs

DAY SEVEN
Lunch

feta cheese, stir-fried in sunflower oil to brown and served with black stoned olives and lemon juice
salad of fresh beansprouts, carrot, celery, watercress, spinach and mixed chopped nuts in classic vinaigrette dressing
white bread

Evening

small amount of extra-lean organic beef, cut into strips and stir-fried in sesame oil with a selection of fresh mixed vegetables, including Chinese leaves, with ginger, garlic, and soy sauce
egg-thread noodles
fresh fruit salad with yoghurt

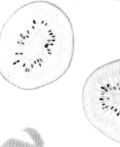
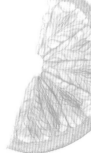
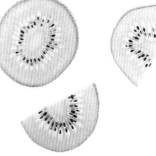

SIXTIES PLUS

The nutritional needs of older people are not all that much different from those of younger adults. However, the practicalities of eating such a balanced diet seem to become increasingly harder as we get older. This means that many older people in the UK do suffer deficiencies in some areas. Here we look at healthy eating in the later years and suggest ways in which diet can be improved – and enjoyed more.

The average requirements for nutrients in older people are similar to those in younger adulthood. The main differences are that older people require fewer calories (2,330 for males and 1,900 for females aged 65-74, and 2,100 for males and 1,810 for females aged 75+) because their lean-body-mass decreases and lifestyle becomes more sedentary. Older women also need less iron (at 8.7 mg/day compared with 14.8 mg in younger women) due to cessation of periods. Most people, however, will require dietary vitamin D, the RNI for which is set at 10 µg/day for people over 65.

■ Energy and nutrients

Energy requirements decline slightly with age as body metabolism slows down; but, in general, the requirements for the micro-nutrients don't. This can pose a problem, as absorption of some of the vitamins and minerals seems to decrease in older people, added to which many of the elderly are on prescription drugs, which can also hinder absorption.

This means that, if deficiencies aren't to occur, food needs to be selected carefully on the reduced-calorie diet that the average older person will eat.

Fat, protein and carbohydrate can be eaten in similar proportion to that of younger adults (see pages 170-71), with up to 35% calories from fat, up to 15% from protein and the balance made up from carbohydrates.

■ Vitamin D

The National Diet and Nutrition Survey: People aged 65 and over (second edition 2001) revealed that the majority of older people lack enough vitamin D in their diet. Vitamin D is vital to maintain bone health in the elderly. In younger adults, this vitamin is obtained via sunlight on the skin, but older people tend to go out in the sunlight less often, and absorption through the skin may also be less efficient. For these reasons, for those aged 65 plus, vitamin D needs to be taken in the diet. 10μg a day is recommended, an amount it is hard to get in a normal diet, so a daily supplement (e.g. a spoonful of cod liver oil) may be needed. Good dietary sources are margarine, eggs and fatty fish.

▪ Nutritional problems in the elderly

Many older people in the UK suffer nutritional deficiencies, because their eating habits differ considerably from younger people. People over 65 eat considerably less fish, fruit, vegetables, meat and cheese than younger affluent adults, but considerably more bakery goods, including cakes and biscuits, many more beverages and twice the amount of sugar.

According to some surveys, main areas of deficiency seem to be the B vitamins, especially vitamins B6, B12 and folate. There may also be deficiencies in the over-65s in magnesium and potassium; while some older people are likely to be deficient in vitamin C, iron and beta-carotene.

We look at the reasons why the diets of many elderly people are inadequate and offer solutions (right).

▪ Keeping the diseases of age at bay

Over 60% of new cancers occur in people aged 65 plus, and a similar proportion of new cases of CHD and stroke. This means that following the kind of diet which can help to prevent these ills, or minimize their effects, is well worth while, whether one is 40 or 80. Briefly, this means a diet high in antioxidants, fresh fruits and vegetables, plant oils, fibre and oily fish, and low in animal fats. Weight should also be watched. For more information see pages 96 and 118.

TYPICAL EATING HABITS AND HEALTHY SOLUTIONS

Eating habits	Reasons	Problems this may exacerbate	Solutions
High sugar	Easy to eat, tasty, low-cost long shelf-life, no cooking	Weight gain and associated symptoms, e.g. high blood pressure, deficiency in nutrients,* dental problems	Nutrition education, supplements, dental advice
Low-fibre processed foods	Easy to chew and swallow; low-cost	Deficiency in vitamins, minerals, fibre. Constipation, piles, increased risk of bowel cancer	See Easy Eats, (overleaf)
Narrow range of foods	Habit; fear of change, lack of interest in food, loss of appetite; shopping difficulties	Nutritional deficiencies, possible deficiency in energy intake (under-weight)	See Easy Eats and Store-cupboard Stand-bys (overleaf)
High-fat diet	Low-cost, easy to eat, habit, frying cheaper than baking or grilling	Deficiency in nutrients,** obesity, increased risk of CHD/stroke	More bread and potatoes, use reduced-fat items,** exercise if appropriate
Low on fruits and vegetables	Expense, shopping/ storage problems, can be hard to chew/ swallow/digest	Deficiencies in vitamins, e.g. C and beta-carotene, fibre. Constipation; piles; increased risk of CHD; some cancers	Long-life fruit juices, dried apricots, baked beans; see also Easy Eats (overleaf)

* A diet high in sugars and fats means there is less 'room' for other more nutritious foods, unless the person overeats and then obesity will be a problem.

** See Section Four for advice on swapping high-fat foods for lower-fat foods. Slim or thin elderly people can eat a higher-fat diet, but should include more plant fats in their diets e.g. vegetable oils for cooking rather than lard.

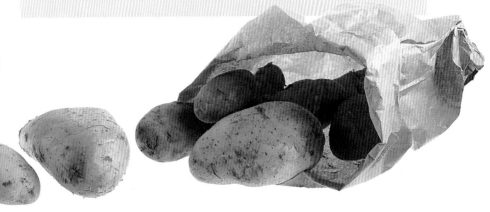

There is evidence that the immune system becomes weaker in old age, which may also lessen immunity against cancer — a diet high in zinc (see page 31 for rich sources list) will help to boost the immune system.

Osteoporosis: adequate calcium (perhaps with supplements, especially for women, who are four times more prone to osteoporosis than men) and vitamin D intake will help to prevent or minimize osteoporosis, which can result in hip and other fractures in the elderly. Smoking is a major factor in loss of bone-density in post-menopausal women — it increases the risk of hip fracture by an amazing 50%. (Smoking before the menopause, however, has little effect.) Body weight is also a factor — thin people are at greater risk of bone fractures. Lack of exercise also increases the risk — if possible, a regular walk will help keep bone-mass intact.

Alzheimer's disease: this is dealt with in full on page 90 but, briefly, research indicates that a Mediterranean-type diet high in antioxidants and essential fats, fruit and veg, and low in saturates (similar to the Healthy Heart Diet on

page 142) may help stall the progress of the disease.

Alcohol: as with younger adults, there is no harm in older people drinking in moderation. All the advice about alcohol (see pages 66 and 86)

STORECUPBOARD STANDBYS

Low-cost storecupboard items —
* Canned sardines, tuna, mackerel, rollmop herrings.
* Canned beans, pulses, carrots, tomatoes.
* Canned fruits.
* Long-life milk, cream, custard, yoghurt.
* Part-baked bread.

Concentrated sources of energy and nutrients —
* For protein and calcium: milk, cheese, eggs, yoghurt, custard.
* For vitamin C: fruit juice.
* For iron, B vitamins: red meat, eggs.
* For calories: full-fat milk, Cheddar, cream cheese, eggs, whole-milk yoghurt, red meat, oily fish.

EASY EATS

For people needing to increase their intake of fruits and vegetables —
* Cooked purées of vegetables, such as swede, parsnip, turnip, carrot, with other vegetables mixed in as appropriate, e.g. peas, spinach, shredded cabbage.
* Canned tomatoes.
* Raw purées of fruits, skinned if necessary, and icing sugar added as necessary, sieved - e.g. strawberries, raspberries, peaches.
* Fruit juices, long-life if necessary.
* Canned fruit salad.
* Baked or stewed fruits — e.g. cooking apples, pears, in season.
* Vegetables added to casseroles and stews.

For people needing to increase their intake of fibre —
* Baked beans on toast or on mashed potato.
* Canned pulses added to casseroles and stews or puréed with meat.
* Ready-to-eat dried apricots.
* Canned stewed prunes or rhubarb.
* Extra fluids to make the extra fibre 'work'.

FISH PIE USING OILY FISH LIKE TUNA, WITH A TOMATO SAUCE, ADDED PULSES AND VEGETABLES, AND MASHED POTATO TOPPING, MAKES EXCELLENT FARE.

applies to older people, although as body-mass and total body fluid content decrease with age, alcohol tolerance may also decrease. It makes sense, if necessary, to drink alcohol in later years at the minimum end of the safety guidelines rather than the maximum, especially if alcohol is bought at the expense of other, nutritious foods.

See also: Alzheimer's Disease (page 90) and Arthritis (page 93).

SAMPLE 3-DAY DIET FOR AN ELDERLY PERSON

This plan represents an ideal food intake for a female aged 75+, assuming she is of reasonable body weight. All portions are medium unless otherwise stated. Overweight females could choose lower-fat versions of the foods marked with a*. Males in the age range could increase portion sizes and add an extra snack a day.

Every day

Allowance of semi-skimmed or full-fat milk * of 250 ml (8 fl oz). Unlimited water, diluted fruit juices. Several cups of tea or coffee allowed a day, with milk from allowance and sugar unless obese. Unlimited salad items, fruits and vegetables in addition to those listed, although the amounts listed should be adequate for provision for vitamin C, fibre, etc.
* Butter if used instead of margarine, have 1 dessertspoon cod liver oil daily.

DAY ONE

Breakfast
glass of orange juice
medium bowl of porridge made with half
milk* and water
milk from allowance to cover
sprinkling of sugar or golden syrup
1 slice of brown bread from cut loaf, with
margarine and jam or marmalade

Light meal
(lunchtime or evening, as preferred)
2 medium eggs scrambled with milk and a
little margarine on 1 slice brown bread from a
cut loaf, toasted. (Chopped tomato stirred in
towards end of cooking, if liked.)
OR
hard-boiled egg and tomato sandwich
1 medium banana

Main meal
(lunchtime or evening as preferred)
chicken casserole made with chopped
tomatoes, tomato purée, chicken stock and
onion
frozen peas
baked potato
thick and creamy fruit yoghurt*

Snack
toasted teacake with margarine
grapes or apple

DAY TWO

Breakfast
glass of orange juice
1-2 Weetabix with milk from allowance
and sugar
1 slice of brown bread from cut loaf with
margarine and jam or marmalade

Light meal (as before)
medium bowlful of ready-made or home-
made lentil soup (preferably green or brown)
1 small roll
OR
baked beans on toast
portion of strawberries with single cream*
and sugar or 1 satsuma with a small piece of
Cheddar cheese

Main meal (as before)
1 portion of cod in butter sauce (ready-made,
frozen)
potato mashed with milk from allowance and
margarine
portion of frozen green beans or spinach
banana, runny honey and single cream*

Snack
handful of ready-to-eat stoned prunes
slice of bread and Marmite

DAY THREE

Breakfast
glass of orange juice
1 boiled egg
2 slices of brown toast, with margarine and
jam or marmalade

Light meal (as before)
sandwich of 2 slices of brown bread with
margarine
filled with canned sardines OR tuna in oil,
drained, plus cress and cucumber if liked
fruit yoghurt

Main meal (as before)
minced lamb* stewed with ready-prepared
stewpack vegetables, lamb stock and tomato
purée, dried pasta shapes added for last 15
minutes of cooking time
carrots
stewed apples and custard

Snack
small slice of fruit cake
grapes or apple

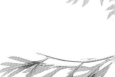

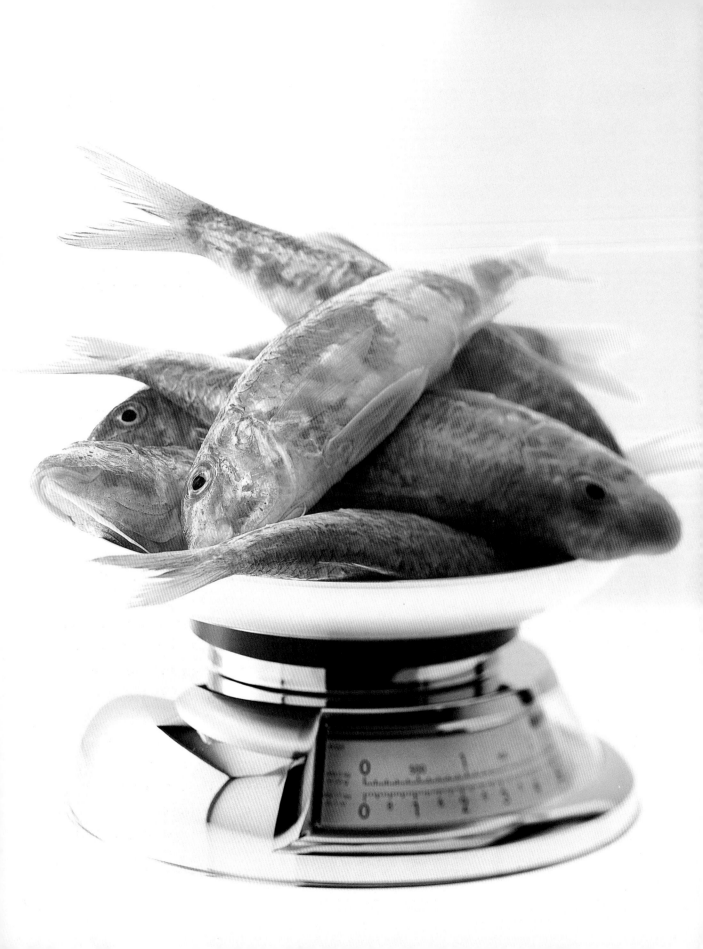

Food for weight control

Average weight in the Western world is on the increase and has been since the 1950s. In the UK since 1980, the proportion of those clinically overweight has risen from 39% to 70% (men) and from 32% to 63% (women), according to a report by the Royal College of Physicians. Of those, one in five are clinically obese (severely overweight). Eight out of ten adults become overweight by their fifties and the average middle-aged man is almost two stones overweight. These figures are worrying because overweight and obesity are linked with many health problems and increased mortality. In fact, obesity has now been declared an endemic disease by the WHO and is recognized as one of the most common avoidable causes of death.

So, with all the health advice on offer, just why are so many of us overweight? It appears that we aren't actually eating any more calories per day than we were. However, we are much less active than we were, taking a third less exercise than we did in the 50s, largely because of a sharp decline in the amount of everyday physical chores. Our hobbies, too, have become more sedentary — we spend an average of four hours a day watching TV rather than walking or playing sport. Decreased activity means that we don't need as many calories — and yet we haven't reduced the amount we eat to compensate. So surplus food is stored as body fat.

The cure, therefore, is not only to eat fewer calories but also to take more exercise, which will redress the balance. It only takes relatively minor regular adjustment to the energy out/energy in balance to achieve steady and healthy weight-loss. In the following pages we will look at how best to achieve this; and will discuss the questions most often asked about diet and weight control.

We will also examine the problems of the minority of people (nevertheless representing millions) who have the opposite dilemma — how to put ON weight.

Your top 20 questions on weight control

To set the scene for this section, here we attempt to answer some of the questions most frequently asked about the whole vexed area of weight control. By doing so, we will to a large extent cover most of the background information you need to know to get to grips with the subject.

1 What is the accepted definition of being overweight?

There is a fairly broad band of 'acceptable weight' for your height, within which you're not, clinically, over- or underweight. The scale used by most professionals to determine acceptable weight is Body Mass Index (BMI). Your BMI is easy to work out with the formula:
BMI = Weight (kg) ÷ height (metres)^2.
The result is then interpreted as follows:
below 20 = underweight
20-25 = acceptable weight range
25-30 = clinically overweight
30-40 = clinically obese
over 40 = morbidly obese
The acceptable range of 20-25 allows, for example, a woman of 1.65 metres (5ft 6in) to weigh anything between 54.5kg (8st 8lb) and 68kg (10st 10lb). An acceptable maximum weight for health, then, is higher than many people realize and means that many people who feel they are overweight aren't really, and a lot of people trying to diet may be having difficulty because they're aiming too low.

Another good indication of genuine overweight is the 'waist circumference' test, because surplus weight around the waist ('central fat distribution') is more likely to be linked with health problems (particularly CHD and non-insulin-dependent diabetes) than surplus weight around the hips, bottom and thighs.

A waist measurement of less than 94cm (37½in) for men and 80cm (32in) for women is all right, from 94cm-101cm (37½-40½in) and 80-87cm (32-34¾in)

respectively indicates further weight gain should be avoided and perhaps weight should be lost; and over 101cm (40½in) and 87cm (34¾in) indicates weight should be lost. If you are 'borderline' on the BMI system (say, just on or over 25), then the waist circumference theory may help you decide, or vice versa.

2 How can I be overweight when I don't overeat?

There is this common idea that overweight people are greedy, but in most cases that is far from the truth. Most people lead fairly sedentary life-styles and calorie (energy) needs may not be great. Eating just a small amount more than those needs will result in a slow but steady weight increase.

For example, the DoH says that an average woman needs 1,940 calories a day to maintain a reasonable weight. Eating just 100 calories a day more than her needs (represented, say, by a banana or one large chocolate biscuit) will result (all other factors being equal) in an annual weight gain of 4.7kg (10lb)!

As we get older, our metabolic rate also slows down a little very gradually (see Q 5), which can result in slow weight-gain in people aged 30 plus.

3 Couldn't my weight problem be due to some reason other than overeating — perhaps hereditary?

'It's my genes!' is an 'excuse' for overweight that doctors have been listening to — with some degree of

scepticism — for years. Now more research is being done to indicate that the tendency to put on weight can certainly be inherited.

After extensive research on twins, it is now known that body-fat distribution is at least 60% inherited (meaning that most people are stuck with their basic body shape and 'fat profile' for life). It also seems possible that our genes control other factors in the weight balancing act, such as how well our body responds to exercise. One leading UK obesity expert says that 25% of obesity may be caused by 'minor gene defects'.

However, all this doesn't mean that it is impossible to stay a reasonable size, even if you have more trouble staying slim than most. What it does mean is balancing your own equation — more exercise, less calories — until you reach a weight that is acceptable. This may be heavier than that considered normal for other people.

In the future it may be possible to reprogram 'faulty' genes so staying slim is no longer a problem. Californian scientists have already isolated a gene (UCP2) that helps burn off excess calories rather than allowing them to convert to fat. Work is also currently being done on the hormone leptin, the product of a defective gene in obese mice.

Lastly it should be pointed out that many people with no inherited tendency to put on weight easily do still get fat, simply by not balancing their energy in/energy out equation correctly (see Q 2).

4 Could I have a slow metabolism?

A lot of overweight people believe that their problem lies in a slow metabolic rate — that they burn up calories slower than slim people. In fact, the opposite is normally true. The most important factor governing energy metabolism is how big you are — the heavier a body is, the more work it has to do, the faster its metabolic rate and the greater its calorie needs. That is why a sixteen-stone woman needs much more to eat than a nine-stone woman in order to maintain weight. Once the sixteen-stone woman begins to lose weight, her metabolic rate will gradually slow down and, if she slims down to nine stone, her metabolic rate (other factors being equal) will be similar to the always-slim nine-stone woman.

However, a small percentage of people do have an underactive thyroid gland, which controls the metabolism. A blood test can diagnose the problem.

5 Isn't it natural to put on weight as you get older?

Our basal metabolic rate (the rate at which we burn up calories when doing no physical activity at all) does very gradually begin to slow down over the years once we reach the age of thirty or so. It is estimated that for every five years older than 30 we are, we need to consume about 50 calories a day less in order to maintain the weight we were then. That means by the age of 60, if you haven't reduced your daily calorie intake to about 300 calories a day less than at 30, you will have slowly put on weight. (After sixty, body fat percentage tends to slowly decrease again, naturally.)

Part of the reason for this slow-down is that we lose lean tissue mass (muscle) as we age. Muscle is more metabolically active than fat and other body tissue. Another reason is that we tend to use up less energy in activity as the years go by. There is also some natural slowing down through the ageing process itself.

The only way to stop or minimize this slowing down of the metabolism is to increase the amount of exercise that you do, and include toning/strengthening exercise to keep muscle mass. It can be done — but, it seems, few manage it.

For your health's sake, a few pounds or even a stone on your slim early-adulthood weight won't harm you, as long as you eat healthily and stay as fit (although plenty of new research indicates that calorie restriction is a key to longer life). Trying to maintain the very slim weight of your youth may be an unrealistic target.

6 I am fat — and happy with my size. Why should I change?

The feminist and politically correct movements have done much in recent years to persuade many overweight people that they shouldn't bow to what they see as social pressure to lose weight. Many overweight people take fitness tests, come through well and see no reason to change. However, the overwhelming majority of evidence demonstrates quite clearly that a high BMI (particularly over 30) is a major cause of ill-health, disease and early death. When people are young and overweight these risks are less evident, and of course there will always be some obese people who live healthy, happy and long lives.

7 So what is the best diet to follow in order to lose weight?

The best diet is one that hardly seems like a diet at all – one where you have a varied diet and at least three meals a day, plus snacks. It needs to be healthy, containing all the major nutrients, fibre and so on. As a rough guide, for men 1,500-1,750 calories a day and for women 1,250-1,500 calories a day are suitable. Very overweight or very active people will be able to eat more than that and still lose weight, particularly if activity levels are stepped up.

8 How do I lose weight quickly?

All recent research has come to the same conclusion — that there is no fast-track to permanent weight loss. There are three main reasons for this. One, in order to stick with a diet, it needs to contain enough calories to ensure you don't feel hungry, get bored or over-restricted in what you can eat. On these calorie levels, you can't lose weight quickly, but it has been shown those who allow themselves a more generous amount of calories do better at weight-loss long-term.

Two, in order to get all the nutrients you need while losing weight, you need a reasonable amount of food, again, meaning you can't lose weight quickly.

Three, there is considerable research to show that people who lose weight quickly are more likely to put the weight back on again, or become serial 'yo-yo' dieters, than those who lose it slowly. There is also some research to show that people who crash-diet are more prone to depression and poorer mental function.

9 Should I count calories or just cut fat?

In effect, the two come to the same thing. In order to lose weight, you have to create a calorie 'deficit', burning up more energy (calories) than you take in as food. On a good calorie-counting diet you will cut down on the high-calorie foods, things like cakes, pastries, desserts, fatty meats, mayonnaise, sugar, alcohol, and so on.

There is no point in cutting down on low-calorie foods like fruit and vegetables, because they are healthy foods your body needs. Neither is there any point cutting out the starchy carbohydrates, such as bread, potatoes, pasta and rice, as these are also healthy foods, although if counting calories you may cut down on portion-size a little.

On a good fat-cutting diet, you will reduce calorie intake by simply avoiding the foods you know to be high in fat, like cream cheese, pastries and fatty meat.

10 Would I have more success on one of the more specialized diets, such as a high-protein one, or the Hay system (food combining)?

There is an appraisal of some of the most popular dieting methods on pages 202–3. For most people, a high-protein diet is not to be recommended for health reasons. There is no scientific evidence to back up the theories behind food combining. More than any fad diet, you need a plan you enjoy and to which you will therefore stick. Two popular diets which are healthy and which do work for many people are the low Glycaemic Index diet (see page 195) and a Mediterranean-style diet (similar to the one on page 142). In one large recent Spanish study, 3,000 adults on Med-style diets found it easier to keep weight off and there was a 40% reduction in obesity.

11 What can I do to control hunger pangs when I diet?

Habit can often be mistaken for hunger — we tend to eat before real hunger manifests itself, if the clock tells us we should eat. If that isn't the case, however, and you follow the guidelines above for sensible slimming (and the Four-week Retraining Programme on page 192), hunger shouldn't be a problem.

Cutting calories by only a little will help prevent hunger, as will following a diet high in foods that have a low Glycaemic Index. More about these appears on pages 194-5, but basically they are carbohydrate foods which have a high 'satiety value' because they are broken down into blood sugars more slowly than other carb foods and keep you feeling full for longer than foods with a high GI. These include pasta, pulses, oats, citrus fruits and natural yoghurt. Each meal should also include a little fat and some protein, both of which have a similar effect on slowing down food absorption as low-GI foods. A diet high in natural fibre will also help control hunger pangs.

Women often feel hungrier in the week before their period. This is a natural occurrence, and such women should eat a little more (healthy foods) at this time, if necessary, reverting to a maintenance diet rather than a slimming diet.

12 What can I do to control specific food cravings, e.g., for chocolate?

A small amount of any food can be included in a healthy diet and so there is no need to give up completely foods you enjoy. Sugary foods can be eaten after a meal. A small bar of chocolate or a chocolate mousse dessert, for instance, after a healthy low-fat main course would be fine, even on a slimming diet.

It is important, when slimming, not to miss meals, go long periods without food or indulge in over-strict calorie control. This could result in low blood-sugar levels producing cravings for sweet and/or high-carbohydrate foods, such as chocolate or biscuits, with the effect of very quickly raising the blood sugar. Such a craving shouldn't be indulged with a sugary snack, though, as excess insulin may be released to cope with the sugary influx and the result may be an even lower dip in blood sugar levels — and another craving for more sweet food!

The way to get off this 'yo-yo' of crave-indulge-crave is to eat regular small meals high in healthy and low glycaemic index foods (see Q 11). These keep blood sugar levels on a more even keel and cravings at bay. Ensure every meal also includes small amounts of protein.

13 Are there any special foods that will help me burn up fat?

Whole books have been written about so-called 'fat-burning' foods, which are said to release enzymes that burn up fat, and whole books have also been written about 'miracle' foods that take more calories to digest than they provide in the first place. Sadly, however, neither theory holds up under scientific examination.

14 So is there any short-cut way to lose weight without dieting?

Unless by surgery (as in liposuction, for example, where melted fat is sucked out of your body), the answer at the moment is no — however many mail-shots you receive telling you otherwise.

Prescription drugs that dull the appetite can help you lose weight, but most doctors will only supply these as a last resort and strict guidelines now apply to their use (and you still need to diet). In the USA, a new pill called Orlistat has been produced (and is awaiting USFDA approval) which causes 30% of the fat in the diet to be excreted without absorption and there are said to be no major safety issues, but side-effects can be unpleasant and vitamin absorption can be affected. It may soon be available on prescription in the UK.

15 How can I eat out and still lose weight?

Much of what you eat when you lunch or dine out isn't really essential to the spirit of the occasion, and that is the best attitude to take if work or a busy social life means that you have to eat out a great deal. If you only eat out occasionally, simply cut back a little for the rest of the day and enjoy yourself, while attempting to eat sensibly.

The pages in Section One on healthy eating out (page 64-5) are useful to provide more background information.

16 How can I stick to a diet when I miss my favourite foods too much?

The re-training programme on the following pages will help you to adapt to healthy tastes. For instance, high-fat savoury foods are often also high in salt — e.g. cheeses, crackers, crisps, savoury snacks and pies. It takes only two weeks to train your taste-buds into disliking high-salt foods. High-sugar foods are often also high in calories and fat — yet, again, it takes only weeks to train yourself to find them far too sweet.

If your favourite foods are things other than those high in sugar and salt, then they can almost certainly form part of your healthy slimming diet. If the re-training approach doesn't suit you, then another method of incorporating favourite foods into a diet is to allow yourself a certain number of 'treat' calories a day and use these up on whatever you like. So that this doesn't lead to a binge, see Q 12.

17 Are the new calorie-free fat products a good idea?

Fat substitutes such as Olestra are used instead of fat in traditionally high-fat foods like ice-creams, desserts, cakes and biscuits. Because of the way Olestra is formulated, the body doesn't absorb it and so calories are saved.

Olestra has been permitted in several products in the USA but not, at the moment, in the UK. This is because of possible depletion of the fat-soluble vitamins A, D, E and K, and carotenoids, and possible side-effects such as loose stools and anal leakage.

Olestra is a sucrose polyester, but other types of fat substitute are also available. Simplesse is made from milk protein and used in a wide range of products for a smooth, creamy taste. It is not calorie-free but, at just over l calorie per gram, is much lower in calories than fat (9 calories a gram) or sugar (3.75 calories a gram). Various other products are available in various countries and more of these fat substitutes are likely to appear in our foods all the time.

There is, though, some evidence that, overall, such highly processed low-fat products don't help us to eat any less or indeed to stay slim, because of their low content of essential fatty acids — natural oils found in plants and fish. This may apply to processed low-fat products in general, not just those containing fat substitutes.

18 Why does weight-loss slow down after a while on a slimming regime?

In the short term, this is because when you begin a slimming diet in the first week or two you will lose several pounds of weight which are fluid, not fat. After this, weight loss will be mostly fat.

For long-term slimmers, the main reason is that when you lose weight, your metabolic rate gradually slows down simply because you are getting smaller. As explained in Q 4, when you are overweight you will have been eating more than average to maintain that weight. For example, a woman of 12 stone may well have been eating 2,500 calories or so a day rather than the 'average' of 1,940. All she needs to do is cut down to, say, 1,750 calories a day for a daily 'deficit' of 750 calories, which will result in a weekly weight loss of 1½ pounds. At ten stone, however, she will be a fairly average weight and a daily diet of 1,750 calories is only slightly under the normal calorie intake (1,940) for a woman of her weight. To continue with good weight-loss, a diet of, say, 1,250 calories a day would be more appropriate. That would result in a daily calorie deficit of 690 calories and a loss of just under 1½ pounds a week.

For weight-loss to continue at a steady rate throughout any diet, therefore, you need gradually to cut the calorie content of the diet accordingly. In practical terms it is probably best to be happy with slower weight-loss as you near target-weight and to increase your exercise levels a little to compensate.

Other reasons why weight-loss may slow down are that you have reached a reasonable body weight (you may have been aiming too low; check your BMI) or that you have begun eating more calories again — check your diet carefully. Also, weight does fluctuate from day to day and week to week for a variety of reasons, including hormones, fluid levels, etc. Most women in the week before a

period won't lose weight at all and may indeed put a little on; this will disappear within days of the start of menstruation.

19 How often should I weigh myself?

As we've seen in Q 18, weight does fluctuate on a daily — and sometimes weekly — basis and so frequent scale-hopping is not advised as the results may not present a true picture. For men, a weekly weigh-in is plenty. For women of menstruating age, it is probably more sensible to limit the weigh-in to once a month, directly after a period.

20 Why is maintaining a new slim body so hard?

It is true that, often, keeping weight off is harder than losing it in the first place. Research indicates that a high percentage of successful dieters do, eventually, put the weight back on again. However, this seems more to do with social, lifestyle and psychological factors rather than being, as so many people believe, a consequence of dieting having artificially lowered the metabolism.

Research at the UK's leading centre for research into obesity, the Dunn Clinical Nutrition Centre, clearly demonstrated that people who were once overweight and who slim down, have a similar metabolic rate to other people of the same (slim) weight who have never been fat.

However, a slim person's basal metabolic rate, as explained in Qs 4 and 18, is always going to be lower than that of an overweight person. In other words, once you are slim, you can't eat as much as you did when you were fat. People who do manage to keep weight off long-term seem to be those who followed a sensible healthy diet to lose the weight slowly, including behaviour modification and exercise, and who continue to eat healthily and take regular exercise once target weight is reached.

Four-week retraining course

For all those people who have battled with their weight for some time, yet another quick-fix diet really isn't ever going to be the answer... but this easy-to-follow four-week eating retraining course could be just what is needed to change things for good.

The four-week course is designed so that by the end of it most people will have little trouble in sticking to a healthy reduced-calorie programme until they are down to a reasonable weight. Each week we will examine different aspects of eating for weight control, including strategies for behaviour modification and practical dietary advice.

At the end of the four weeks, two diet plans are laid out as a sample of how you could be eating to slim.

For the course, all you will need is enough time to give to the programme, a notebook, and a degree of enthusiasm! Once the course is over and whenever you have reached a suitable weight, the Basic Healthy Diet and all the information in Section One will help you to maintain that weight; along with the behaviour modification you will learn in the four-week course.

Week one – getting started

Goals for the week:
* Read Section One and understand what makes a healthy diet.
* Decide on sensible targets.
* Check out motivation (see box on the right).
* Cut calories and fat in snack foods.

If you have tried, and failed, to lose weight on various 'fad' or 'crash' diets in the past, don't be deterred. The basis of any good weight-loss diet is varied and healthy eating. Any diet which isn't

based on such principles is likely to fail, certainly in the long term.

During Week One, don't think about 'dieting' as such at all. All you need to do is read through Section One and spend the week preparing practically and mentally to begin adjusting your eating accordingly. Sort out your larder and shop for a healthier range of foods; look through the recipe section and find a few recipes that appeal to your taste-buds. Try one or two.

Meanwhile, also work out your own BMI (see Question 1, page 188), work out what weight will achieve a sensible BMI, then decide on a sensible time-scale for achieving your ideal BMI.

Example: you are 1.65 m (5ft 6in) tall and 75.5 kg (12 stone) now with a BMI of 28. You decide you will be happy with a BMI of 24, which will be achieved when you weigh 64.8 kg (10 stone 4lb). You have 11 kg (24lb) to lose. You can adjust this target later — a good gauge of being a reasonable size is the waist circumference test (Question 1, page 188).

You lead a busy lifestyle and eat out regularly, so it would be sensible to achieve that weight-loss slightly more slowly than average. Allowing 0.5-1.5 kg (1-1½ lb) a week loss on average it will take you 16-24 weeks to achieve.

FACT:

To gain 0.5 kg (1 pound) of weight you need to eat around 3,500 calories more than you need. That is represented by just seven standard chocolate snack bars and seven bags of crisps.

■ Take a look at your snacking habits.

One major cause of slow-but-sure weight-gain is wayward snacking habits. We live in an era when grabbing food on the run has become normal; busy lives mean that it seems easier to eat a pie or bag of crisps than bother with healthier food. On other occasions, a quick snack fills a gap between meals and we don't stop to consider what a large contribution such items can make to the total calories in the diet. Just one unwise snack a day could put over half a pound on your waistline every week — and do more damage to a slimming diet than

MOTIVATING YOURSELF

Use this week to complete a list of all the reasons why you would like to be a reasonable body weight. Divide them into health reasons (check the index for all the ailments linked with overweight), practical reasons (e.g. getting into favourite clothes, being able to do your favourite sport better) and social and other reasons. Most people should be able to come up with a list of at least twenty reasons they would like to lose weight.

If you have tried and failed previously to lose weight and/or keep it off, agree with the following three statements:
* I didn't fail on past diets, the diets failed me.
* I will not dwell on my past disappointments.
* Now I am willing to take responsibility for what I eat.

you may think. Take a look at your snacking habits — use your notebook to write a list of all the 'non-meal' foods you eat this week. Analyse your reasons for eating that particular food (e.g., nothing else available when hungry, speed, ease of eating) and think of better alternatives for each occasion.

However, don't try to give up snacks altogether; simply swap them for better alternatives. One or two small but nutritious 'mini-meals' a day will help to keep hunger at bay (see Week 2) and will provide useful nutrients. Ten low-calorie, yet filling, snacks are listed below. Fresh fruits, dried fruits and small amounts of shelled raw nuts are always easy to eat — plan ahead and carry some with you.

The box on the right shows three examples of how high in calories snack foods can be. Most are high-calorie because they are high in fat (and sometimes sugar) and yet, because you don't think of them as a 'meal' (and neither should you because useful

nutrient content tends to be low), they are eaten as 'extras'. Instead of each of the snacks — eaten in a few mouthfuls — you could have a complete slimmer's meal, as the illustration shows.

Alternatively, for many calories less, you could have a more balanced snack that would fit in well with a reduced-calorie diet. (See the Ten Low-calorie Healthy Breakfasts box below.)

CALORIES AND FATS IN COMMON SNACKS

High-calorie snack	Low-calorie slimmer's meal
1 standard Mars bar (65g)	1 medium banana; 50 g (1¾oz) ready-to-eat dried peaches; 1 dark rye crispbread spread with 15 g (½oz) Tartex yeast pâté, with herbs
295 calories and 11.4 g fat	229 calories and 6g fat
1 buffet size pork pie	1 x 50 g (1¾oz) wholemeal roll; 22 g (¾oz) Camembert cheese; 80 g (2⅞oz) homemade coleslaw (made using 40g white cabbage, 10g each grated carrot and onion; 5 g sultanas and 1 tablespoon 70% fat-free mayonnaise); 75 g (2¾oz) tomato, cucumber and celery salad; 1 small red apple
275 calories and 20 g fat	275 calories and 8 g fat
1 x 50 g bag of dry roasted salted peanuts	Sandwich of 2 slices of bread from a large sliced wholemeal loaf spread with 7 g (¼oz) low fat spread; 1 small hard-boiled egg, sliced; 10 g (³⁄₈oz) 70% fat-free mayonnaise; plenty of salad greens and sliced tomato
295 calories and 24g fat	265 calories and 10.5 g fat

TEN LOW-CALORIE HEALTHY SNACKS
(All around 100-150 calories each and none contains more than 6g fat.)

* 2 dark rye crispbreads spread with 25 g (¾oz) hummus; 1 satsuma.
* 1 small slice of whole-grain bread with a little low-fat spread and Marmite; 5 ready-to-eat dried apricot halves.
* 1 small pot of bio yoghurt; 10 g (¼oz) chopped walnuts.
* 1 traditional oatcake; 1 apple.
* 6 shelled almonds; 1 kiwi fruit, 1 plum.
* 1 orange; 1 Weetabix with skimmed milk.
* Ready-made fresh fruit salad; 1 small pot of bio yoghurt.
* 1 small banana; 1 dark rye crispbread with 1 tablespoon cottage cheese.
* Portion of Baba Ganoush (page 215) with mini pitta
* Mango and Peach Booster (page 253).

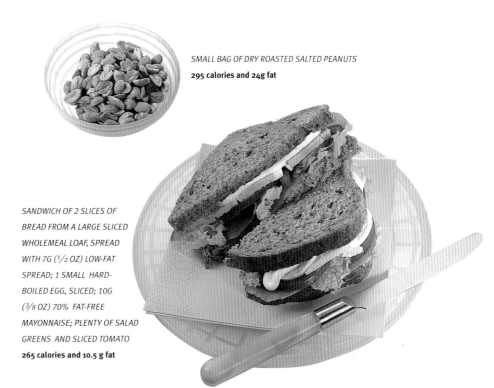

SMALL BAG OF DRY ROASTED SALTED PEANUTS
295 calories and 24g fat

SANDWICH OF 2 SLICES OF BREAD FROM A LARGE SLICED WHOLEMEAL LOAF, SPREAD WITH 7G (½ OZ) LOW-FAT SPREAD; 1 SMALL HARD-BOILED EGG, SLICED; 10G (³⁄₈ OZ) 70% FAT-FREE MAYONNAISE; PLENTY OF SALAD GREENS AND SLICED TOMATO
265 calories and 10.5 g fat

Week two – taking control

Goals for the Week:

* Learn that you — and only you — have control over what you eat, despite outside influences.
* Learn how to avoid hunger while reducing your overall calorie intake.
* Start retraining your taste-buds to like less salt.
* Examine your breakfast eating habits.
* Begin to build more activity into your life.

If you want to be slimmer, you need to control your food intake. Nobody else can do that for you. Though often it does seem that almost everyone is trying to influence what, when, where and how much you eat, and it is for precisely that reason that you need to make that positive decision that you are going to eat what YOU want, what is good for YOU.

This week, take note of every time you are offered food or drink that you hadn't planned on eating. You'll be surprised how often it happens. You'll also be surprised how the typical reaction is to accept the food.

This week, start to say 'no' to food you don't want, food you don't need and food that isn't going to do your body much good. Keep a diary and note your achievements.

Also take note of how many times during the week you eat something you hadn't intended to eat because hunger

FACT:

If you removed from your diet all food that you didn't actually eat through genuine hunger and pre-planned decision, most people would save enough calories in a week to lose weight steadily without doing one other thing.

THE ANTI-HUNGER FOODS

Many people dislike the idea of slimming because they fear hunger. In fact, on a sensible diet such as that outlined in the answer to Question 11 on page 190, hunger is much less likely to be a problem than on faddy diets or diets too low in calories.

An anti-hunger diet, just like a normal healthy diet, will contain plenty of complex carbohydrates, adequate protein and some fat. A normal non-slimming diet should contain 30-35% fat; a slimming diet can reduce this to around 25%, the rest of the diet being made up from up to 20% protein and 55% carbohydrate. An extremely low-fat diet, such as is sometimes recommended, can exacerbate hunger and is also very impractical to follow.

Importantly, a hunger-free diet will contain plenty of the carbohydrate foods that have a low Glycaemic Index. The Glycaemic Index was invented to help professionals treat diabetics and it measures the rate at which blood glucose levels rise when a particular carbohydrate food is eaten. Given that glucose itself has a GI rating of 100, then the nearer to 100 a food's rating is, the quicker it will be absorbed, and the lower a food's rating is the slower it will be absorbed. Foods with a low GI rating will help you to feel full for longer than high-GI foods and will help keep your blood sugar levels constant.

Protein and fat aren't measured on the glycaemic index, but both have the effect of lowering a food's GI rating when eaten at the same time, which is why each meal and snack that you eat should contain a small to moderate amount of protein and a small amount of fat. See the Glycaemic Index, opposite.

has taken you by surprise. Most high-fat snack foods are eaten this way. In the quest to control your own eating, it helps to plan ahead as much as you can. Decide where and what you're going to eat in advance. Make sure you are well stocked up with healthy easy-to-prepare food items so that you aren't tempted by others.

Lastly, take note of all the times that you eat simply because food is there in front of you — reasons of habit and availability (e.g. in the newsagents, while you are preparing food for others). This all, too, is food you don't really need. When you have time on your hands, food 'surplus to requirements' can easily find its way into your mouth. Waiting on a station and

the train is late, you get a chocolate bar from the vending machine; sitting at home waiting for guests to arrive, you nibble at a bowl of salted nuts.

BOILED EGG; 1 SLICE OF WHOLE-GRAIN BREAD WITH A LITTLE LOW-FAT SPREAD;

■ Salt reduction

Most of us eat much more salt than we need (see page 33) and many of the high-salt foods are also those that contain a lot of fat. In order to give your taste-buds a better chance to enjoy natural foods, you need to retrain them to need less salt. This is very easy to do.

✱ This week, stop adding salt to food at the table and cut down by half all the salt that you add in cooking. If you see low-salt versions of products you usually buy (e.g. baked beans), buy those instead.

■ Better breakfasts

Mid-morning can be difficult for many slimmers. Hunger pangs creep up and that doughnut can be very tempting. This is usually because many people skip breakfast when trying to lose weight.

As we saw in Section One, breakfast is important for everyone, but particularly so for weight control and avoidance of hunger. A sensible breakfast for slimmers will contain 250-300 calories a day and consist of some carbohydrate, some protein and a little fat. The following healthy low-calorie breakfasts will all keep hunger away until it is time for a 'legitimate' snack or lunch. Carbohydrate-only breakfasts, based on white or wholemeal bread and marmalade, are high-GI and should be avoided. This week improve your breakfast habits and their quality.

✱ 175 g (6oz) baked beans on 1 medium slice of whole-grain bread with a little low-fat spread.
✱ Half a grapefruit; low-fat natural yoghurt; teaspoon of fructose; medium slice of whole-grain bread with a little low-fat spread; yeast extract.
✱ Old-fashioned porridge oats made into porridge with skimmed milk and water; teaspoon of honey; orange or nectarine.
✱ Citrus fruit, apple and grape salad; low-fat yoghurt; 2 tablespoons of muesli.
✱ Boiled egg; 1 slice of rye bread with a little low-fat spread; apple.

■ Begin some exercise

Start doing a daily walk of at least 20 minutes. Try to build more activity into your normal routine, e.g. stair climbing, washing the car by hand, using the stairs rather than the lift. A slimming programme can't be successful long-term without regular exercise.

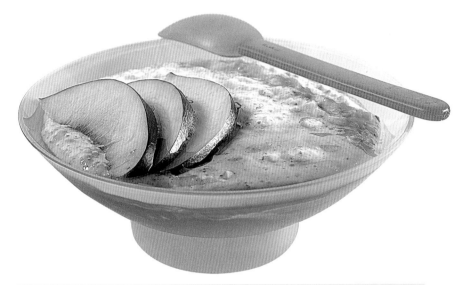

OLD-FASHIONED PORRIDGE MADE FROM ROLLED OATS WITH SKIMMED MILK AND WATER; TEASPOON OF HONEY; NECTARINE SLICES

THE GLYCAEMIC INDEX

Low-GI foods (long-term energy; try to include plenty of these in your diet):

All pulses including lentils, soya beans, kidney beans, chickpeas, butter beans,baked beans.
Barley.
Apples, dried apricots, peaches, grapefruit, plums, cherries.
Avocado, courgettes, spinach, peppers, onions, mushrooms, leafy greens, leeks, green beans, broad beans, Brussels sprouts, mange-tout peas, broccoli, cauliflower.
Natural yoghurt, sweetened yoghurt, milk, peanuts.

Medium-GI foods (medium-term energy; eat freely):

Sweet potatoes, boiled potatoes, yams, raw carrots, sweetcorn, peas.
White pasta, wholewheat pasta, oats, porridge, oatmeal biscuits, All Bran, noodles.
Whole-grain rye bread (pumpernickel), pitta bread, buckwheat, bulgar, white and brown rice.
Grapes, oranges, kiwi fruit, mangoes, beetroot, fresh dates, figs, apple-and-date bars.

High-GI foods (quick-release, short-term energy; eat as part of a meal containing protein/fat/low-GI foods):

Glucose, sugar, honey, pineapple, bananas, raisins, watermelon.
Baked potatoes, mashed potatoes, parsnips, cooked carrots, squash, swede.
Rye crispbreads, wholemeal bread, white bread, rice cakes, couscous, bread sticks.
Cornflakes, Bran Flakes, instant oat cereal, puffed cereal, popcorn, wheat crackers, muffins, crumpets.
Orange squash, watermelon, dried dates.

Week three – eating to slim

Goals of the week:

* Learn to listen to body signals about food.
* Build up a more detailed picture of how to cut calories sensibly.
* Retrain taste-buds to prefer less sugar.
* Look at your main meals and see how they can be re-balanced to provide fewer calories.
* Continue with exercise and control techniques.

If, for years, you have been eating from habit, overeating just because food is there, eating without paying attention to what you were doing, then this week you need to get back in touch with what your body is telling you about its needs.

Few of us actually feel genuine hunger any more — mealtimes and snack-times come around well before real hunger has time to set in. This week see if, instead of eating exactly by the clock, you can get that slightly hungry feeling before tucking in. If you find it is lunch-time and you don't have that hunger, but you can't eat later because of, say, your work, just have a little and save some more for mid-afternoon.

Few of us are truly in tune with the moment when we feel full and should stop eating. Instead, we just eat all that is on the plate because it is there, and usually there is more of it than we would genuinely need to satisfy hunger.

This week pay attention when you eat. Chew thoroughly, take your time — and decide to stop when you feel full enough. If you do this a few times and find you always have food left on your plate, give yourself smaller portions, especially of the high-fat foods.

If you don't override your body signals, soon you will get back in tune with your real needs and weight-loss should become much more natural.

■ Calorie-cutting without pain

By cutting surplus fat from the diet, in the form of high-fat snacks, high-fat meats, high-fat dairy produce and too much fat used in cooking, and by following the behaviour techniques you have learned so far, it is likely that you can be saving enough calories to effect a steady weight-loss without having to do much else. If that doesn't prove to be the case, though, sugars and alcohol should be cut next because these provide calories with virtually no nutrients.

You can retrain a sweet tooth in just the same way as a salty tooth — by gradually cutting back: firstly on sugar added to drinks and cereals, then on sweet drinks themselves, then on sugary items such as cakes, biscuits and confectionery. High-calorie desserts are best avoided by slimmers except now and then. Nutritious desserts based on fruit and low-fat dairy produce are ideal. Artificial sweeteners save calories by replacing sugar, but do little to help a sweet tooth long-term.

If calories still need to be saved you need, finally, to look at the amount of protein and starchy foods on your plate. An overall slight reduction in portion size can save enough calories in a day to make a difference.

Remember that many protein foods are also high in fat — cut these down first — and also remember not to add too much fat to carbohydrate foods — e.g., butter to a baked potato, and so on.

The chart on the right shows an ideal breakdown of a day's calorie and fat intake for two different slimming levels. A diet of about 1,250 calories a day, such as that on page 200, is suitable for people with less than a stone to lose, for most women, for small men and towards the end of a diet. A diet of about 1,500 calories a day, such as that on page 201, is suitable for people with a lot of weight to lose, for many men, and at the start of most diets.

There is no need to stick rigidly to these amounts (it would be very hard to do so anyway) but they provide a blueprint on which to build. Calorie and fat content of many foods is listed in the Food Charts at the end of the book and more information is contained in Section One. The recipes in Section Five are calorie- and fat-counted, too, and indicated suitable for slimmers as appropriate, to help you incorporate them into a slimming plan.

■ Salt

This week try to reduce salt in your diet further by cutting the amount you add while cooking to just a few grains. The addition of fresh herbs and spices may help you miss the salt less. Check out the list of high-salt foods on page 33 and start cutting back on the amount of those that you eat. In general, processed food contains a lot of salt.

DIET INTAKE LEVELS

1,250 calories a day

	Calories	Fat (g) *
Breakfast	250	5
Lunch	350	8
Main meal	350	12
Snack	100	5
Snack/Treat	100	5
Milk allowance	100	trace
	1,250	35

1,500 calories a day

	Calories	Fat (g)
Breakfast	300	6
Lunch	400	10
Main Meal	400	14
Snack	150	6
Snack/treat	150	6
Milk allowance	100	trace
	1,500	42

* based on 25% of total calorie intake.

CALORIE-CUTTING MAIN MEAL – CHICKEN

Chicken in the traditional manner

Chicken-leg portion, lean and skin, total weight 300 g (10¹/₂oz), edible portion 150 g (5oz), grilled; 125 g (4¹/₂oz) new potatoes; 10 g (¹/₂oz) butter; 115g (4oz) salad of lettuce, cucumber and tomato (50 g/1¹/₂oz) lettuce, 20 g/¹/₂oz cucumber, 40 g/1¹/₄oz tomato) ; 10 g (¹/₄oz) mayonnaise.

530 calories and 26g fat. Total weight of meal 410g (14¹/₂oz).

Chicken is a favourite with slimmers, but a typical weight-watcher's slimming chicken meal isn't always as low-calorie as it may seem. The meal described on the left looks innocent enough, with its small portion of potatoes and

Calorie-cutting chicken ★ ★ ★ ★ ★

1 portion of Lemon Chicken (page 230); 175 g (6oz), cooked weight, egg-thread noodles; 165 g (5¹/₂oz) mixed vegetables (50 g/1¹/₂oz carrot, 25 g/³/₄oz courgette, 20 g/¹/₂oz green beans, 50g/1¹/₂oz broccoli, 20 g/¹/₂oz beansprouts) stir-fried in 1 teaspoon of oil.

382 calories and 12g fat. Total weight of meal 470 g (1lb 1oz).

salad. In fact, it contains nearly one-third more calories than the bigger, and heavier, plateful on the right.

CALORIE-CUTTING MAIN MEAL – STEAK

High-calorie, high-fat steak meal

225 g (8oz) sirloin steak (including part-trimmed fat); 200 g (7oz) deep-fried frozen chips; 50 g (1³/₄oz) fried mushrooms; 50 g (1³/₄oz) peas.

1,152 calories and 62 g fat. Total weight of meal 525 g (1lb 2¹/₂oz).

A generous and satisfying steak meal needn't be off the menu for most weight-watchers. The plateful on the right contains approximately half the number of calories and one-third the fat of the plateful on the left simply

Reduced-calorie, reduced-fat steak meal ★ ★ ★ ★ ★

200 g (7oz) sirloin steak, trimmed of fat; 200 g (7oz) potato wedges brushed with oil and baked; l medium tomato, grilled, 60 g (2oz) peas.

599 calories and 20g fat. Total weight of meal 540 g (1lb 3oz).

because the amount of fat has been quite drastically reduced. Remember, when you're cutting fat, add more vegetables, then you will still have plenty to eat.

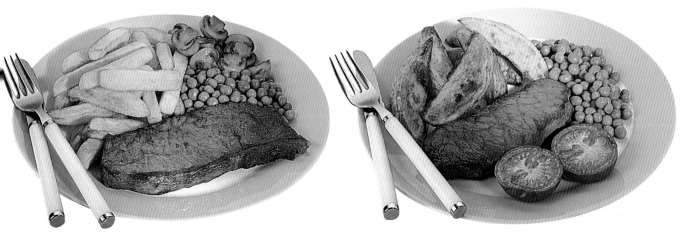

1,152 CALORIES AND 62G FAT. TOTAL WEIGHT OF MEAL 525G (1LB 2 ¹/₂ OZ).   *599 CALORIES AND 20G FAT. TOTAL WEIGHT OF MEAL 540G (1LB 3OZ).*

Week four – getting back to nature

Goals for the Week:

✻ Treat your body with respect and give it high-quality fuel.
✻ Discover a taste for natural foods.
✻ Learn to manage 'treat' foods within your diet.
✻ Lunch-time make-over.
✻ Consider long-term success.

It is hard to over-eat on a diet high in natural wholesome foods, and that is why the two main keys to long-term success with weight-watching are:

1 To recognize that your body is important and that it deserves the best fuel you can give it.

2 For this reason to give it good-quality, nutritious and fresh food.

In this last week of the retraining course you should be fully appreciating the flavours, textures and colours of your food. Instead of tasting just salt or sugar, you should be enjoying the subtleties of every type of food that you choose. This week try to:

✻ Eat as much unadulterated fresh food as possible. Eat fruits and vegetables raw or very lightly cooked.
✻ Try a variety of new foods, such as different breads, fishes, fruits, salad leaves.
✻ Expand on the idea that 'treating yourself' doesn't have to mean with something 'naughty' (as in cream cakes or chocolate), but can just as easily mean enjoying something nutrient-dense and light, such as a slice of perfect cantaloupe melon, or six grade-one oysters on ice.
✻ Also consider the low-cost 'top-quality' foods such as brown lentils, bulgar, pot barley, chickpeas, and enjoy them as much as you may enjoy that feast of shellfish.
✻ Get more quality, not quantity, into your diet. Think of having one beautiful glass of delicious wine rather than several glasses of plonk. Think of having a small organic fillet steak rather than a large plateful of dubious origin.
✻ Think of yourself as a 'foodie' rather than a gourmand.
✻ Long-term, vow not to put any item of food or drink in your mouth that doesn't serve a useful purpose for your body or provide you with pure unadulterated pleasure.

By following these tips and ideals you will be able to control your weight not by feeling deprived and miserable (as you will agree has been the case previously, which is why it didn't work) but by feeling in control, by enjoying your daily diet and by feeling proud that you care enough about your body to provide for it well.

The diet plans that follow here are samples of how you may like to eat to slim now that the four-week course is over. (See page 196 for some guidelines on whether to try Diet 1250 or Diet 1500.)

■ Healthy low-calorie lunches

✻ Any of the soups from the recipe section (pages 216-19) with some slices of whole-grain bread and an average portion of fruit.
✻ Chickpea Salad with Peppers and Tomatoes (page 220); apple
✻ Thai Salmon Salad (page 222)
✻ Panzanella (page 222); banana.
✻ Hummus; wholemeal mini pitta; orange.
✻ ½ avocado pear, sliced, with dressed

MANAGING 'TREAT' FOODS

Most people who undertake a four-week course such as this find that, however much they enjoyed items such as confectionery, crisps, cakes and so on at the start, by the end of week 4 their tastes have changed and these foods no longer hold such appeal.

However, if you still want to include such items in your diet, you can do so even while slimming. The 1,250 calories-a-day plan overleaf allows 100 calories a day for a 'treat', and the 1,500-a-day plan allows 150. Treats should be eaten or drunk with or after a meal, not on their own or when you are hungry (when you might easily eat more). Suggested options appear below:

100 calorie treats: one 140 ml (¼ pint) glass of wine; 1 wrapped chocolate biscuit bar; 1 double measure of spirits; 2 small chocolate digestive biscuits.

150 calories treats: 1 standard bag of crisps; 1 small slice of sponge cake; 25 g (¾oz) salted peanuts or cashew nuts.

crab and olive-oil French dressing; slice
of wholemeal bread,green salad.
* Seafood and Tropical Fruit Salad (page
224); average portion of cooled cooked
brown rice.

■ Long-term weight-watching
Once your desired body-weight is
reached, maintain your weight by
following all the ideas you have learnt
in the preceding weeks. You can eat
more than you did while slimming —
about 1,940 calories a day for women
and 2,500 for men. As we have seen in
the Question and Answer session, your
metabolic rate is likely to be normal for
a person of your size and age.

The Basic Healthy Diet on page 53 is
a good sample diet to follow; the food
charts and recipes will help you build an
enjoyable and satisfying diet for life.

Regular exercise is a vital key to
long-term weight control. Try to ensure
that you indulge in regular walking,
cycling or swimming, as well as
generally building more activity into
your daily life.

Try to combine such aerobic exercise
with muscle-toning exercise such as
window-cleaning or circuit-training.
because the higher your muscle-to-fat
ratio the more calories you will burn.

LUNCH MAKEOVER

Within a busy life, lunch is often the one meal of the day that is eaten without any thought or planning.
Most people believe that they 'hardly eat a thing' at lunch-time and yet, when what they do actually eat
is analysed, it turns out to be much higher in calories and fat than they imagined.
The example below is typical. The cheese and biscuits 'snack' actually contains more calories and much
more fat than the satisfying, healthy and tasty (yet still quick) lunch on the right. Such a lunch will keep
hunger pangs at bay and provide a better range of nutrients than the cheese snack.

High-calorie Snack	*Low-calorie Meal* ★★★★★
60 g (2oz) Cheddar cheese;	100 g (3¹/₂oz) tuna (canned in water, drained) flaked with 1 medium chopped
3 cream crackers;	tomato, 70 g (2¹/₂oz) cooked butter beans, 4 spring onions, chopped,
7 g (¹/₄oz) soft margarine.	1 tablespoon French dressing made with olive oil, 35 g (1¹/₄oz) dark rye bread,
	1 peach
391 calories and 29.7g fat	360 calories and 10 g fat

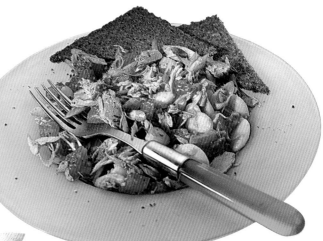

*PROVING THAT YOU DON'T HAVE TO STARVE TO SLIM, THIS SLIMMER'S LUNCH WEIGHS
MORE THAN THE SNACK BELOW AND IS MUCH MORE SATISFYING.*

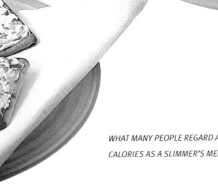

*WHAT MANY PEOPLE REGARD AS A SMALL SNACK, YET CONTAINS AS MANY
CALORIES AS A SLIMMER'S MEAL.*

DIET 1250

Eat everything in the diet below plus:

* Daily 275 ml (10 fl oz) skimmed milk for use on its own or in tea and coffee.
* One extra snack/treat to the value of 100 calories to be eaten with or after a meal.
* Unlimited — fresh salad items, leafy green vegetables, lemon juice, fresh herbs and spices, water, mineral water.
* Tea and coffee — up to four cups a day altogether. No sugar or sweeteners.

Meals should be spaced out as evenly as possible. The daily snack should either be eaten mid-morning, mid- to late-afternoon or shortly before bedtime. Calorie content works out at an approximate average of 1,250 per day, fat content averages 35 g a day maximum. Note: recipes for the dishes that are capitalized appear in Section 5.

DAY ONE
Breakfast
125 ml (4fl oz) natural bio yoghurt
25 g (³/₄ oz) All Bran
125 g (4¹/₂ oz) fresh fruit, chopped
Lunch
Broad Bean Soup
2 slices of Oatbread, with a little low-fat spread
Evening
Chicken Cacciatore
175 g (6oz), cooked weight, pasta shapes
large green salad
Snack
60 g (2 oz) dried ready-to-eat apricots

DAY TWO
Breakfast
25 g (³/₄ oz) traditional porridge oats, made into porridge using half water and half skimmed milk from allowance
1 orange
1 slice of Oatbread with 1 teaspoon honey
Lunch
Feta and Pepper Spread
1 wholemeal pitta
1 apple
Evening
Rice and Beans
large mixed salad with oil-free French dressing
Snack
1 large banana

DAY THREE
Breakfast
¹/₂ pink grapefruit
1 medium free-range boiled or poached egg
1¹/₂ slices of Oatbread or whole-grain bread with a little low-fat spread
Lunch
Chickpea Salad with Peppers and Tomatoes
1 apple
Evening
Seared Tuna with Lemon Grass, large portion of green beans, 75 g (2³/₄ oz) new potatoes
Snack
One 25g (³/₄ oz) slice of whole-grain bread OR Oatbread, little low-fat spread and 1 teaspoon honey

DAY FOUR
Breakfast
40 g (¹/₄ oz) no-added-sugar muesli
125 ml (4 fl oz) skimmed milk extra to allowance, apple chopped in
Lunch
Sandwich of two 40 g (¹/₄ oz) slices of dark rye bread with a little low-fat spread filled with plenty of salad items, plus 1 portion Cannellini Bean and Basil Spread
Evening
Turkish Aubergines
large green salad with 1 dessertspoon French dressing
Summer Fruits Compote
Snack
Banana and Strawberry Smoothie

DAY FIVE
Breakfast
As Day 1
Lunch
medium slice of cantaloupe melon
50 g (1³/₄ oz) Parma or Serrano ham
100 g (3¹/₂ oz) slice of Ciabatta bread
green salad
Evening
Tabbouleh
Mushroom and Red Pepper Skewers
Snack
60 g (2oz) ready-to-eat dried apricots

DAY SIX
Breakfast
As Day 2
Lunch
Baba Ganoush
1 wholemeal pitta bread
1 apple
Evening
1 small chicken breast fillet, seasoned with black pepper and herbs, grilled or baked
Cannellini Beans with Hot Tomato Vinaigrette
large green salad
Snack
1 large banana

DAY SEVEN
Breakfast
As Day 3
Lunch
Spinach, Parsley and Garlic Soup
50 g (1³/₄ oz) French bread
1 apple
Evening
One 200 g (7 oz) shark steak, grilled or dry-fried
Fresh Pepper Coulis
75 g (2³/₄ oz), cooked weight, bulgar wheat
broccoli
Snack
1 slice of Oatbread with 1 teaspoon honey

Diet 1500

Eat everything in the diet below plus:

* Daily milk allowance of 275ml (10fl oz) for use on its own or in tea and coffee.
* One extra daily snack or treat to value of 150 calories, with or after a meal.
* Unlimiteds as diet 1250.
* Up to 4 cups of tea or coffee a day altogether.

Instructions as diet opposite. Provides an average 1,500 calories a day and 42g fat.

DAY ONE
Breakfast
40 g (1¼ oz) Grapenuts with skimmed milk from allowance

1 orange

one 30 g (1 oz) slice of whole-grain bread with a little low-fat spread and 1 teaspoon honey
Lunch
Skordalia, selection of crudités

two 30g (1oz) slices of dark rye bread or Oatbread
Evening
Parcels of Tilapia, Tomatoes and Olives

125 g (4½ oz), cooked weight, pasta
large green salad
Snack
30 g (1 oz) ready-to-eat dried apricots
1 large banana

DAY TWO
Breakfast
1 medium free-range egg, boiled or poached

2 slices of Oatbread or whole-grain bread with a little low-fat spread

1 peach or orange
Lunch
Carrot and Orange Soup

1 average whole-grain or rye roll

2 level tablespoons cottage cheese
Evening
Potato and Mediterranean Vegetable Bake
green salad
Snack
1 medium banana; 1 traditional oatcake

DAY THREE
Breakfast
1 apple and date bar, ½ pink grapefruit, 100g (3½ oz) tub of natural fromage frais
Lunch
½ medium avocado sliced with tomato, onion and iceberg lettuce, oil-free French dressing, 1 medium whole-grain roll

1 kiwi fruit
Evening
Spiced Chicken and Greens

75 g (2¾ oz), cooked weight, brown rice
Snack
2 traditional oatcakes with 1 teaspoon honey

DAY FOUR
Breakfast
25 g (¾ oz) traditional porridge oats, made with half water and half skimmed milk (extra to allowance), 1 medium banana
Lunch
Seafood and Tropical Fruit Salad

100 g (3½ oz) natural bio yoghurt
Evening
Pasta with Milanese Sauce
large green salad
Snack
1 Oaty Flapjack

DAY FIVE
Breakfast
40 g (¼ oz) no-added-sugar muesli

125 ml (4fl oz) skimmed milk extra to allowance, 1 apple chopped in
Lunch
Roast Tomato, Garlic and Pepper Soup

90 g (3¼ oz) slice of ciabatta bread

1 orange
Evening
100 g (3½ oz) turkey escalope or steak, peppered and grilled, Mango Salsa

125g (4½ oz), cooked weight, brown rice
medium portion of green beans
Snack
125 g (4½ oz) natural bio yoghurt

DAY SIX
Breakfast
As Day 1
Lunch
Cucumber and Mint Soup

Sandwich of two 30g (1 oz) slices of dark rye bread filled with a little low-fat spread and 1 tablespoon cottage cheese, plus plenty of salad
Evening
Chickpea and Vegetable Crumble, broccoli
Snack
Citrus Granita

DAY SEVEN
Breakfast
As Day 3
Lunch
175 g (6 oz), cooked weight, pasta, cooled and mixed with 175 g (6 oz) selection of raw thinly sliced vegetables and tossed in 1 tablespoon tofu mayonnaise

1 apple
Evening
One 90 g (3¼ oz) fillet of wild salmon

Tomato and Bean Salsa

125 g (4½ oz) new potatoes
Snack
2 traditional oatcakes, 45 g (1½ oz) grapes

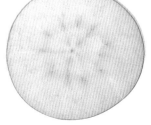

Popular dieting methods evaluated

You may have been tempted to follow one or more of the popular diet methods that receive much publicity. Here we examine the theory behind each method, appraise its advantages and drawbacks and rate each for various qualities (the more of the blank circles that are filled in, the better).

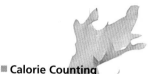

■ The Hay Diet (food combining)

Theory: says if we mix 'protein' and 'carbohydrate' foods at the same meal, they are incompletely digested, leading to toxicity and weight problems, therefore meals generally must not contain both. Vegetables and fruit form a large part of the diet, but fruit must be eaten in isolation. Only whole-grain or unprocessed starches should be eaten. Four hours should elapse between meals. Milk is restricted and there are many other rules.

Typical lunch: cheese with green salad; yoghurt.

Appraisal: there is no scientific evidence or reason to believe the 'protein fights carbohydrates' theory. In normal health, our digestive systems can happily cope with both protein and starch. The theory falls down, anyway, because many foods contain both — e.g. the starchy foods like pulses, grains and potatoes all contain protein too. For many people, the complicated rules may be hard to grasp and stick to, and don't fit in well with other people's eating habits. Weight-loss may be achieved simply because the system restricts calories.

Score: Ease ●○○○ Palatability ●●○○ Satiety level ●●○○ Safety ●●●○ Short-term effectiveness ●●●○ Long-term effectiveness ●●○○ Healthy eating basis ●●●○ Scientific basis ○○○○

Total score: 15/32

■ High-protein Diet

Theory: protein content of the diet is doubled, or more, to 30% or more of total calories. Carbohydrates and fats are restricted. There are various well-known diets based on the high-protein principle; each varies in its explanation of how they work. One, for instance, explains that a high-carbohydrate diet blocks utilization of calories and fat because of various hormonal reactions, therefore restricting carb intake will increase fat loss.

Typical lunch: grilled skinless chicken, broccoli.

Appraisal: high-protein, low-carb flies in the face of all current nutritional knowledge. Restricting carbohydrates will also restrict fibre intake, which can cause constipation, bowel cancer and other problems; and eating a diet high in protein can damage the liver, increase excretion of calcium from the body (which could lead to increased chance of osteoporosis). High-protein diets work to slim because they restrict overall calorie consumption rather than by hormonal reactions. On a high-protein, low-carb diet, ketosis may occur — characterized by acetone-smelling breath.

Score: Ease ●●○○ Palatability ●●○○ Satiety level ●●○○ Safety ●○○○ Short-term effectiveness ●●●○ Long-term effectiveness ●●○○ Healthy eating basis ○○○○ Scientific basis ●○○○

Total score: 13/32

■ Calorie Counting

Theory: all food contains calories (energy); weight-loss is based on calorie restriction — by taking in less calories than the body needs to maintain its weight, stored body fat has to be used for energy and weight-loss results. With a guide to the calorie content of all foods, it is possible to include any food within a diet as long as it fits in with the overall chosen calorie level — usually between 1,000 and 1,500 calories a day.

Typical lunch: prawn sandwich with low-calorie mayonnaise; apple, small chocolate biscuit.

Appraisal: although the scope for including any food in a calorie-controlled diet may sound appealing to most people, the system doesn't necessarily teach healthy eating habits. Foods often need to be weighed or measured to ensure accuracy, which can be time-consuming and boring. With the right dietary advice, however, a calorie-controlled diet can be tailored to suit anyone and will work.

Score: Ease ●●○○ Palatability ●●●● Satiety level ●●○○ Safety ●●●○ Short-term effectiveness ●●●○ Long-term effectiveness ●●○○ Healthy eating basis ●●○○ Scientific basis ●●●●

Total score: 22/32

■ High-fibre, High-carbohydrate, Low-fat

Theory: a diet high in fibre and carbohydrate helps the dieter to feel full for longer, while taking in fewer calories, because high-fibre foods take more chewing, swallowing and digesting, and keep blood sugar levels more constant than many other types of diet. Calorie count will be restricted in such a diet, because fat levels are also controlled.

Typical lunch: baked beans on wholemeal toast; orange, a few prunes.

Appraisal: sensible, works well and is similar in approach to a basic healthy diet (page 53). It tends to have more long-term success than many other diets, but results may be slow. A similar type of diet, which can be included in this category, is a low Glycaemic Index diet (see pages 194–5), moderate in fat and with the carb content based around low or moderate GI foods.

Scores: Ease ●●●○ Palatability ●●○○ Satiety level ●●●● Safety ●●●● Short-term effectiveness ●●○○ Long-term effectiveness ●●●● Healthy eating basis ●●●● Scientific basis ●●●○

Total score: 26/32

■ Very-low-fat Diet

Theory: fat is the nutrient highest in calories — at 9 calories per gram compared with 4 for protein and 3.75 for carbohydrate — therefore more calories can be cut by avoiding fat than by any other method. Also, a high-fat diet is linked with some illnesses, so fat-cutting is healthy too, the theory goes.

Fat content of all foods is listed in various guides and the theory is if fat is avoided as far as possible but normal quantities of carbohydrate and low-fat protein are allowed then weight-loss must follow without the need to count calories.

Typical lunch: vegetable soup made without added fat; skinless turkey breast sandwich (no fat spread) with salad; fat-free fruit fromage frais.

Appraisal: a reduced-fat diet can be healthy if it is mostly saturated fat that is reduced, but some very-low-fat diets also disallow the healthy fats found in

items like nuts, plant oils and oily fish, and such diets may be short of essential fatty acids and of the fat-soluble vitamins A, D, E and K. There is evidence that the EFAs can help weight-loss rather than hinder it, and there are many links between adequate intake of omega-3 oils and long-chain omega-6 oils and protection from major diseases such as CHD, cancer, arthritis, Alzheimer's and diabetes.

A very-low-fat diet can be quite unpalatable — less than around 25% of total calories is almost unworkable in most people's lives. There is also some evidence that people on a low-fat diet tend to eat more of the carbohydrate foods to make up the 'lost' calories and so it isn't a guaranteed route to success.

Scores: Ease ●●●○ Palatability ●●○○ Satiety level ●●●○ Safety ●●○○ Short-term effectiveness ●●○○ Long-term effectiveness ●●○○ Healthy eating basis ●●○○ Scientific basis ●●○○

Total score: 18/32

■ Meal Replacement

Theory: one, two or three meals a day are replaced with a manufactured calorie-counted meal, such as a milk shake or a bar containing protein, vitamins, minerals, fibre, and so on. The idea is that this takes away the need to think about preparing reduced-calorie meals and provides all the nutrients the dieter needs while containing an exact stated low number of calories.

Typical lunch: 1 serving of meal-replacement chocolate milk-shake, glass of water

Appraisal: research shows that many people do well on meal-replacement diets if used to replace one or two meals a day and the remaining meal(s) is/are healthy and balanced.

Long term, replacement diets can be boring and critics say that the replacement meals don't provide phytochemicals, and that it is hardly

possible to get the recommended five portions of fruit and vegetables or enough carbohydrate every day on such a regime. Also meal replacements do little to help re-educate people to long-term healthy eating. Although guidelines for usage are given on packs, over-fast weight-loss could result if used to replace too many meals. However, using the meals as a one-a-day replacement does work well for some people, even in the long term.

Score: Ease ●●●● Palatability ●○○○ Satiety level ●●○○ Safety ●●○○ Short-term effectiveness ●●●○ Long-term effectiveness ●●○○ Healthy eating basis ●●○○ Scientific basis ●●●●

Total score: 21/32

■ Fasting

Theory: existing on nothing but water (some 'fasts' allow fruit and vegetable juices, too) for days or weeks at a time encourages rapid fat-loss; hunger pangs disappear within 2-3 days of the start of the fast and the faster may feel highly energetic, clear-headed and calm.

Typical lunch: water

Appraisal: on a fast, a high percentage of lean body tissue (muscle) can be lost, including that from the vital organs such as the heart, meaning that such a regime can be dangerous, especially if vigorous activity is undertaken while fasting. Headaches, dizziness, faintness, constipation and bad breath (as a result of ketosis) are common side-effects. Undertaken regularly or for weeks at a time, deficiency in various vitamins and minerals will occur.

Score: Ease ●●○○ Palatability ○○○○ Satiety level ○○○○ Safety ○○○○ Short-term effectiveness ●●●● Long-term effectiveness ○○○○ (unsafe for long term) Healthy eating basis ○○○○ Scientific basis ●●○○

Total score: 8/32

Weight gain

Approximately 5% of, or one in twenty, adults in the UK are underweight — with a BMI of less than 20. Though underweight is hardly ever mentioned, due to the national preoccupation with obesity, it is, in fact, also linked with poor health. According to most research, the greater the degree of underweight, the greater the risks of malnutrition, heart attacks, sexual and reproductive problems, osteoporosis and reduced life-span.

New research linking calorie restriction with increased life-span contradicts much of these traditionally accepted statistics and so more research is needed, but it may be that BMIs at the lower end of 'average' (i.e., 20-21) are healthy, while those under 20 are not.

Why do some adults have trouble maintaining their body fat? Just like obese people, hereditary factors may be one reason for some. This could cause a predisposition to burning off the calories in food more quickly than average. Although not a great deal of research has

SNACKS FOR WEIGHT GAIN

Healthy high-fat snacks: fresh nuts, seeds, muesli, Greek yoghurt.
Healthy high-carbohydrate snacks: muesli bars, Flapjacks, bread, oatcakes.
Healthy high-calorie drinks: full-fat or semi-skimmed milk, milky malt drinks; hot chocolate, fruit juice, 1-2 glasses wine or stout a day.

Examples of adding 500 calories' worth of snacks to the daily diet:
* 1 large slice of white bread with a little butter and jam; 300 ml (1/2 pint) semi-skimmed milk; 1 large banana
* 2 small slices of malt loaf with a little butter; 100 g (3 1/2 oz) portion of vanilla ice-cream; average portion of corn-flakes with a little semi-skimmed milk
* 1 portion Complan; 2 digestive bis-cuits; 1 Flapjack

been carried out on underweight people, it does seem that the main reason for underweight is the most obvious one — that low-weight people take more exercise and/or eat fewer calories.

In one recent study, people who thought they were naturally thin were fed a controlled high-calorie diet and, much to their surprise, every one of them put on the amount of weight that would be expected. They just hadn't been eating as much as they thought. It seems slim people prefer lower-calorie foods, such as fruits and vegetables, and are less tolerant of large, calorie-dense meals.

Some slim people also tend to be more active than normal-weight people, 'fidgeting' more and perhaps even sleeping for fewer hours, perhaps with a natural inclination towards active hobbies.

Lastly, almost anyone can become too thin during or as a result of illness.

For everyone, a high-calorie diet can restore a suitable BMI. The trick is to offer a diet which the recipient will actually eat and doesn't find too daunting.

■ The Weight-gain Diet

Nutritionists have found that an increment of 500 calories a day on average is about right in order to help most thin people put on weight. More than this may over-face most people; less means weight-gain would be slow. This amount is only a guide — it depends on starting weight and other factors. For instance, a very thin person who has been eating only a few hundred calories

a day will probably gain weight on a diet which is lower in calories than a normal average diet (1,940 for women, 2,550 for men), but someone who is thin because they exercise a lot could need more than 500 calories a day above average.

The extra calories should be added to the diet so that the balance of nutrients is still healthy — with not too much fat, plenty of carbohydrate and enough protein. Although fat is the most calorie-dense of the nutrients, at 9 calories a gram, it isn't suitable to offer the extra 500 calories in nothing but high-fat foods as this would increase the fat content to unacceptably high levels. However, it is reasonable to offer a diet a little higher in fat than would be provided in the diet long-term (especially if mostly in the form of the essential fatty acids), as thin people with poor appetite often have difficulty in managing enough high-bulk foods, such as starchy carbohydrates, to provide enough extra calories, although sugars are easy to eat and digest.

IDEAL CALS FOR GAIN (females)

Daily milk and fruit juice allowance :	280 calories
Breakfast:	400 calories
Mid-morning snack:	200 calories
Lunch (or evening meal):	550 calories
Mid-afternoon snack:	150 calories
Evening meal (or lunch):	700 calories
Bedtime snack:	150 calories
Total:	2,430 calories

Sample weight gain diet for women

This sample diet gives an average of around 2,450 calories a day, divided up roughly as the blueprint opposite.
Daily allowance: 275ml (10fl oz) full-fat milk; 275ml (10fl oz) orange, or other fruit, juice.
Unlimited: fresh or frozen vegetables; salad; fresh fruit.
Note: recipes for dishes that are capitalized appear in Section 5.

DAY ONE
Breakfast
2 Weetabix with 1 teaspoon brown sugar and 1 dessertspoon sunflower seeds sprinkled over
140 ml (5 fl oz) semi-skimmed milk to cover (extra to allowance)
1 medium slice of white bread with a little butter and 1 teaspoon honey
1 apple or peach
Mid-morning
1 portion of ice-cream
Lunch
Smoked Mackerel Pâté, salad
Mid-afternoon
1 Flapjack
Evening
Pasta with Basil and Ricotta
tomato salad
1 banana
Bedtime
mug of Horlicks and 1 rich tea biscuit

DAY TWO
Breakfast
poached egg on large slice of toast with a little butter
1 large slice of toast and butter with marmalade
1 satsuma
Mid-morning
20 g (½ oz) shelled Brazil nuts and 5 halves of ready-to-eat dried apricots
Lunch
Squash, Potato and Butter Bean Soup
medium brown roll with a little butter
Mid-afternoon
small slice of sponge cake
Evening
Seafood Risotto with Ginger
fresh fruit salad with 1 dessertspoon crème fraîche
Bedtime
mug of hot semi-skimmed milk
chocolate digestive biscuit

DAY THREE
Breakfast
As Day One
Mid-morning
As Day 1
Lunch
Brown Rice and Citrus Salad
Mid-afternoon
1 Flapjack
Evening
Avocado and Turkey Tortillas
Peach and Banana Fool
Bedtime
As Day 1

DAY FOUR
Breakfast
As Day 2
Mid-morning
As Day 2
Lunch
Home-baked Beans
large slice of crusty bread with a little butter
Mid-afternoon
As Day 2
Evening
Steak and Spinach Stir-fry
Raspberry Gratin
Bedtime
As Day 2

DAY FIVE
Breakfast
50 g (1¾ oz) muesli with 15 g (½ oz) chopped almonds added
125 ml (4 fl oz) semi-skimmed milk to cover
1 pear or nectarine
Mid-morning
As Day 1
Lunch
Salad of Tuna, Avocado and Tomato
1 large slice of brown bread
1 apple
Mid-afternoon
As Day 1
Evening
Almond, Chickpea and Raisin Pilaf
green salad
Bedtime
mug of semi-skimmed hot milk
small slice of malt loaf

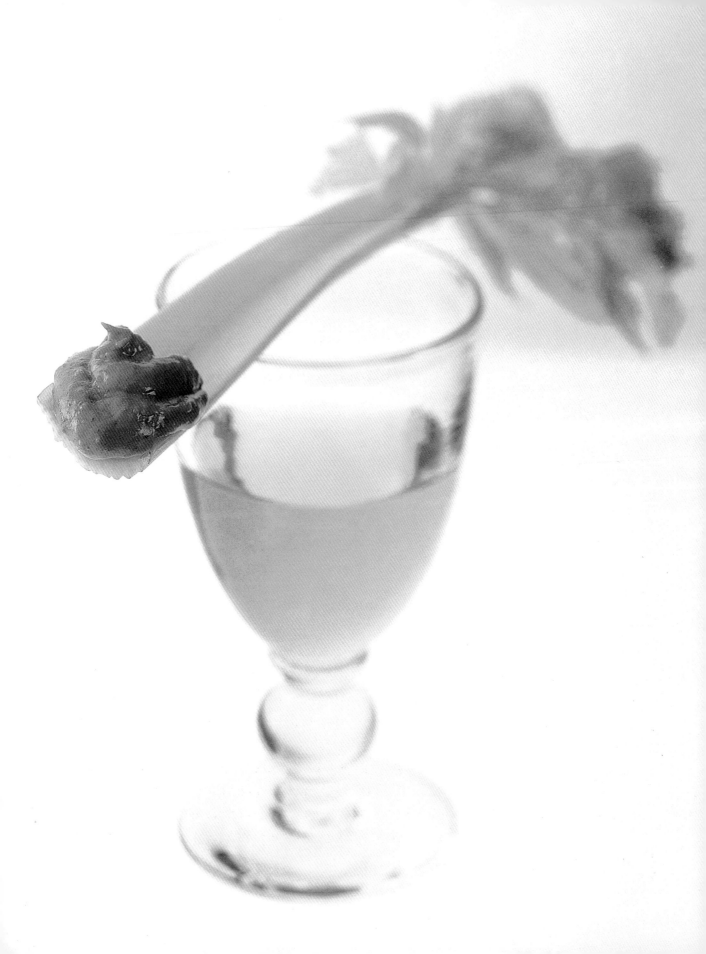

Food for health and pleasure

Knowing what foods to eat for your continuing good health is, of course, what this book is all about. Almost as important, however, is knowing how to put it all together. Apart from those occasions when you eat out, the kitchen is where you put all your knowledge into practice. Cooking well is important for two main reasons. Firstly, it is quite possible to turn decent healthy basic ingredients into less than healthy meals, and so a basic knowledge of healthy cooking is vital. Secondly, you need to provide meals you and your family actually want to eat. No amount of diet theory will work unless you can convert it into tempting dishes that you really enjoy and which fit into your lifestyle and budget.

This section sets out to provide you with enough good ideas in the form of tips, healthy cooking charts and carefully thought-out recipes to do just that.

Healthy Cooking Guidelines

The nutritional content of healthful ingredients and basic foods can be enhanced by careful cooking — or debased by poor cooking. For example, some cooking methods rob food of vital vitamins while others help to retain them.

Throughout the book more detailed guidance is given on food and diets for specific ailments and conditions. The chart on the right shows the benefits and drawbacks of each common cooking method.

Using the recipes that follow:

The 100 or so recipes that follow give you a wide selection of ideas on how to incorporate all the healthy foods into your regular diet and that of your family.

Most of the recipes are also featured within the various specialized diet plans. They can also be used in the same way as you would the recipes in a general healthy cookery book. To help you, each has a panel of symbols above it which will guide you to the recipe that is right for your purposes. For example, if searching for recipes suitable for someone with high blood-cholesterol, look for the ♥ symbol.

The Nutrition Panels

Each recipe has a nutrition panel giving information on the nutrient content per serving. For more information on all these nutrients, see Section One.

* Total fat is given in grams. Sometimes you may think a recipe looks very high in fat, but serving suggestions are given where appropriate and, if followed, will bring the total meal into a good balance of the macro-nutrients — i.e. protein, fat and carbohydrate.

Also bear in mind that it is saturated fat that most people should be limiting in their diets and that the seemingly high-fat recipes in fact contain high levels of the protective unsaturated fats and low levels of saturates.

COMMON COOKING METHODS COMPARED

* **Raw:** Retains maximum nutrients normally lost through cooking, with exception of carrots.
Not suitable for wide range of foods; may be indigestible.
Cut surfaces quickly lose vitamin C, prepare at last minute.

* **Boiling:** No added fat.
Boiled vegetables lose up to 70% of their water soluble vitamins B and C.
Retain more vitamins by using minimum water and cooking until only just tender.

* **Steaming:** Retains more nutrients than boiling.
Still 30% or more water-soluble vitamin losses.
Use cooking water in sauces, etc. to put back the vitamins.

* **Microwaving:** Retains most water-soluble nutrients if minimum water used.
Quite easy to over-cook or undercook unless care taken. Food thermometer useful.
Reheated food should be stirred and served piping hot.

* **Baking/roasting:** No added fat necessary with meat — use foil; brush vegetables with olive oil.
Heat destroys vitamin C. Poultry needs thorough cooking.
Meat juices from roasting contain B vitamins — use in sauce.

* **Braising/casseroling/stewing:** Tenderizes low-cost meats; vitamins retained within dish.
Can be high in meat fats unless cooled and skimmed of surplus.
Ideal method for root vegetables and pulses.

* **Grilling/barbecuing:** Low-fat way to cook meat; no added fats, plus fats melt and drip out of meat.
Overgrilled, charred meat linked with several types of cancer. Don't serve burned food.

* **Frying (deep- or shallow):** Poor method for slimmers. Frying at very high temperatures releases carcinogens into the atmosphere, particularly true of carb foods such as chips. Foods are best fried occasionally or at moderate temperatures.
Use groundnut oil for high-temp frying – olive oil has too low a smoke point.
Change cooking oils frequently – much-used oils oxidize and may be carcinogenic.

* **Stir-frying:** Retains water-soluble vitamins; little fat used.
Suitable method for only 2-3 people at a time as not much food can be stir-fried correctly in one batch. Cut surfaces of vegetables quickly lose vitamin C — prepare shortly before use.

* Protein content per portion is 'low', 'medium' or 'high'. 'Low' means less than 10% of total calories are in the form of protein; 'medium' 10-15 %; and 'high' over 15%.

* Carbohydrate content per portion is 'low', 'medium' or 'high'. 'Low' means less than 35% of total calories are in the form of carbohydrate; 'medium' 35-50 %; and 'high' over 50%.

SYMBOLS

♥ Anti-heart/-circulatory disease, high blood cholesterol

☻ Anti-cancer

🗲 Immune system boost

🐾 Anti-arthritis

⬌ Bone strength

▼ Dairy-free

✗ Gluten/wheat free

✖ Yeast-free

V Vegetarian

◐ Low-calorie

◕ Quick

▣ Budget

All recipes serve 2 and are low in salt and dietary cholesterol, unless otherwise stated.

Index of Recipes

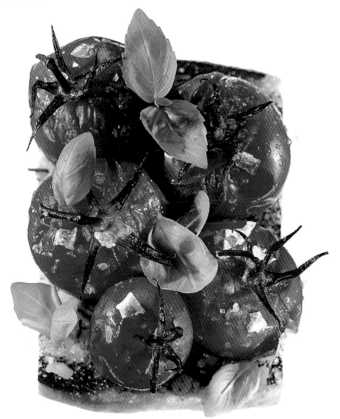

BAKED BABY TOMATOES WITH BASIL

Marinated shiitake mushrooms

Calories: 261	
Total fat: 22g	
Saturated fat: 3.3g	
Fibre: 1.6g	
Protein: low	
Carbohydrate: low	
Vitamins: C	
Minerals: copper	

225 g (8 oz) shiitake mushrooms
4 tablespoons olive oil
2 garlic cloves, crushed
1 small red chilli, deseeded and chopped
2 shallots, finely chopped
1 tablespoon white wine vinegar
1 teaspoon balsamic vinegar
2 tablespoons chopped parsley
1 tablespoon chopped tarragon
1 teaspoon chopped thyme
1 teaspoon sea salt
black pepper

Tear the mushrooms into bite-sized pieces. Heat half the oil in a non-stick pan and stir-fry the garlic, chilli and shallots for a minute or two, until the shallots are softened. Add the mushrooms and stir in the remaining ingredients with the rest of the oil. Serve warm or cold.

Baked baby tomatoes with basil

Calories: 228	
Total fat: 13g	
Saturated fat: 1g	
Fibre: 1.6g	
Protein: low	
Carbohydrate: medium	
Vitamins: C, E, carotenoids	

325 g (11½ oz) baby tomatoes (about 12)
1 fresh juicy garlic clove, chopped
2 tablespoons olive oil
1 teaspoon sea salt
black pepper
1 teaspoon rosemary leaves
handful of fresh basil leaves, torn if large
two 40 g (1½ oz) slices of French bread

Preheat oven to 200°C/ 400°F/ gas 6.
Arrange the tomatoes in a small ovenproof dish. Sprinkle with the garlic, half the olive oil, the salt, pepper and rosemary. Bake for 25 minutes, or until the tomatoes are soft.
Arrange on serving plates with the juices, topped with the remaining olive oil and basil leaves. Serve with the bread.

Smoked mackerel pâté salad

Calories: 571	
Total fat: 40g	
Saturated fat: 8.5g	
Fibre: 2.4g	
Protein: high	
Carbohydrate: low	
Vitamins: B₁, B₂, nicotinic acid, B6, B12, D, E, folate	
Minerals: selenium, iodine, calcium, magnesium, potassium, iron, copper	

225 g (8 oz) hot-smoked mackerel fillets
140 ml (5 fl oz) natural low-fat bio yoghurt
2 tablespoons tomato paste
dash of Worcestershire sauce
1 tablespoon chopped fresh parsley, plus more parsley sprigs to serve
black pepper
50 g (1¾ oz) mixed green salad leaves
4 oatcakes to serve

In a large bowl, flake the mackerel with a fork. Add the yoghurt, tomato paste, Worcestershire sauce, chopped parsley and black pepper to taste. Combine well.
Arrange the leaves and parsley sprigs on plates, spoon over the pâté and serve with the oatcakes.

Mushroom and red pepper skewers

🐚 ⊙ ✄ ❢ ✂ ⋁ ⬓ ☖

Calories:	111
Total fat:	6.4g
Saturated fat:	1g
Fibre:	3.2g
Protein:	medium
Carbohydrate:	medium
Vitamins:	A, nicotinic acid, B6, folate, C
Minerals:	copper

2 medium red peppers, halved and deseeded (about 200 g / 7 oz)
1 tablespoon olive oil
1 fresh juicy garlic clove
1 teaspoon sea salt
½ small fresh red chilli, deseeded and chopped
2 teaspoons balsamic vinegar
8 small chestnut (brown-cap) mushrooms (about 115 g / 4 oz)

Preheat the grill to medium-hot and place the pepper halves on the grill tray, skin side up. Brush them with a little of the olive oil, and grill on both sides until softened but not black.

Remove the pepper halves from the grill and, when they have cooled a little, cut them into bite-sized squares.

Using a pestle and mortar, pound the garlic with the salt until well combined and creamy. Beat in the remaining olive oil, chilli and the vinegar.

Thread the pepper squares and mushrooms alternately on 2 skewers (soaked in water if wooden) and brush with the garlic oil mixture.

Grill under a medium heat, turning a few times and basting with remaining sauce until the mushrooms are cooked through, about 5 minutes. Serve hot.

MUSHROOM AND RED PEPPER SKEWERS

Turkish aubergines

🐚 ⊙ ✄ ❢ ✕ ⋁ ⬓ ☖

Calories:	186
Total fat:	7.1g
Saturated fat:	1.1g
Fibre:	12g
Protein:	medium
Carbohydrate:	high
Vitamins:	A, B1, nicotinic acid, B6, folate, C, E
Minerals:	potassium

1 tablespoon olive oil, plus more for the baking tray
1 large aubergine (about 250 g / 9 oz)
1 medium red pepper, deseeded and chopped small
1 red onion, finely chopped
1 level teaspoon ground cumin
1 teaspoon sea salt
black pepper
2 medium tomatoes, halved
25 g (¾ oz) couscous (dry weight)
4 tablespoons boiling water

Preheat the oven to 180°C/ 350°F/ gas 4 and oil a baking tray.

Halve the aubergine and scoop out all but the last 1 cm (½ inch) of flesh. Turn the shells upside down on the oiled baking tray and bake for 25 minutes, or until the shells are just tender.

Meanwhile, heat the remaining olive oil in a non-stick frying pan. Chop the aubergine flesh and add it to the pan, together with the red pepper, onion, cumin and seasoning. Stir-fry for a few minutes until soft.

Squeeze the tomato halves to remove the pips, then chop them roughly and add to the aubergine mixture.

Soak the couscous in the boiling water until all water is absorbed, about 10-15 minutes. Stir the aubergine mixture into the couscous and adjust the seasoning.

Pile the mixture into the aubergine shells and return to the oven to warm through. Serve at once.

All the following eight simple recipes are very versatile: they can be used as dips with crudités, bread or crispbreads, they are good on toast or bruschetta, and some also as sandwich fillings. Some make excellent accompaniments to meat or fish or can be added by the spoonful to soups or casseroles to enrich them healthily. Individual usage notes appear below the recipes where appropriate.

Note re PORTIONS: It is hardly worth making these eight recipes in quantities to serve two, so each complete recipe will serve 4-6, depending on appetite.

They will all keep well, covered, in the fridge for several days. Filming the top with a little olive oil is a good way of keeping them from drying out and prolonging their lives.

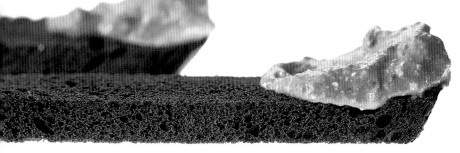

FETA AND PEPPER SPREAD

Feta and pepper spread

Calories: 179	
Total fat: 15g	
Saturated fat: 7.5g	
Fibre: 0.7g	
Protein: high	
Carbohydrate: low	
Vitamins: nicotinic acid, B12, C, A, carotenoids	
Minerals: calcium	

1½ tablespoons olive oil
1 medium red pepper, deseeded and chopped
½ fresh red chilli, deseeded and chopped
dash of chilli sauce (such as Tabasco)
200 g (7 oz) Greek feta cheese, roughly mashed

Heat the oil in a non-stick frying pan and stir-fry the pepper and chilli until soft but not browned. Add the chilli sauce.

Place the cheese in a blender or food processor followed by the contents of the pan and blend until you have a smooth spread. Serve at room temperature.

This is a lower-calorie, calcium-rich alternative to basic cheese, ideal for sandwiches.

Hummus

Calories: 186	
Total fat: 13g	
Saturated fat: 1.8g	
Fibre: 3.3g	
Protein: medium	
Carbohydrate: low	

one 400-g (14-oz) can of good-quality chickpeas, well drained and rinsed
juice of 1 lemon
3 tablespoons extra-virgin olive oil
1 tablespoon light tahini (sesame seed paste)
1 garlic clove, crushed
1 teaspoon sea salt
black pepper or paprika to taste

Put all ingredients in a blender or food processor and blend until you have a smooth but textured purée. Adjust the seasoning.

Cannellini bean and basil spread

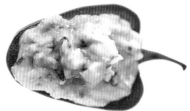

Calories: 86	
Total fat: 3g	
Saturated fat: 0.5g	
Fibre: 4.3g	
Protein: high	
Carbohydrate: medium	

one 400-g (14-oz) can of cannellini
   beans, drained and rinsed
2 garlic cloves, crushed
1 tablespoon olive oil
2 teaspoons lemon juice
1 teaspoon sea salt
black pepper
1 average pack or pot of basil leaves

Place all ingredients except the basil in
a blender or food processor and blend
until you have a pâté which is still
slightly rough — don't over-blend.

Add the basil leaves, fork them
through and blend for 2 seconds. Check
seasoning.

You could use butter beans for a
similar result.

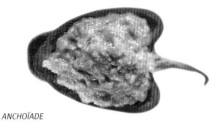

CANNELLINI BEAN AND BASIL SPREAD

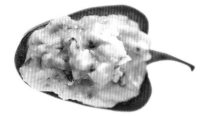

ANCHOÏADE

Anchoïade

Calories: 195	
Total fat: 20g	
Saturated fat: 2.9g	
Fibre: 0.4g	
Protein: low	
Carbohydrate: low	
Vitamins: B12	

4 fresh juicy garlic cloves, peeled
12 canned anchovy fillets in oil, drained
12 good plump green olives, stoned
about 100 ml (3½ fl oz) extra-virgin
   olive oil
dash of white wine vinegar

Put the garlic, anchovies and olives in
a blender or food processor and blend
until puréed. Pour in half the oil and the
vinegar and blend again.

Add as much more of the oil as you
need to make a paste or purée or sauce,
depending upon its intended use.

Good as a dip, as a quick sauce for a
pasta starter, as a topping for crostini
or as a side sauce with eggs.

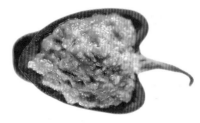

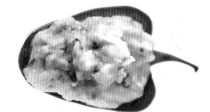

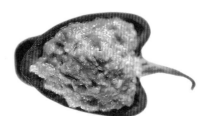

Rouille

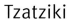

Calories:	129
Total fat:	8.5g
Saturated fat:	1.2g
Fibre:	0.3g
Protein:	low
Carbohydrate:	low

50 g (1¾ oz) slightly stale rough white breadcrumbs
100 ml (3½fl oz) semi-skimmed milk
pinch of saffron
little hot water
2 fresh juicy garlic cloves, crushed
1-2 fresh red chillies, deseeded and chopped
1 teaspoon sea salt
3 tablespoons olive oil

In a bowl, add the bread to the milk, stir and leave for a few minutes. In another small bowl, infuse the saffron in the hot water. Press out any surplus milk from the bread.

Using a pestle and mortar, blend together the garlic, chillies and salt. Add the soaked bread and saffron infusion to the mortar and pound, gradually adding the olive oil to make a well blended purée.

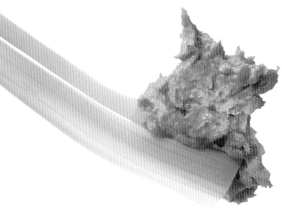

ROUILLE

Tzatziki

Calories:	96
Total fat:	6.9g
Saturated fat:	3.9g
Fibre:	0.5g
Protein:	high
Carbohydrate:	low
Vitamins:	B2

½ fresh tasty cucumber
4 fresh juicy garlic cloves, crushed
little sea salt
300 g (10½ oz) strained Greek-style yoghurt
2 teaspoons white wine vinegar

Peel the cucumber and then grate it on a medium-coarse grater. Wrapping it in a clean tea towel, remove as much moisture from the cucumber as you can.

Place the cucumber in a bowl, add the crushed garlic and salt and combine thoroughly. Add the yoghurt and vinegar and combine well again. Serve chilled. **Ideal as a dip** or with grilled meats. More garlic can be added to taste.

Skordalia

Calories: 204
Total fat: 18g
Saturated fat: 2.5g
Fibre: 3.3g
Protein: low
Carbohydrate: low
Vitamins: folate, C

sea salt
300 g (10½ oz) celeriac root, peeled and cut into small cubes
125 g (4½ oz) potato suitable for boiling, cubed
3 fresh juicy garlic cloves, crushed
100 ml (3½ fl oz) skimmed or semi-skimmed milk
100 ml (3½ fl oz) olive oil

Bring a pan of lightly salted water to the boil, add the celeriac and potato and boil until tender, about 20 minutes. Drain until absolutely dry.

In a blender or food processor, blend the vegetables until smooth. Add the garlic and 1 teaspoon of salt and blend again.

Warm the milk and mix it with the olive oil, then pour this into the blender slowly, with the machine still running. The resulting purée should be smooth and silky. Adjust the seasoning.

Baba ganoush (aubergine purée)

Calories: 76
Total fat: 5.7g
Saturated fat: 0.9g
Fibre: 4g
Protein: medium
Carbohydrate: low
Vitamins: folate

2 large aubergines (about 675 g / 1½ lb in total)
1 teaspoon freshly ground cumin seed
1-2 garlic cloves, crushed
1 tablespoon light tahini (sesame seed paste)
2 teaspoons olive oil
juice of ½ lemon
1 teaspoon sea salt
black pepper

Preheat the oven to 200°C/ 400°F/ gas 6. Prick the aubergines and bake them for 40 minutes or until soft right through.

Allow them to cool a little, then halve them and scoop their flesh into the bowl of a blender or food processor.

Add the remaining ingredients and blend until you have a purée. Check seasoning.

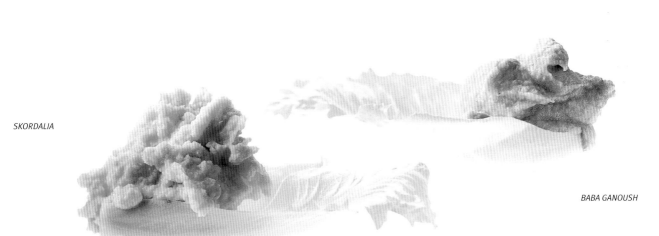

SKORDALIA

BABA GANOUSH

Cucumber and mint soup

Calories: 131	
Total fat: 8.4g	
Saturated fat: 1.8g	
Fibre: 1.8g	
Protein: medium	
Carbohydrate: low	
Vitamins: E	

½ cucumber (about 250 g / 9 oz)
1 tablespoon sunflower oil
1 medium onion, finely chopped
450 ml (¾ pint) good-quality vegetable
    stock
handful of fresh mint
1 teaspoon sea salt
black pepper
2 tablespoons reduced-fat Greek yoghurt

Cut a 2-cm (¾-inch) chunk off the cucumber, chop it and set this aside. Peel the remaining cucumber, halve it lengthwise and scoop out the seeds. Chop the flesh.

Heat the oil in a pan and sauté the onion until soft. Stir in the cucumber. Add the stock, a couple of mint leaves and seasoning. Simmer for 15 minutes.

Purée the soup in a blender or food processor, then leave to cool.

Chop the remaining mint leaves. Before serving, stir the chopped mint and yoghurt into the soup and garnish with the reserved chopped cucumber.

Carrot and orange soup

Calories: 109	
Total fat: 4.8g	
Saturated fat: 0.7g	
Fibre: 3.6g	
Protein: low	
Carbohydrate: high	
Vitamins: B6, folate, A, C, E, carotenoids	

2 teaspoons corn or groundnut oil
1 small onion (about 75 g / 2¾ oz),
    finely chopped
1 small garlic clove, crushed
225 g (8 oz) carrots, peeled and
    chopped
125 g (4½ oz) good-quality canned
    chopped tomatoes (with their liquid)
juice of 1 large orange, freshly squeezed
½ teaspoon ground cumin seeds
1 teaspoon sea salt
black pepper
200 ml (7 fl oz) good-quality vegetable
    stock
fresh green herbs, such as parsley, to
    garnish

Heat the oil in a saucepan and sauté the onion until soft, adding the garlic towards the end of cooking time.

Add the carrots and stir for a minute, then add the remaining ingredients except the herbs for garnish. Stir and bring to simmer. Cook for 30 minutes or until the carrots and onions are tender.

Liquidize the contents of the pan in a blender or food processor until smooth.

Adjust the seasoning, reheat and serve garnished with the herbs.

CARROT AND ORANGE SOUP

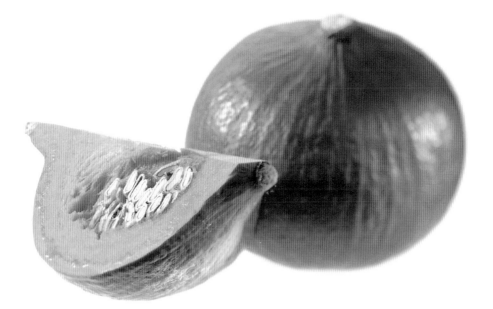

Squash, potato and butter bean soup

🐑 🌣 🥚 🍷 🍴 🚫 🅥 🅞 🖨

Calories: 252
Total fat: 6.5g
Saturated fat: 0.8g
Fibre: 7.3g
Protein: medium
Carbohydrate: high
Vitamins: B1, nicotinic acid, B6, folate, A, carotenoids, C, E
Minerals: magnesium, potassium, iron, copper

1 tablespoon olive oil
1 small onion (about 75 g / 2¾ oz), finely chopped
400 g (14 oz) orange-fleshed squash, such as onion squash or butternut, peeled and cut into cubes
1 medium potato, cubed
1 garlic clove, chopped
1 teaspoon fresh thyme leaves
1 teaspoon sea salt
black pepper
300 ml (½ pint) good vegetable or chicken stock
100 g (3½ oz) drained canned butter beans

Heat the oil in a non-stick frying pan and sauté the onion until soft.

Add the vegetables and stir. Add the rest of the ingredients except the butter beans, bring to a simmer and cook for 30 minutes, adding the butter beans towards the end of cooking time.

When the vegetables are tender, purée the soup in a food processor. Adjust the seasoning. If the soup is too thick, add some water or stock and blend again. Reheat gently to serve.

Roast tomato, garlic and pepper soup

🐑 🌣 🥚 🍷 🍴 🚫 🅥 🅞 🖨

Calories: 223
Total fat: 11g
Saturated fat: 1.8g
Fibre: 7.5g
Protein: medium
Carbohydrate: medium
Vitamins: B1, nicotinic acid, B6, folate, A, carotenoids, C, E
Minerals: magnesium, potassium, iron

8 fresh juicy garlic cloves, peeled
8 tasty ripe tomatoes (about 450 g / 1 lb) halved and deseeded
1 medium red pepper, halved and deseeded, then quartered
1⅔ tablespoons olive oil
1 teaspoon sea salt
black pepper
400 ml (14 fl oz) good vegetable stock
100 g (3½ oz) pre-cooked (e.g. canned) butter beans, well drained
handful of fresh basil leaves

Preheat the oven to 200°C/ 400°F/ gas 6. Arrange the garlic, tomatoes and red pepper quarters on a baking dish and drizzle the oil over them, then sprinkle on the salt and pepper. Bake for 20-30 minutes, or until the vegetables are soft. (If the garlic looks like over-cooking, remove it from the baking dish and set it aside).

Now transfer the contents of the baking dish, together with the stock and beans, to a blender or food processor and purée until smooth. Pour into a pan and reheat, adding the basil at the last minute. Adjust the seasoning.

Lentil and coriander soup

Calories: 269	
Total fat: 8.4g	
Saturated fat: 1.8g	
Fibre: 6.8g	
Protein: high	
Carbohydrate: medium	
Vitamins: B1, nicotinic acid, B6, folate, A	
Minerals: magnesium, potassium, iron, copper, selenium	

1 tablespoon groundnut oil
1 medium red onion, finely chopped
1 garlic clove, finely chopped
500 ml (18 fl oz) good-quality vegetable stock
100 g (3½ oz) (dry weight) brown or Puy lentils
1 medium carrot (about 100 g / 3½ oz), peeled and chopped
1 teaspoon sea salt
black pepper
2 tablespoons chopped fresh coriander
1 tablespoon reduced-fat Greek-style yoghurt

Heat the oil in a saucepan and sauté the onion until soft. Add the garlic and stir for a minute. Add the stock, lentils and carrot and bring to simmer.

Cook for 30 minutes or until the lentils are tender.

Add seasoning to taste, stir in the coriander and serve with the yoghurt stirred in.

Broad bean soup

Calories: 184	
Total fat: 9.4g	
Saturated fat: 2.1g	
Fibre: 7.9g	
Protein: high	
Carbohydrate: low	
Vitamins: nicotinic acid, folate, C	
Minerals: copper	

1 tablespoon corn oil
1 medium onion (about 125 g / 4½ oz), finely chopped
225 g (8 oz) shelled fresh (or frozen) tender broad beans
500 ml (18 fl oz) good-quality vegetable stock
1 tablespoon chopped mint, plus more leaves for garnish
1 teaspoon sea salt
black pepper
2 tablespoons reduced-fat Greek-style yoghurt

Heat the oil in a pan and sauté the onion until soft and translucent.

Add the beans and stock and simmer for 20 minutes.

Add the chopped mint, salt and pepper and blend in a blender or food processor until the soup is smooth. Adjust the seasoning, reheat and stir in the yoghurt before serving, garnished with mint leaves.

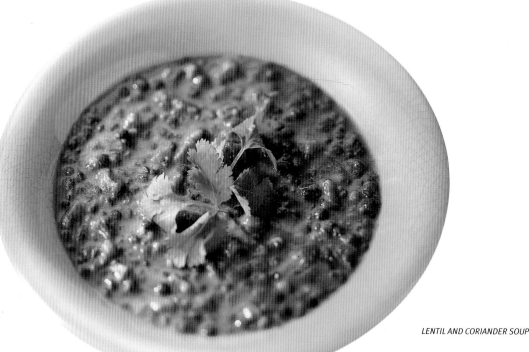

LENTIL AND CORIANDER SOUP

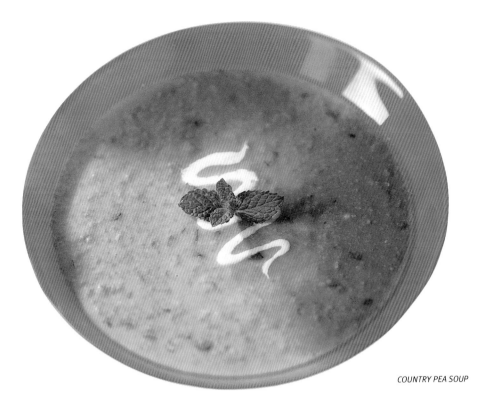

COUNTRY PEA SOUP

Country pea soup

🐟 🌀 🥚 🍷 🍴 🐚 Ⓥ ⓞ ◕ 🗓

Calories: 225	
Total fat: 7.4g	
Saturated fat: 1g	
Fibre: 8.8g	
Protein: high	
Carbohydrate: high	
Vitamins: B1, nicotinic acid, B6, folate, C, E	
Minerals: magnesium, potassium, iron	

1 tablespoon sunflower oil
1 medium onion (about 125 g / 4½ oz),
    finely chopped
1 potato (about 100 g / 3½ oz),
    chopped
275 g (10 oz) fresh peas
    (shelled weight)
300 ml (½ pint) good-quality chicken
    stock
1½ tablespoons chopped fresh mint
1 teaspoon sea salt
1 tablespoon bio yoghurt

Heat the oil in a non-stick pan and
sauté the onion until soft.
   Add the potato, peas, stock, 1
tablespoon of the mint and the salt,
and simmer for 30 minutes.
   Process the soup in a blender or food
processor to a rough purée.
   Reheat and serve with the remaining
chopped mint and the yoghurt stirred in
at the last minute.

Spinach, parsley and garlic soup

🐟 🌀 🥚 🍴 🐚 Ⓥ ⓞ 🗓

Calories: 150	
Total fat: 9g	
Saturated fat: 2g	
Fibre: 4.7g	
Protein: high	
Carbohydrate: low	
Vitamins: B1, nicotinic acid, B6, folate, A, carotenoids, C, E	
Minerals: calcium, magnesium, potassium, iron	

1 tablespoon olive oil
1 medium onion, finely chopped
3 garlic cloves, crushed
1 leek, thinly sliced (to produce about
    100 g / 3½ oz when prepared)
1 fresh stalk of celery (about 50 g / 1¾
    oz), chopped
200 g (7 oz) baby spinach leaves
good handful of chopped fresh flat-
    leaved parsley
400 ml (14 fl oz) vegetable stock
sea salt and black pepper
1 tablespoon freshly grated Parmesan

Heat the oil in a saucepan and sauté
the onion, garlic, leek and celery until
softened. Add the spinach, parsley, stock
and seasoning, then simmer for a few
minutes.
   Blend the soup using a blender or
food processor. Adjust the seasoning.
   Reheat and serve with the Parmesan
sprinkled over.

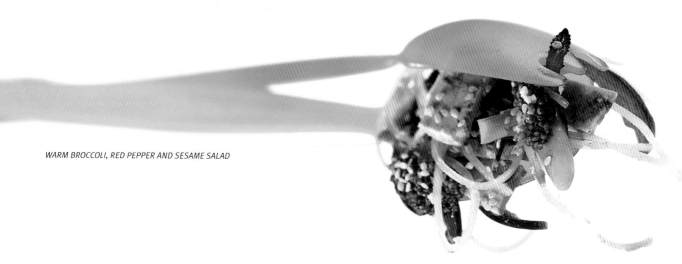

WARM BROCCOLI, RED PEPPER AND SESAME SALAD

Warm broccoli, red pepper and sesame salad

Calories: 229	
Total fat: 15g	
Saturated fat: 2.3g	
Fibre: 4.5g	
Protein: medium	
Carbohydrate: low	
Vitamins: nicotinic acid, B6, folate, A, carotenoids, C, E	
Minerals: potassium, iron	

2 tablespoons sesame oil
2 red peppers, deseeded and thinly
  sliced (about 200 g / 7 oz)
125 g (4½ oz) broccoli, cut into small
  florets
1 garlic clove, crushed
100 g (3½ oz) silken tofu, sliced
2 teaspoons light soy sauce
½ teaspoon chilli sauce
1 teaspoon honey
½ teaspoon freshly grated root
  ginger
1 teaspoon sesame seeds

Heat half the oil in a frying pan and stir-fry the peppers and broccoli for 5 minutes, until the peppers are tinged golden and slightly soft.

Add the rest of the ingredients except the remaining oil and the sesame seeds and stir-fry for a minute.

Turn out on serving plates and serve warm with the sesame oil drizzled over and the sesame seeds sprinkled on top.

Chickpea salad with peppers and tomatoes

Calories: 300	
Total fat: 15g	
Saturated fat: 2.1g	
Fibre: 7.8g	
Protein: medium	
Carbohydrate: medium	
Vitamins: nicotinic acid, B6, folate, A, carotenoids, C, E	
Minerals: magnesium, potassium, iron	

250 g (9 oz) well-drained canned
  chickpeas
2 medium ripe tomatoes
2 whole red canned or bottled red
  peppers, well drained and thinly
  sliced
1 tablespoon each finely chopped fresh
  mint, coriander and parsley
2 tablespoons extra-virgin olive oil
2 tablespoons lemon juice
pinch of sugar
pinch of mustard powder
1 teaspoon sea salt
black pepper
pinch of ground chilli powder

Put the chickpeas in a serving bowl.

Halve the tomatoes and squeeze out the pips, then roughly chop the flesh and add to the bowl together with the red pepper and fresh herbs.

Combine the olive oil with the remaining ingredients and pour over the chickpea salad. Toss and serve.

Spiced lentils with mixed green vegetables

Calories: 272
Total fat: 7.8g
Saturated fat: 1.5g
Fibre: 8.5g
Protein: high
Carbohydrate: medium
Vitamins: B1, B2, nicotinic acid, B6, folate, A, C, E
Minerals: calcium, magnesium, potassium, iron, zinc, copper, selenium, iodine

1 tablespoon groundnut oil
1 medium onion, thinly sliced
1 teaspoon each freshly ground cumin seeds and ginger
1 small red chilli, deseeded and finely chopped
1 teaspoon sea salt
black pepper
one 400-g (14-oz) can of green lentils, well drained and rinsed
200 g (7 oz) mixed young dark green leafy vegetables (such as spinach, chard or spring greens), torn
juice of ½ lemon
2 tablespoons low-fat natural bio yoghurt

Heat the oil in a non-stick pan and sauté the onion until soft. Add the spices, chilli and seasoning and sauté for a further minute.

Add the lentils and stir for a minute or two, then add the leaves and stir again for a minute until slightly wilted.

Add the lemon juice and drizzle over the yoghurt before serving slightly warm or at room temperature.

Brown rice and citrus salad

Calories: 545
Total fat: 14g
Saturated fat: 1.9g
Fibre: 4.4g
Protein: high
Carbohydrate: medium
Vitamins: B1, nicotinic acid, B6, folate, C
Minerals: magnesium potassium, copper

1 large orange
300 g (10½ oz) pre-cooked brown rice
3 ready-to-eat dried apricots, chopped
1 tablespoon chopped walnuts or brazils
200 g (7 oz) cooked lean chicken, sliced
1 tablespoon chopped fresh mint
1 tablespoon sultanas
1 tablespoon walnut or sesame oil
1 teaspoon sea salt
black pepper

Peel and segment the orange above a plate, retaining all the juices.

Place the rice, orange segments, apricots, nuts, chicken, mint and sultanas in a serving bowl.

Pour the retained orange juice into a bowl and combine with the walnut or sesame oil, salt and pepper and mix in with the rice salad.

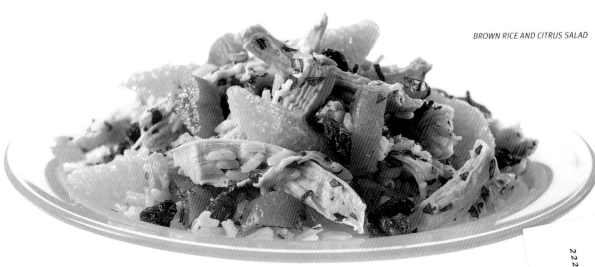

BROWN RICE AND CITRUS SALAD

FOOD FOR HEALTH A

Panzanella

Calories: 272
Total fat: 15g
Saturated fat: 2.2g
Fibre: 4.6g
Protein: medium
Carbohydrate: low
Vitamins: B1, nicotinic acid, B6, folate, A, carotenoids, C, E
Minerals: calcium, magnesium, iron, selenium

2 slightly stale ciabatta rolls
3 medium tasty ripe tomatoes
4 cm (1½ inch) piece of cucumber, diced
1 small red onion (about 75 g / 2¾ oz), thinly sliced
6 black olives, stoned and halved
8 capers, well rinsed and drained
1 fresh juicy garlic clove
1 teaspoon sea salt
1⅔ tablespoons tomato juice or passata
2 tablespoons olive oil
1 tablespoon red wine vinegar
black pepper
1 tablespoon chopped fresh basil
1 tablespoon chopped fresh flat-leaved parsley

Tear the bread into small bite-sized pieces and place these in a serving bowl.

Halve the tomatoes and gently squeeze out the pips, retaining any juice that comes out. Roughly chop the tomatoes and add to the bread. Add the cucumber, onion, olives and capers to the dish.

Pound the garlic and salt with a pestle in a mortar until you have a paste. Gradually add the tomato juice or passata, olive oil, vinegar and black pepper until you have a pouring dressing. Pour this over the salad. Add the chopped herbs and stir in lightly.

Leave for up to an hour for the bread to absorb the dressing.

A more substantial dish can be made with the addition of some diced Mozzarella cheese or by grating some fresh Parmesan over the top before serving.

This would add to the calcium, calorie and fat content.

Thai salmon salad

Calories: 315
Total fat: 17g
Saturated fat: 3g
Fibre: 2.9g
Protein: high
Carbohydrate: low
Vitamins: B1, B2, nicotinic acid, B6, B12, folate, A, C, D, E
Minerals: magnesium, potassium, iron, copper, selenium, iodine

2 medium salmon fillets (about 115 g / 4 oz each)
2 tablespoons teriyaki marinade
100 g (3½ oz) mango
5-cm (2-inch) piece of cucumber
1 courgette
100 g (3½ oz) fresh beansprouts
2 teaspoons groundnut oil
juice of 1 fresh juicy lime
2 teaspoons Thai fish sauce
1 garlic clove, crushed
1 small green chilli, deseeded and chopped
pinch of caster sugar
few mint or coriander leaves, chopped
2 lime wedges, to serve

Place the salmon fillets in a dish and pour the teriyaki marinade over them, coating well. Leave, covered, in the fridge for at least 30 minutes but no more than 1 hour.

Meanwhile, make the salad. Peel and stone the mango and slice into thin strips. Peel the cucumber and cut it into thin strips. Slice the courgette similarly. Combine the mango, cucumber, courgette and beansprouts.

When the salmon is ready, preheat the grill to high and put a good-quality baking tray underneath it. Remove the salmon from the marinade and brush with a little of the oil. Put on the baking tray under the grill and cook for about 5 minutes, depending upon the thickness of the salmon. (If the baking tray is good and hot, there's no need to turn the fish as the underside will cook nicely.)

While the salmon is cooking, mix together any remaining oil with the lime juice, fish sauce, garlic, chilli, sugar and herbs and combine with the salad.

Arrange the salad on serving plates and when the salmon is cooked, cut it into chunks and serve on the salad with the lime wedges.

Seafood risotto with ginger

Calories: 604	
Total fat: 22g	
Saturated fat: 7.3g	
Fibre: 2.5g	
Protein: high	
Carbohydrate: high	
Vitamins: B1, B2, nicotinic acid, B6, folate, C	
Minerals: calcium, magnesium, potassium, iron, zinc, copper	

500 ml (18 fl oz) good-quality fish stock
1 sachet (about 1 teaspoon) of real
  saffron
15 g (½ oz) butter
1 tablespoon light olive oil
12 shallots, finely chopped
1-cm (½-inch) root ginger, grated
175 g (6 oz) risotto rice
1 medium fresh dressed crab (about
  150 g / 5 oz crab meat)
2 tablespoons dry white wine or sherry
1 tablespoon chopped fresh coriander
1 teaspoon sea salt
black pepper
1 tablespoon freshly grated Parmesan

Heat the stock in a pan. Ladle a small amount into a small bowl when hot and infuse the saffron in this.

Heat the butter and oil in a non-stick frying pan and add the shallot. Sauté until soft, then add the ginger and stir for half a minute. Add the rice, stirring for a minute to coat all the grains.

Add one-quarter of the stock in the pan, stir and bring to gentle simmer, stirring frequently. When all the stock is absorbed, add more and repeat, using the saffron stock towards the end of cooking.

When the rice is plump and cooked but still with a moist and creamy texture, add the crab meat, wine or sherry, coriander and seasoning. Serve at once, with the Parmesan cheese sprinkled over.

Salad of tuna, avocado and tomato

Calories: 409	
Total fat: 23g	
Saturated fat: 4.3g	
Fibre: 10g	
Protein: high	
Carbohydrate: low	
Vitamins: B1, B2, nicotinic acid, B6, B12, folate, A, C, D, E	
Minerals: magnesium, potassium, iron, copper, selenium, iodine	

150 g (5 oz) fresh tuna steak
2 tablespoons extra-virgin olive oil
8 asparagus tips
2 beef tomatoes (about 250 g / 9 oz)
150 g (5 oz) pre-cooked cannellini or
  lima beans, rinsed and drained
1 medium mild onion, thinly sliced
1 small ripe avocado (about 150 g / 5 oz)
1 tablespoon lemon juice
1 tablespoon chopped fresh oregano
1 teaspoon sea salt
black pepper

Brush the tuna steak with a little of the olive oil and grill or dry-fry for about 3 minutes on each side, until the outside is golden but the inside is still pink.

Meanwhile, steam or microwave the asparagus tips until just tender. Halve the tomatoes and squeeze out the pips, then chop roughly.

Arrange the beans on serving plates with the tomato, asparagus and onion. Peel and slice the avocado and add to the plates.

Mix together the oil, lemon juice, most of the oregano and seasoning. Pour most of it over salad. Slice tuna and add. Drizzle over remaining dressing. Garnish with rest of oregano.

SALAD OF TUNA, AVOCADO AND TOMATO

Prawns, rice and avocado

Calories: 619	
Total fat: 28g	
Saturated fat: 8.3g	
Fibre: 6.4g	
Protein: high	
Carbohydrate: medium	
Vitamins: B1, B2, nicotinic acid, B6, B12, folate, A, C, E	
Minerals: magnesium, potassium, iron, zinc, copper, selenium, iodine	

125 g (4½ oz) (dry weight) quick-cook brown rice
1 tablespoon olive oil
1 medium onion, finely chopped
1 garlic clove, finely chopped
200 g (7 oz) large raw prawns
1 red pepper, deseeded and chopped
1 medium courgette (about 100 g / 3½ oz), sliced across into rounds and then these halved
1 medium avocado
1 tablespoon lemon juice
2 tablespoons half-fat crème fraîche
dash of chilli sauce (Tabasco)
1 teaspoon sea salt
black pepper

Cook the rice in lightly salted boiling water until tender. Drain and reserve, keeping warm.

Heat the oil in a non-stick frying pan and sauté the onion until soft. Add the garlic, prawns, pepper and courgette and stir-fry for a further 2-3 minutes.

Peel, stone and chop the avocado and place in a bowl. Add the lemon juice, crème fraîche, chilli sauce and seasoning, and mix roughly together.

Pour this mixture into the frying pan and stir into the prawns, etc. Finally, toss the cooked rice through and serve still warm.

Seafood and tropical fruit salad

Calories: 251	
Total fat: 5.2g	
Saturated fat: 0.8g	
Fibre: 4.1g	
Protein: high	
Carbohydrate: medium	
Vitamins: nicotinic acid, B6, B12, folate, A, C, E	
Minerals: calcium, magnesium, potassium, iron, copper, selenium, iodine	

10 large raw prawns (about 250 g / 9 oz)
2 teaspoons lime juice
1 teaspoon balsamic vinegar
2 teaspoons corn oil
1 teaspoon chilli sauce (such as Tabasco)
pinch of caster sugar
1 pink grapefruit
1 small ripe mango
1 small banana
2 passion fruit

Preheat a hot grill or barbecue. Peel the prawns but leave their tails on.

In a small bowl, mix together the lime juice, vinegar, oil, chilli sauce and sugar. Brush the prawns with a little of the mixture, then thread them on skewers (soaked in water if wooden) and grill for 5 minutes, turning once.

Peel and slice the grapefruit and mango, adding any juice that runs out to the dressing and mixing well.

Arrange the sliced fruit on serving plates. Peel the banana and cut in half, then into long slices, and add to the plates. Spoon the flesh out of the passion fruit and add to the salad, then top with the prawns and remaining dressing.

If using pre-cooked prawns, flash under the grill for only 2-3 minutes.

SEAFOOD AND TROPICAL FRUIT SALAD

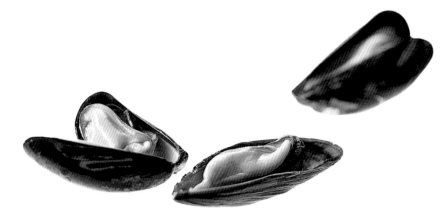

Tiger prawns with rice noodles

Calories: 413	
Total fat: 6.7g	
Saturated fat: 1.3g	
Fibre: 1.3g	
Protein: high	
Carbohydrate: medium	
Vitamins: nicotinic acid, B6, B12, A, C, E	
Minerals: calcium, magnesium, potassium, iron, zinc, copper, selenium, iodine	

1 small red pepper (about 100 g / 3½ oz), deseeded and chopped
1 fresh juicy garlic clove, chopped
1 tablespoon chopped flat-leaved parsley
juice of ½ lemon
1 tablespoon groundnut oil
2 teaspoons chilli paste
1 teaspoon honey
12 raw large tiger prawns (about 30 g / 1 oz each), tails left on
115 g (4 oz) rice noodles
2 spring onions, chopped
2-cm (¾-inch) piece of cucumber, deseeded and chopped
1 tablespoon coconut milk

In a shallow dish, combine the pepper, garlic, parsley, lemon juice, oil, chilli paste and honey well. Place the prawns in the dish and toss to coat with the mixture. Leave to marinate for up to 1 hour.

Cook the noodles and mix with the spring onions and cucumber.

Meanwhile preheat a hot grill and remove prawns from marinade, leaving some on each. Grill for 5 minutes or so, turning once or twice, until cooked.

While the prawns are cooking, heat the remaining marinade in a small pan with the coconut milk, stirring well. Serve the prawns with the sauce and noodles.

Scallops and mussels in the pan

Calories: 361	
Total fat: 9.5g	
Saturated fat: 1.9g	
Fibre: 3.3g	
Protein: high	
Carbohydrate: medium	
Vitamins: B1, B2, nicotinic acid, B6, B12, folate, A, C, E	
Minerals: magnesium, potassium, iron, zinc, copper selenium, iodine	

1 medium red onion, finely chopped
1 small green chilli, deseeded and chopped
1 small yellow pepper, deseeded and chopped
2 tomatoes, deseeded and chopped
1-cm (½-inch) piece of fresh root ginger, peeled and grated
good handful of fresh coriander leaves
juice of 1 lime
1 teaspoon sea salt
black pepper
150 ml (¼ pint) vegetable or fish stock
50 g (1¾ oz) (dry weight) couscous
1 tablespoon groundnut oil
250 g (9 oz) good-quality scallops
1 garlic clove, chopped
200 g (7 oz) shelled mussels

In a bowl, combine the onion, chilli, pepper, tomatoes, ginger, coriander, lime juice, salt and pepper. Set aside for at least 30 minutes. Heat the stock and place in a bowl with the couscous. Set aside.

Heat the oil in a non-stick frying pan over a medium heat and cook the scallops (halved if very big) and garlic for a minute or two. Add the mussels and onion mixture and stir for 2 minutes.

Fluff up the couscous and serve with the scallop and mussel dish.

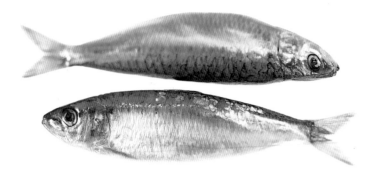

Speedy herbed swordfish

Calories: 260	
Total fat: 13g	
Saturated fat: 2.4g	
Fibre: 0.4g	
Protein: high	
Carbohydrate: low	
Vitamins: B1, B2, nicotinic acid, B6, B12	
Minerals: magnesium, potassium, selenium, iodine	

2 mild shallots, finely chopped
1 level tablespoon each of chopped fresh flat-leaved parsley and dill
1 teaspoon fresh thyme leaves
juice of ½ lemon
1 tablespoon olive oil
2 medium swordfish steaks, each about 175g (6 oz)
1 tablespoon fresh breadcrumbs

In a blender or food processor, mix together the shallots, herbs, lemon juice and olive oil. Place the fish steaks in a shallow dish and cover with the blended mixture. Leave for 1-2 hours.

When you are ready to eat, preheat the grill with a good-quality baking tray underneath it. Remove the swordfish steaks from the marinade (using a knife to return most of the marinade to the dish) and place on the hot baking tray. Quickly mix the remaining marinade with the breadcrumbs and use to coat the tops of the swordfish steaks. Grill for a few minutes until the steaks are cooked and the topping browned. (If the baking tray is good and hot, the underside of the fish will cook nicely so there's no need to turn it.)

Sardines with redcurrant glaze

Calories: 230	
Total fat: 11g	
Saturated fat: 3.2g	
Fibre: negligible	
Protein: high	
Carbohydrate: low	
Vitamins: B2, nicotinic acid, B6, B12, D	
Minerals: selenium, iodine	

8 fresh sardines (about 75 g / 2¾ oz each), cleaned and heads removed
1 teaspoon sea salt
black pepper
1 tablespoon chopped fresh parsley
lemon wedges, to serve
for the redcurrant glaze:
1 tablespoon redcurrant jelly
grated zest of 1 lemon
1 tablespoon medium-dry sherry

First make the redcurrant glaze: in a small bowl, mix together the redcurrant jelly, lemon zest and sherry.

Make several diagonal cuts across the flesh of each sardine and season with the salt and pepper. Brush the redcurrant glaze over the sardines and in the cavities.

Preheat the grill to medium-high and grill the sardines for about 8 minutes, turning them once, until they are cooked through. Garnish with the parsley and serve immediately with the lemon wedges.

You could use cranberry jelly for the sauce, for a slightly more piquant change.

Spanish-style baked trout with chard

Calories: 471

Total fat: 19g

Saturated fat: 3g

Fibre: 5.4g

Protein: high

Carbohydrate: low

Vitamins: B1, B2, nicotinic acid, B6, B12, folate, A, carotenoids, D, C, E

Minerals: magnesium, potassium, iron, copper, selenium, iodine

2 teaspoons olive oil

225 g (8 oz) potatoes, sliced and parboiled

1 beef tomato, sliced

1 large or 2 small trout or sea bass or mackerel (total weight about 450 g / 1 lb), cleaned

4 black olives, stoned and halved

1 tablespoon pine nuts

1 tablespoon sultanas

250 g (9 oz) tender Swiss chard leaves or spinach, pre-cooked and thoroughly drained

1 teaspoon sea salt

black pepper

3 tablespoons dry white wine

juice of ½ lemon

Preheat the oven to 200°C/ 400°F/ gas 6 and brush a baking dish that will hold the fish snugly with the oil.

Cover the base of the dish with the sliced potatoes, then with the tomatoes. Lay the fish on top.

Scatter round the olives, pine nuts, sultanas and Swiss chard, season with salt and pepper and drizzle over the white wine and the lemon juice.

Bake, uncovered, for 30 minutes, or until the fish is tender.

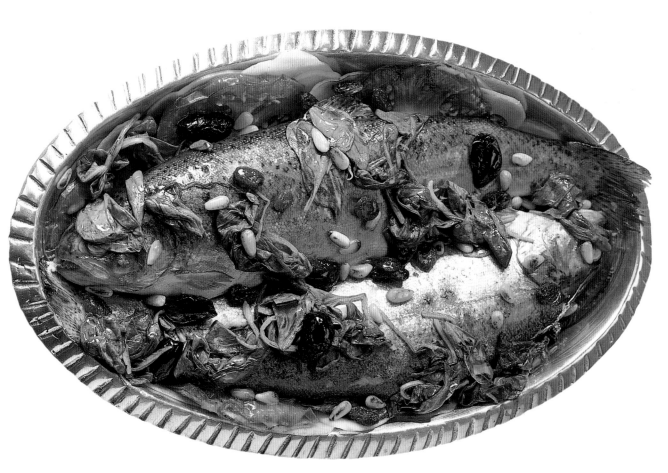

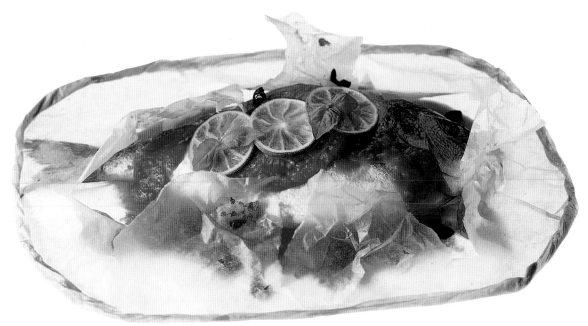

PARCEL OF TILAPIA, TOMATO AND OLIVES

Parcels of tilapia, tomato and olives

Calories: 225
Total fat: 8.3g
Saturated fat: 1.3g
Fibre: 2g
Protein: high
Carbohydrate: low
Vitamins: nicotinic acid, B6, B12, C, E
Minerals: calcium, potassium, iron, copper, selenium, iodine

1 teaspoon olive oil
2 tilapia fish or small trout, cleaned
½ recipe-quantity of Tomato Sauce (see page 247)
1 medium tomato, sliced
1 fresh juicy lime, sliced
6 stoned black olives, roughly chopped
2 tablespoons chopped fresh basil

Preheat the oven to 180°C/ 350°F/ gas 4. Brush two large sheets of foil with the oil and place the fish in the centre of each. Spoon the sauce over each fish, then arrange the tomato and lime slices on top. Sprinkle over the olives and basil and seal up the foil tightly, though leaving plenty of air in the parcels.

Cook the parcels on a baking tray in the oven for about 30 minutes.

Serve the fish parcels still closed so that when they are opened at the table their full aroma will hit!

Seared tuna with lemon grass

Calories: 216
Total fat: 6.8g
Saturated fat: 1.7g
Fibre: 0.3g
Protein: high
Carbohydrate: low
Vitamins: B1, nicotinic acid, B6, B12, D
Minerals: magnesium, potassium, iron, copper, selenium, iodine

2 tuna steaks, each about 150 g (5 oz)
2 tablespoons teriyaki marinade
1 tablespoon black bean sauce
1 teaspoon chilli sauce
1 stalk of lemon grass, bashed with a rolling pin to release aroma and chopped
1 tablespoon chopped fresh coriander

Place the tuna steaks in a shallow dish. Mix together the remaining ingredients and spoon over the steaks. Leave to marinate for 1 hour or so.

Remove the tuna from the marinade, preheat the grill and, when it is very hot, cook the steaks for about 4 minutes, turning once (depending upon the thickness of the steaks, which should be served rare).

If you can't get teriyaki marinade just use soy sauce.

Salmon and broccoli risotto

Calories: 634
Total fat: 25g
Saturated fat: 5g
Fibre: 3.3g
Protein: high
Carbohydrate: medium
Vitamins: B1, B2, nicotinic acid, B12, folate, C, E
Minerals: calcium, magnesium, potassium, iron, zinc, copper, selenium, iodine

2 tablespoons light olive oil
1 medium onion, finely chopped
1 garlic clove, finely chopped
140 g (4¾ oz) risotto rice
700 ml (1¼ pints) good-quality fish stock, warmed
150 g (5 oz) broccoli, separated into small florets
50 g (1¾ oz) smoked salmon, cut into small pieces
150 g (5 oz) salmon fillet, cubed
1 teaspoon sea salt
black pepper
1 tablespoon freshly grated Parmesan cheese

Heat the oil in a large non-stick frying pan and sauté the onion until soft. Add the garlic and rice and stir for a minute or two to coat the rice well.

Add the fish stock, one-quarter of the volume at a time, stirring to absorb each quantity before adding more.

Meanwhile, blanch the broccoli for 1 minute in boiling water. About 5 minutes before the end of cooking time (when the rice is tender, moist and creamy), add the two salmons and the broccoli and seasoning.

Serve the risotto topped with the cheese.

Herring fillets with ginger and coriander

Calories: 383
Total fat: 26g
Saturated fat: 6.6g
Fibre: negligible
Protein: high
Carbohydrate: low
Vitamins: B2, nicotinic acid, B6, B12, D
Minerals: potassium, iron, copper, selenium, iodine

4 herring fillets, each about 100 g (3½ oz)
2 teaspoons soy sauce
2 teaspoons lemon juice
1 teaspoon freshly grated root ginger
little sea salt to taste
black pepper
2 teaspoons chopped fresh coriander

Arrange the herring fillets on a plate and place this in a Chinese bamboo steamer (if you have one, otherwise use a conventional steamer). Sprinkle the fillets with the soy sauce, lemon juice, ginger, salt and pepper. Steam for a few minutes over boiling water until cooked through.

Serve the fillets with the juices poured over, and garnished with the coriander and a small amount of ground sea salt if you wish.

HERRING FILLETS WITH GINGER AND CORIANDER

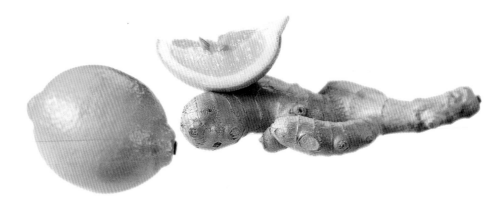

Chicken cacciatore

🟡 ⚪ 🔶 ▼ ✖ 🔵 🔴 🔋

Calories: 214

Total fat: 12g

Saturated fat: 2.4g

Fibre: 1g

Protein: high

Carbohydrate: low

Vitamins: nicotinic acid, B6, C, E

Minerals: copper

1 tablespoon olive oil
4 chicken thighs, part-boned and
    skinned
1 fresh juicy garlic clove, crushed
few sprigs of fresh thyme, tarragon and
    oregano or 1 teaspoon each of the
    dried herb
100 ml (3½ fl oz) dry white wine
1 small can (200 g / 7 oz) of chopped
    tomatoes
black pepper
6 stoned black olives, halved
6 capers, rinsed and drained

Heat the oil in a flameproof casserole
or heavy frying pan with a lid and brown
the chicken on all sides.

Turn the heat down a little and add
the garlic and herbs together with the
wine. Stir for a minute or two. Add the
tomatoes with their liquid and some
pepper. Bring to simmer and cook
covered, for 20 minutes or until the
chicken is tender.

Add the olives and capers, stir well
and cook for a further 2-3 minutes,
uncovered, until you have just a little
thick sauce left. Adjust the seasoning
and add a little sea salt if necessary.

Lemon chicken

🟡 ⚪ 🔶 🍖 ▼ ✖ 🐟 🔵 🔴 🔋

Calories: 189

Total fat: 6.9g

Saturated fat: 1.2g

Fibre: negligible

Protein: high

Carbohydrate: low

Vitamins: nicotinic acid, B6

2 medium chicken breast fillets,
    skinned
1 garlic clove
1 teaspoon sea salt
1 teaspoon grated zest and juice of
    1 good juicy lemon
1.5-cm (¾-inch) piece of fresh root
    ginger, peeled and grated
1 tablespoon sesame or groundnut oil

Put the chicken pieces in a shallow
dish. Mash together the garlic and salt
until you have a purée. Mix this with the
lemon zest and juice, the ginger and the
oil and coat the chicken pieces. Leave to
marinate for 30 minutes if possible.

Either bake the chicken in the dish
in an oven preheated to 180°C/ 350°F/
gas 4 for 25 minutes or, if you prefer,
grill the pieces under a preheated
medium-hot grill or griddle, or dry-fry
them on a non-stick pan or griddle.

Spiced chicken and greens

Calories: 314
Total fat: 13g
Saturated fat: 13g
Fibre: 3.9g
Protein: high
Carbohydrate: low
Vitamins: B1, B2, nicotinic acid, B6, folate, A, carotenoids, C, E
Minerals: calcium, magnesium, potassium, iron, selenium

200 g (7 oz) tender young green leaves of choice (pak-choi, Cos lettuce, Chinese leaves, tender spring greens, spinach or well-rinsed seaweed, or a mixture)
2 medium chicken breast fillets, skinned
1 tablespoon groundnut oil
1 medium onion, finely chopped
2 garlic cloves, finely chopped
1 green fresh chilli, deseeded and finely chopped
½ teaspoon each ground turmeric and cumin seeds
2 large tomatoes (about 150 g / 5 oz in total), halved and deseeded
100 ml (3½ fl oz) natural Greek-style yoghurt or whole-milk bio yoghurt
about 3 tablespoons chicken stock
sea salt and black pepper

Chop the green leaves into thin slices. Slice each chicken breast across the grain into 4 pieces.

Heat the oil in a non-stick frying pan and sauté the onion until soft. Move the onion to one side and add the chicken pieces. Cook until they have turned slightly golden — if the onion is also slightly golden by now that is fine.

Reduce the heat and add the garlic, chilli and spices, stirring everything in well for a minute or two. Chop the tomatoes and add to the pan, then cook for a further 2 minutes. Add the greens and stir for 2 minutes more, then spoon in the yoghurt and bring to simmer.

Using the chicken stock, thin the sauce down a little. Adjust the seasoning with a little sea salt and black pepper.

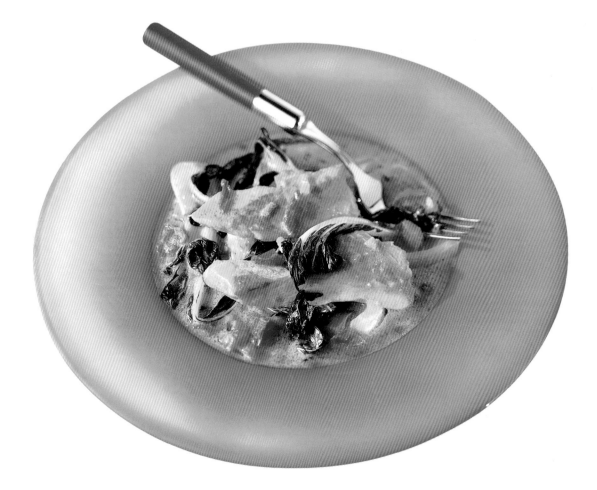

Avocado and turkey tortillas

Calories:	534
Total fat:	13g
Saturated fat:	
2.9g	
Fibre:	5.9g
Protein:	high
Carbohydrate:	
medium	
Vitamins: B1, B2,	
nicotinic acid, B6,	
folate, E	
Minerals:	
magnesium,	
potassium, iron,	
copper,	
selenium	

4 wheat-flour tortillas
1 small avocado
2 teaspoons lime juice
200 g (7 oz) smoked turkey, sliced
sea salt and black pepper
for the salsa:
2 medium tomatoes, deseeded and
    chopped
2 spring onions, chopped
2-cm (¾-inch) piece of cucumber,
    deseeded and chopped
50 g (1¾ oz) ready-cooked black-eye
    beans
1 tablespoon lime juice
1 tablespoon chopped fresh coriander
1 teaspoon chilli sauce

First make the salsa: in a bowl, combine all the ingredients and set aside for an hour or so, if you can.

When you are ready to serve, heat the tortillas in the oven preheated to 180°C/350°F/gas 4, wrapped in foil or baking parchment.

Peel and stone the avocado and mash it with seasoning and lime juice. Fill the warm tortillas each with some smoked turkey, salsa and avocado.

You could use smoked chicken instead of the turkey.

Thai guinea fowl, cashew and pineapple

Calories:	416
Total fat:	28g
Saturated fat:	
6.1g	
Fibre:	2.2g
Protein:	high
Carbohydrate:	
low	
Vitamins: B1,	
folate, C	
Minerals:	
magnesium, iron,	
copper	

2 guinea fowl breasts, skinned
1 tablespoon sesame oil
1 heaped teaspoon each ground
    coriander seeds, cumin seeds and
    fresh chopped chilli
pinch of ground galangal or ginger
4 spring onions, finely chopped
juice of 1 lime
1 garlic clove, crushed
1 tablespoon groundnut oil
4 baby sweetcorn, blanched
1 tablespoon Thai fish sauce
2 tablespoons coconut milk
2-cm (¾-inch) piece of cucumber,
    diced
3 rings of fresh pineapple, diced
40 g (1½ oz) shelled roasted
    cashew nuts

Cut the guinea fowl breasts across the grain into bite-sized strips and place them in a shallow dish. Mix together the sesame oil, spices, spring onions, lime juice and garlic and coat the chicken with this. Set aside for 30 minutes if you can.

Heat the groundnut oil in a non-stick frying pan and add the chicken and its marinade. Stir-fry for a few minutes.

Add the sweetcorn and Thai fish sauce and stir for a few more minutes. Add the coconut milk, cucumber, pineapple and cashews and stir again for a minute or two. Serve immediately.

You can use corn-fed chicken or turkey breast fillets in this recipe if you prefer. Thai fish sauce is now available from many better supermarkets, health-food shops and Oriental stores; if you can't find any, use good-quality soy sauce.

AVOCADO AND TURKEY TORTILLAS

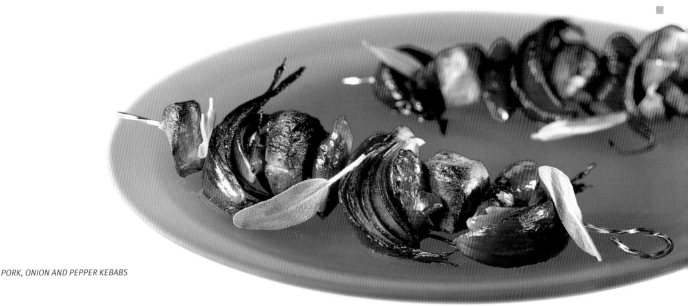

PORK, ONION AND PEPPER KEBABS

Pork, onion and pepper kebabs

Calories: 275

Total fat: 11g

Saturated fat: 2.5g

Fibre: 3.8g

Protein: high

Carbohydrate: low

Vitamins: B1, B2, nicotinic acid, B6, B12, folate, A, carotenoids, C, E

Minerals: magnesium, potassium, zinc, copper, selenium

200 g (7 oz) fillet of pork, cubed
1 garlic clove, crushed
juice of 1 lemon
1 teaspoon sea salt
black pepper
1 red pepper, deseeded and cut into
*   squares*
1 red onion, cut into wedges
2 teaspoons olive oil
½ recipe-quantity Tomato Sauce
*   (see page 247)*
1 teaspoon chopped fresh sage

Put the pork in a shallow dish. In a small bowl, roughly blend the garlic into the lemon juice with the salt and pepper. Tip this mixture over the pork. Cover and set aside for an hour if you can.

When ready to cook, preheat the grill. Thread the pork pieces on 2 kebab sticks alternating them with pieces of red pepper and red onion. Brush with olive oil and grill for 8 minutes, turning occasionally.

Heat the tomato sauce and stir in the sage. Serve the kebabs with the sauce.
An alternative sauce would be Tzatziki (see page 214).

Pork tenderloin in chinese sauce

Calories: 237

Total fat: 12.4g

Saturated fat: 2.6g

Fibre: 0.6g

Protein: high

Carbohydrate: low

Vitamins: B1, B2, nicotinic acid, B6, B12

Minerals: zinc

200 g (7 oz) pork fillet, cut into thin
*   rounds*
1 fresh juicy garlic clove, crushed
1.5-cm (¾-inch) piece of peeled fresh
*   root ginger*
2 teaspoons runny honey
2 teaspoons light soy sauce
1 tablespoon dry sherry
1 tablespoon sesame oil
2 teaspoons yellow bean sauce
2 teaspoons toasted sesame seeds

Preheat the oven to 200°C/ 400°F/ gas 6.

Place the pork fillets in a shallow baking dish which is just big enough to hold them in a single layer, overlapping them slightly.

Combine all the remaining ingredients except the sesame seeds in a small saucepan and heat through, stirring to mix well. Pour over the pork fillets and combine well.

Cover the pork loosely with a piece of foil and bake for 20 minutes or until tender, basting two or three times.

Sprinkle with the toasted sesame seeds to serve.

Turkish lamb stew

Calories: 407	
Total fat: 13g	
Saturated fat: 4.7g	
Fibre: 12g	
Protein: high	
Carbohydrate: medium	
Vitamins: B1, B2, nicotinic acid, B6, B12, folate, C, E	
Minerals: magnesium, potassium, iron, zinc, copper	

1 tablespoon olive oil

225 g (8 oz) lean fillet of lamb, cut into cubes

1 large onion, thinly sliced

1 garlic clove, crushed

1 medium potato (about 175 g / 6 oz), peeled and cubed

4 canned tomatoes, drained

1 medium green pepper, deseeded and sliced

100 g (3½ oz) pre-cooked chickpeas

1 small aubergine, topped and tailed and cut into chunks

about 200 ml (7 fl oz) good-quality beef stock

black pepper

1 tablespoon red wine vinegar

1 teaspoon each chopped fresh thyme, rosemary and oregano

4 black olives, stoned and halved

little sea salt

Heat the oil in a flameproof casserole or heavy-based saucepan and brown the lamb over a fairly high heat.

Turn the heat down a little, add the onion and garlic and sauté for a few minutes until soft.

Add the remaining ingredients except the olives and sea salt. Stir well to combine, bring to simmer and cook, covered, for 1-1½ hours, or until everything is tender.

Add the olives and sea salt and simmer, uncovered, for a further 15 minutes.

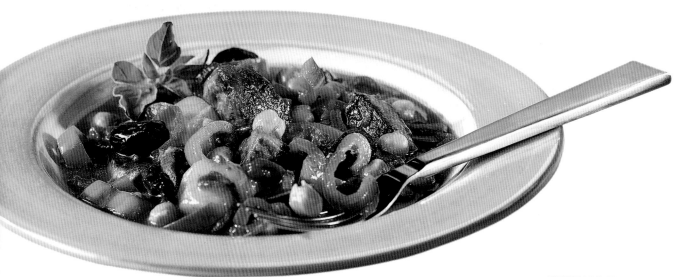

TURKISH LAMB STEW

Steak and spinach stir-fry

Calories: 482	
Total fat: 18g	
Saturated fat: 5.3g	
Fibre: 6.3g	
Protein: high	
Carbohydrate: medium	
Vitamins: B1, B2, nicotinic acid, B6, B12, folate, A, carotenoids, C, E	
Minerals: calcium, magnesium, potassium, iron, zinc, copper	

200 g (7 oz) fillet or lean rump steak
1 tablespoon black bean sauce
2 teaspoons red wine vinegar
2 teaspoons light soy sauce
2 teaspoons oyster sauce
1 teaspoon chilli sauce
100 g (3½ oz) (dry weight) egg-thread noodles
1 tablespoon groundnut oil
40 g (1½ oz) broccoli, broken into small florets
1 red pepper, deseeded and thinly sliced
4 spring onions, halved lengthwise
100 g (3½ oz) fresh beansprouts
150 g (5 oz) fresh baby spinach leaves

Slice the beef across the grain into thin bite-sized strips and place in a shallow dish. Mix together the black bean sauce, vinegar, soy sauce, oyster sauce and chilli sauce, and pour evenly over the beef. Set aside, covered, for an hour if you can.

Cook the noodles according to packet instructions, drain and leave in their pan with a little of the cooking liquid to keep them warm and moist.

Heat the oil in a wok or large non-stick frying pan. Remove the beef from the marinade (some will cling to the pieces of beef, but that is fine) and add it to the wok. Stir-fry for 2 minutes.

Remove the beef from the pan and add the broccoli and red pepper. Stir-fry for 3 minutes.

Add the spring onions, beansprouts and spinach, and return the beef to the pan. Stir-fry again for 1 minute. Add the marinade and stir-fry some more.

If the mixture is too dry for you, add a little water or beef stock.

Toss the drained noodles into the pan to warm through and combine. Serve immediately.

Pasta with chicken livers

Calories: 477	
Total fat: 15g	
Saturated fat: 5.6g	
Fibre: 2.3g	
Protein: high	
Carbohydrate: medium	
Vitamins: B1, B2, nicotinic acid, B6, B12, folate, A, C	
Minerals: magnesium, iron, zinc, copper	

150 g (5 oz) tagliatelle
little sea salt
1 tablespoon light olive oil
200 g (7 oz) chicken livers, trimmed and halved
2 garlic cloves, crushed
100 ml (3½ fl oz) good-quality chicken stock
2 tablespoons half-fat crème fraîche
juice of ½ lemon
black pepper
2 teaspoons chopped fresh parsley

Cook the tagliatelle in plenty of lightly salted boiling water until just tender. Drain well.

Meanwhile, heat the oil in a non-stick frying pan and, when very hot, add the chicken livers, stirring gently. When the outsides are browned but the insides still pink, remove with a slotted spoon and drain on some kitchen paper. Keep warm.

Add the garlic to the pan and stir for a minute or two, but don't let it burn.

Add the stock and bring to a simmer. Cook for a few minutes until the stock is reduced by about half, breaking the garlic up well with the back of a spoon to distribute.

Add the rest of the ingredients and the livers to the pan, stir to combine and cook gently for a minute or two. Adjust the seasoning if necessary. Serve the pasta with the chicken livers as soon as it is cooked and drained.

Pasta with olives and sardines

Calories: 541	
Total fat: 23g	
Saturated fat: 5.4g	
Fibre: 2.7g	
Protein: high	
Carbohydrate: medium	
Vitamins: nicotinic acid, B6, B12, D	
Minerals: calcium, magnesium, iron, copper, selenium, iodine	

150 g (5 oz) penne pasta
1 teaspoon sea salt, plus more for cooking the pasta
6 fresh sardines
2 tablespoons extra-virgin olive oil
6 black olives, stoned and chopped
juice of 1/2 lemon
1 tablespoon chopped fresh flat-leaved parsley
black pepper
1 tablespoon freshly grated Parmesan cheese

Cook the pasta in plenty of lightly salted boiling water until just tender. Drain well.

Meanwhile, grill the sardines, turning once, until cooked (about 3 minutes per side). Carefully remove the central bone and any other bones you can see and chop the flesh into bite-sized pieces.

When the pasta is cooked and the sardines ready, add the olive oil, sardines, olives, lemon juice, parsley and seasoning to the pasta in its pan. Stir well and heat through for 2 minutes over a low heat.

Serve with the Parmesan cheese sprinkled over.

Pasta with broccoli and anchovies

Calories: 505	
Total fat: 20g	
Saturated fat: 3g	
Fibre: 6.6g	
Protein: medium	
Carbohydrate: medium	
Vitamins: B1, nicotinic acid, B6, B12, folate, A, carotenoids, C, E	
Minerals: calcium, magnesium, potassium, iron, copper, selenium	

150 g (5 oz) pasta shells or fusilli
300 g (10 1/2 oz) broccoli
1 fresh juicy garlic clove
1 teaspoon sea salt
1 small red chilli, deseeded and chopped
4 large canned anchovies in oil, drained (reserving the oil) and chopped
juice of 1/2 lemon
2 tablespoons extra-virgin olive oil
2 tablespoons slightly stale breadcrumbs

Cook the pasta in plenty of lightly salted boiling water until just tender. Drain well.

Meanwhile, break the broccoli into small florets and blanch for 1 minute, then drain.

Using a pestle and mortar, mash together the garlic, salt and chilli into a paste. Blend 2 teaspoons of the reserved oil from the anchovies and the lemon juice into this.

Heat 1 tablespoon of the olive oil in a non-stick frying pan and add the breadcrumbs. Cook, stirring occasionally until the crumbs are golden. Remove the crumbs and reserve.

Add the remaining oil to the pan and stir-fry the broccoli for a few minutes. Add the garlic mixture and stir for another minute, then add the anchovies.

Lightly toss the broccoli mixture with the drained pasta and serve sprinkled with the breadcrumbs.

PASTA WITH OLIVES AND SARDINES

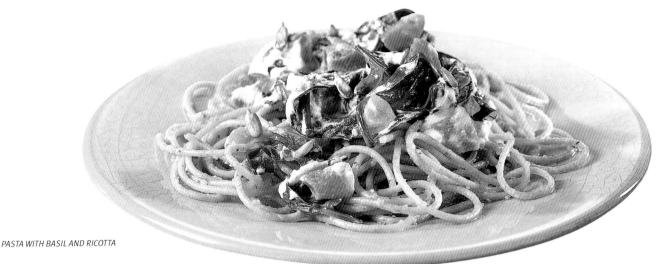

PASTA WITH BASIL AND RICOTTA

Pasta with milanese sauce

Calories: 445	150 g (5 oz) spinach tagliatelle
Total fat: 12g	salt
Saturated fat: 1.9g	1 tablespoon olive oil
Fibre: 5.8g	2 tender celery stalks (about 100 g / 3½ oz), chopped
Protein: high	1 red pepper, deseeded and chopped
Carbohydrate: high	1 garlic clove, crushed
Vitamins: B1, B2, nicotinic acid, B6, folate, A, C, E	100 g (3½ oz) mixed mushrooms of choice (such as chestnut, oyster, porcini), chopped
Minerals: magnesium, potassium, iron, zinc, copper	75 g (2¾ oz) extra-lean ham, chopped
	½ recipe-quantity Tomato Sauce (see page 247)
	1 tablespoon chopped flat-leaved parsley

Cook the pasta in plenty of lightly salted boiling water until just tender. Drain well.

Meanwhile, heat the oil in a non-stick frying pan and stir-fry the celery, pepper and garlic for a few minutes until softened.

Add the mushrooms, ham and tomato sauce. Stir well and leave to simmer for 20 minutes, adding a little chicken stock, water or white wine if the sauce gets too thick.

Serve the sauce on top of the tagliatelle and the parsley sprinkled over.

Pasta with basil and ricotta

Calories: 601	150 g (5 oz) wholemeal spaghetti
Total fat: 31g	1 teaspoon sea salt, plus more for cooking the pasta
Saturated fat: 6.3g	1 fresh juicy garlic clove
Fibre: 9.5g	2 tablespoons pine nuts
Protein: medium	1 pack or pot (15 g / ½ oz) of fresh basil
Carbohydrate: medium	2 tablespoons extra-virgin olive oil
Vitamins: B1, B2, nicotinic acid, B6, folate, A, E	1 tablespoon sunflower seeds
Minerals: calcium, magnesium, potassium, iron, zinc, copper	40 g (1½ oz) ready-to-eat dried apricots, chopped
	40 g (1½ oz) young spinach or sorrel leaves
	100 g (3½ oz) ricotta cheese

Boil the pasta in a large pan of lightly salted water until just tender and then drain.

Meanwhile, using a pestle and mortar, crush the garlic with the sea salt until well combined. Add the pine nuts and blend again. Add most of the basil and crush, adding the olive oil until you have a rich sauce.

Toss the drained pasta with the basil sauce and all remaining ingredients while the pasta is still warm.

Serve garnished with the remaining basil leaves.

Potato and mediterranean vegetable bake

Calories: 463	
Total fat: 18g	
Saturated fat: 2.6g	
Fibre: 13g	
Protein: medium	
Carbohydrate: high	
Vitamins: B1, nicotinic acid, B6, folate, C	
Minerals: magnesium, potassium, iron, copper	

2 medium waxy potatoes (about 350 g / 12 oz in total)
1 teaspoon sea salt, plus more for cooking the potatoes
2 courgettes (about 200 g / 7 oz in total)
2 medium red peppers (about 250 g / 9 oz in total)
1 large aubergine (about 275 g / 10 oz)
1⅔ tablespoons olive oil
1 recipe-quantity Tomato Sauce (see recipe page 247)
black pepper
2 teaspoons chopped fresh oregano leaves

Preheat the oven to 200°C/ 400°F/ gas 6.

Peel the potatoes and cut them into 0.5-cm (¼-inch) slices, then parboil these in lightly salted water until almost tender. Drain and reserve.

Meanwhile, top and tail the courgettes and slice them thinly at an angle. Deseed the pepper and cut it into quarters, then halve these. Top and tail the aubergine and slice it into 1-cm (½-inch) rounds. Place all the vegetables except the potatoes on a baking tray, brush them with one-third of the olive oil, sprinkle on the tablespoon of sea salt and bake for 25 minutes, or until soft and turning golden.

Brush a suitable baking dish (small lasagne dish or similar) with a little of the remaining olive oil and put half the potato slices in the bottom. Arrange the baked vegetables over the potatoes, then pour on the tomato sauce to coat evenly.

Arrange the remaining potatoes evenly on top, sprinkle with pepper and oregano and drizzle over the last of the oil.

Return to the oven for 20 minutes before serving.

Potato gnocchi with cheese and cauliflower

Calories: 779	
Total fat: 23g	
Saturated fat: 9.7g	
Fibre: 6.7g	
Protein: high	
Carbohydrate: high	
Vitamins: B1, B2, nicotinic acid, B6, B12, folate	
Minerals: calcium, magnesium, potassium, zinc, copper, iodine	

1 rounded tablespoon (25 g / ¾ oz) sunflower spread
500 g (1 lb 1½ oz) ready-made potato gnocchi
1 small cauliflower, broken into florets
1 rounded tablespoon plain flour (25 g / ¾ oz)
400 ml (14 fl oz) skimmed milk
40 g (1½ oz) reduced-fat farmhouse Cheddar cheese, grated
1 teaspoon sea salt
black pepper
1 medium tomato, sliced and halved
40 g (1½ oz) Fontina cheese
1 tablespoon freshly grated Parmesan cheese

Brush a two-serving size gratin dish with a little of the sunflower spread. Cook the gnocchi in boiling water according to packet instructions, drain and place in the gratin dish.

Cook the cauliflower florets in a very little boiling water (or steam or microwave) until tender, then carefully add them to the gnocchi, spreading them around the dish evenly.

Heat the remainder of the sunflower spread in a saucepan and add the flour. Stir well to cook for a minute, then add the milk. Bring to a simmer, stirring until you have a pouring sauce. Add the grated Cheddar, salt and pepper, and stir for a minute.

Preheat a hot grill.

Pour the sauce over the gnocchi and cauliflower and arrange the tomato pieces around the surface. Cut the Fontina cheese into small pieces and dot over the top, then sprinkle on the Parmesan.

Grill the dish until the top is bubbling and turning golden, then serve.

Winter squash with lentils and ginger

Calories:	388
Total fat:	7.8g
Saturated fat:	1.3g
Fibre:	13g
Protein:	high
Carbohydrate:	high
Vitamins: B1, nicotinic acid, B6, folate, A, carotenoids, C, E	
Minerals: calcium, magnesium, potassium, iron, zinc, copper, selenium	

450 g (1 lb) orange-fleshed squash (see note)
1 tablespoon groundnut oil
1 medium onion, thinly sliced
1 garlic clove, chopped
2-cm (¾-inch) piece of fresh root ginger, grated
1 tablespoon black bean sauce
one 400-g (14-oz) can of pre-cooked green or brown lentils, drained and rinsed
about 150 ml (¼ pint) good-quality vegetable stock
1 tablespoon chopped fresh coriander

Peel the squash, deseed it and cut the flesh into medium chunks.

Heat the oil in a flameproof casserole or heavy frying pan which has a matching lid and sauté the onion until just turning golden.

Add the garlic and ginger and stir for a minute. Add the squash and sauté until the chunks are tinged golden, then add the black bean sauce and lentils and give everything a good stir. Pour in enough stock barely to cover the squash, bring to a simmer and cook, covered, for 20 minutes or until squash is tender.

Adjust the seasoning. adding a little sea salt if necessary, then serve garnished with the coriander.

NOTE: suitable squashes for this sort of treatment include butternut, onion squash, Sweet Mama or Crown Prince, or any with firm deep orange flesh. Watery pale pumpkins or squashes aren't suitable for this dish.

WINTER SQUASH WITH LENTILS AND GINGER

Rice and beans

Calories: 356	
Total fat: 3.1g	
Saturated fat: 0.8g	
Fibre: 5.3g	
Protein: medium	
Carbohydrate: high	
Vitamins: B1, nicotinic acid, B6, folate, A, C	
Minerals: magnesium, potassium, copper	

125 g (4½ oz) basmati rice
1 teaspoon sea salt, plus more for cooking the rice
4 tablespoons coconut milk
1 green chilli, deseeded and chopped
1-cm (½-inch) piece of fresh root ginger, chopped
1 red pepper, deseeded and chopped
2 spring onions, finely chopped
half a 400-g (14-oz) can of mixed pulses, drained and rinsed
black pepper
1 tablespoon chopped fresh coriander

Cook the rice in 250 ml (9 fl oz) boiling lightly salted water in a pan covered with a tight-fitting lid until tender.

Meanwhile, put the coconut milk, chilli, ginger, pepper and spring onions in a small saucepan and simmer for a few minutes.

When the rice is cooked, toss the rice, coconut sauce, pulses, seasoning and coriander together and serve.

Almond, chickpea and raisin pilaf

Calories: 714	
Total fat: 30g	
Saturated fat: 4.6g	
Fibre: 7.3g	
Protein: medium	
Carbohydrate: high	
Vitamins: B1, B2, nicotinic acid, B6, folate, E	
Minerals: magnesium, potassium, iron, zinc, copper	

275 ml (10 fl oz) vegetable stock
1 sachet (about 1 teaspoon) of real saffron threads
150 g (5 oz) brown rice
1 tablespoon groundnut oil
35 g (1¼ oz) unsalted cashews
35 g (1¼ oz) flaked almonds
1 medium onion, finely chopped
½ teaspoon each ground coriander seeds and cumin seeds
100 g (3½ oz) pre-cooked chickpeas
40 g (1½ oz) raisins
1 tablespoon chopped fresh coriander

Heat the vegetable stock in a saucepan and add the saffron. Add the rice, bring to simmer and cook, covered, for 30 minutes or until the rice is tender and all the stock absorbed (add more stock or water if rice dries out before it is tender).

Heat a non-stick frying pan and brush the base with a little of the groundnut oil. Add the cashews and almonds and stir-fry until golden. Remove from the pan and reserve.

Add the rest of the oil to the pan and sauté the onion until soft and just turning golden.

Add the ground coriander and cumin seed and stir-fry for a minute, then add the chickpeas and raisins and stir-fry for another minute. Add the rice, toasted nuts and chopped coriander and stir together gently to combine.

ALMOND, CHICKPEA AND RAISIN PILAF

Rice and greens

Calories: 516	
Total fat: 21g	
Saturated fat: 0.8g	
Fibre: 5.3g	
Protein: medium	
Carbohydrate: high	
Vitamins: B1, nicotinic acid, B6, B12, folate, A, carotenoids, C, E	
Minerals: calcium, magnesium, potassium, iron, zinc, copper	

1 medium leek (about 100 g / 3 1/2 oz), sliced into rounds
1 medium courgette (about 100 g / 3 1/2 oz), sliced into rounds
100 g (3 1/2 oz) broccoli, broken into small florets
handful of fresh basil leaves
2 tablespoons extra-virgin olive oil
1 teaspoon sea salt
1 tablespoon pine nuts
2 tablespoons fresh grated Parmesan cheese
black pepper
150 g (5 oz) risotto rice
400 ml (14 fl oz) good-quality vegetable stock
100 g (3 1/2 oz) young leaf spinach
handful of rocket leaves (about 10 g / 1/3 oz), finely sliced

Blanch the leek, courgette and broccoli in boiling water for 1 minute, drain well.

Using a blender or food processor, blend the basil, half the oil, the salt, pine nuts, Parmesan and pepper into a paste.

Heat the remaining oil in a non-stick frying pan, add the rice and stir to coat.

Heat the stock to a simmer. Add one-quarter of the stock to the rice with the blanched vegetables, stir and bring to simmer. Stir from time to time and, when the stock is all absorbed, add another similar quantity, continuing like this until all the stock is used up and the rice is tender and moist. (Add extra stock if you need to.)

When the dish is nearly cooked, add the spinach and rocket and the basil sauce and stir gently for a minute or two so that the spinach wilts. Adjust the seasoning and serve immediately.

Asparagus can be used instead of broccoli in this dish.

Chickpea and vegetable crumble

Calories: 374	
Total fat: 14g	
Saturated fat: 3.4g	
Fibre: 10g	
Protein: high	
Carbohydrate: medium	
Vitamins: B1, nicotinic acid, B6, B12, folate, A, C, E	
Minerals: calcium, magnesium, potassium, iron, copper	

1 tablespoon olive oil
1 medium onion, finely chopped
1 garlic clove, chopped
100 g (3 1/2 oz) spinach or Swiss chard
2 medium carrots (about 200 g / 7 oz), peeled, diced and parboiled
2 medium tomatoes, deseeded and chopped
juice of 1/2 lemon
200 g (7 oz) pre-cooked chickpeas
1 tablespoon chopped fresh flat-leaved parsley
1 red chilli, deseeded and chopped
1 teaspoon sea salt
black pepper
3 tablespoons passata
1 medium slice of stale bread
1 level tablespoon coarse oatmeal
2 tablespoons freshly grated Parmesan

Preheat the oven to 180°C/ 350°F/ gas 4.

Heat the olive oil in a non-stick frying pan and sauté the onion until soft and slightly golden.

Add the garlic and stir for a minute. Add the spinach or chard and carrots and stir for a few minutes, then add the tomatoes, lemon juice, chickpeas, parsley, chilli, seasoning and passata. Stir well, bring to simmer and transfer everything to a suitably sized gratin dish.

Chop the bread into small pieces or coarsely grate it. Mix this with the oatmeal and Parmesan and sprinkle over the chickpea mixture.

Bake for 30 minutes or until the top is golden.

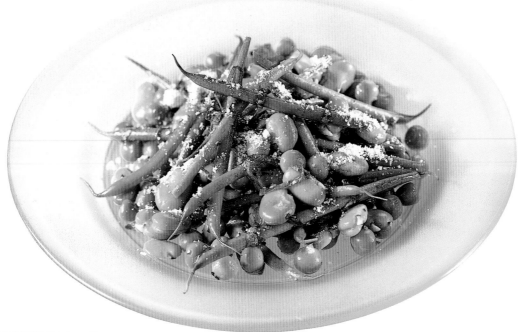

SUMMER VEGETABLES WITH MINT

Summer vegetables with mint

Calories: 136

Total fat: 7g

Saturated fat: 1.8g

Fibre: 6g

Protein: high

Carbohydrate: low

Vitamins: B1, nicotinic acid, folate, C

100 g (3½ oz) fresh broad beans
100 g (3½ oz) (shelled weight) peas
50 g (1¾ oz) fine beans, topped and
tailed
sea salt
2 teaspoons extra-virgin olive oil
1 tablespoon chopped fresh mint
black pepper
2 teaspoons lemon juice
1 tablespoon freshly grated Parmesan

Simmer the broad beans, peas and beans in a little lightly salted water until just tender.

Drain and add to a small frying pan with the oil, mint, seasoning and lemon juice. Stir for a minute so that the flavours combine. Serve with the grated cheese sprinkled over.

Stir-fried pak-choi with almonds

Calories: 108

Total fat: 9.2g

Saturated fat: 1.1g

Fibre: 2.3g

Protein: medium

Carbohydrate: low

Vitamins: folate, C

1 tablespoon sesame oil
1-cm (½-inch) piece of peeled fresh root
ginger, grated
1 garlic clove, chopped
300 g (10½ oz) pak-choi leaves, any
tough stalks discarded, thinly sliced
1 teaspoon soy sauce
2 teaspoons toasted chopped
almonds

Heat the sesame oil in a wok or non-stick frying pan and add the grated ginger and chopped garlic, stirring for 30 seconds.

Add the sliced pak-choi leaves and the soy sauce and stir-fry for 2 minutes.

Add the toasted chopped almonds, stir through and serve immediately.

Aubergine and okra sauté

🌸 🌀 🥩 🍴 🍽 🐟 V 🌑 🌓 🗓

Calories: 137	
Total fat: 6.9g	
Saturated fat: 1.1g	
Fibre: 7.1g	
Protein: high	
Carbohydrate: medium	
Vitamins: B1, B6, folate, C, E	
Minerals: magnesium, potassium, copper	

1 tablespoon olive oil
1 medium red onion, finely chopped
1 fresh juicy garlic clove, chopped
100 g (3½ oz) trimmed okra
50 g (1¾oz) baby sweetcorn
1 medium aubergine
200 g (7 oz) canned chopped tomatoes
1 teaspoon chopped fresh thyme
1 teaspoon salt
black pepper
about 3 tablespoons vegetable stock
1 tablespoon chopped fresh coriander

Heat the oil in a non-stick saucepan (which has a tight-fitting lid) and sauté the onion until soft.

Add the garlic and stir for a minute. Add the okra and sweetcorn and stir to combine.

Chop the aubergine into small cubes and add to the pan with the tomatoes and their liquid, the thyme, seasoning and stock. Mix well and bring to simmer. Cook for 15 minutes, covered, then for a further 15 minutes uncovered, until you have a rich vegetable stew.

Serve sprinkled with the coriander.

Peas and lettuce

🌸 🌀 🥩 🍢 🍽 V 🌑 🌓 🗓

Calories: 134	
Total fat: 6g	
Saturated fat: 3.1g	
Fibre: 5.6g	
Protein: high	
Carbohydrate: medium	
Vitamins: B1, nicotinic acid, folate, C, A	
Minerals: iron	

200 g (7 oz) (shelled weight) fresh small peas
1 Little Gem lettuce, cut lengthwise into 8 pieces
4 spring onions, chopped
10 g (½ oz) butter
1 teaspoon balsamic vinegar
1 teaspoon chopped fresh parsley
1 teaspoon chopped fresh mint
1 teaspoon sea salt
black pepper

Put all the ingredients in a saucepan with 3 tablespoons of water and bring to a simmer.

Cook uncovered for a few minutes until the peas are tender.

AUBERGINE AND OKRA SAUTÉ

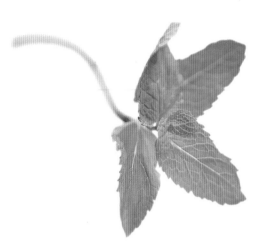

Green lentils with herbs

Calories: 220	
Total fat: 7.2g	
Saturated fat: 0.9g	
Fibre: 4.9g	
Protein: high	
Carbohydrate: medium	
Vitamins: B1, nicotinic acid, B6, folate	
Minerals: magnesium, iron, copper, selenium	

100 g (3½ oz) green lentils
1 small mild onion (about 75 g / 2¾ oz)
400 ml (14 fl oz) vegetable stock
1 tablespoon extra-virgin olive oil
juice of ½ lemon
2 tablespoons fresh mixed herbs, such as
    oregano, mint, marjoram, thyme,
    sage and parsley
1 teaspoon sea salt
black pepper

Put the lentils in a pan with the onion and stock. Bring to a simmer and cook for 45 minutes, or until lentils are tender.

Drain off any remaining stock and stir the olive oil, lemon juice, herbs and seasoning into the lentils. Serve hot.

Spinach, broccoli and walnut stir-fry

Calories: 107	
Total fat: 8.5g	
Saturated fat: 0.8g	
Fibre: 3.1g	
Protein: high	
Carbohydrate: low	
Vitamins: folate, A, carotenoids, C, E	
Minerals: calcium, magnesium, iron	

125 g (4½ oz) broccoli, broken into
    florets
2 teaspoons walnut oil
125 g (4½ oz) baby spinach leaves
1 tablespoon chopped walnuts
1 teaspoon sea salt
black pepper
2 tablespoons vegetable stock

Blanch the broccoli in boiling water for 1 minute.

Drain and refresh in cold water. Dry on kitchen paper.

Heat the oil in a small non-stick frying pan and stir-fry the broccoli for 2 minutes.

Add the spinach, walnuts and seasoning and stir-fry for a minute, adding the stock towards the end of cooking time.

Tabbouleh

Calories: 299	
Total fat: 12g	
Saturated fat: 1.7g	
Fibre: 2.6g	
Protein: low	
Carbohydrate: high	
Vitamins: B1, nicotinic acid, folate, A, C	
Minerals: magnesium, iron, copper	

100 g (3½ oz) bulgar
1 large tomato, skinned, deseeded and
    chopped
6-cm (2½-inch) piece of cucumber,
    chopped
handful of chopped fresh flat-leaved
    parsley
1 tablespoon chopped fresh mint
2 spring onions, chopped
2 tablespoons olive oil
1 teaspoon sea salt
black pepper
juice of ½ lemon

Put the bulgar in a large bowl, pour over boiling water and leave to soak for 30 minutes, or according to packet instructions, until plumped up. Drain.

Mix the bulgar with all the other ingredients in the bowl. Allow to stand, covered, for up to an hour before serving.

Home-baked beans

Calories: 361
Total fat: 13g
Saturated fat: 1.6g
Fibre: 12g
Protein: medium
Carbohydrate: high
Vitamins: B1, nicotinic acid, B6, folate, E
Minerals: calcium, magnesium, potassium, iron, copper

one 400-g (14-oz) can of pre-cooked
    haricot beans
1 tablespoon sunflower oil
1 medium onion, finely chopped
1 level teaspoon English mustard
    powder
2 teaspoons soft brown sugar
1 teaspoon black treacle
2 teaspoons lemon juice
1 teaspoon Worcestershire
    sauce
1 teaspoon sea salt
1 recipe-quantity Tomato Sauce
    (see page 247)

Preheat the oven to 150°C/ 300°F/ gas 2. Rinse the haricot beans well, and drain them and place them in a small casserole dish.

Heat the oil in a non-stick frying pan and sauté the onion until soft and just turning golden. Add the rest of the ingredients to the pan and stir well to heat through.

Pour the sauce over the beans, put the lid on and bake in the oven for 1 hour, stirring once or twice.

If the mixture begins to look dry at any time, add a little water or tomato passata and stir.

Adjust the seasoning with salt, sugar, lemon juice and Worcestershire sauce to taste and serve.

Cannellini beans with hot tomato vinaigrette

Calories: 223
Total fat: 12g
Saturated fat: 1.8g
Fibre: 8g
Protein: high
Carbohydrate: medium

250 g (9 oz) pre-cooked cannellini
    beans
1 good-sized (about 100 g / 3½ oz)
    juicy tomato
2 tablespoons olive oil
2 teaspoons red wine vinegar
pinch of English mustard powder
pinch of caster sugar
1 teaspoon sea salt
black pepper
2 teaspoons chopped fresh basil

Rinse the beans well and drain them. Place them in a saucepan.

Blanch the tomato and skin it; halve it and deseed, then chop, retaining any juices that come out during this process.

In a bowl, mix together the oil, vinegar, tomato (with juices), mustard, sugar and seasoning.

Pour this over the beans in the pan and heat gently, stirring, until all is warmed through.

Add the basil and serve warm.

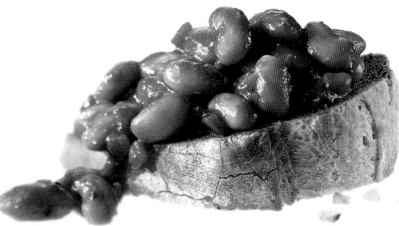

HOME-BAKED BEANS

Sauces serve from 2-4, depending upon use. Nutrition details given are per portion, based upon each recipe serving two. Halve these nutritional details if you are serving four.

Mango salsa

🍷 ☕ 🥄 🍴 ❗ 🎉 ❌ Ⅴ ⊘ ◑ 📅

Calories:	64
Total fat:	0.2g
Saturated fat:	
negligible	
Fibre:	2.9g
Protein:	low
Carbohydrate:	
high	
Vitamins: A, carotenoids, C	

1 ripe mango
1 small red onion
1 tablespoon lime juice
2 teaspoon chopped fresh mint
pinch of sea salt

Peel and stone the mango flesh, then chop the flesh, reserving any juice. In a bowl, combine this with all the remaining ingredients and leave in the fridge for 30 minutes.

Serve cold with poultry, game or fish.

Tofu mayonnaise

🍷 ☕ 🥄 🍴 🍽 ❗ 🎉 ❌ Ⅴ ⊘ ◑ 📅

Calories:	33
Total fat:	1.6g
Saturated fat:	
0.2g	
Fibre: negligible	
Protein: high	
Carbohydrate:	
low	

100 g (3½ oz) silken tofu, mashed
1 small garlic clove, crushed
2 teaspoons white wine vinegar
1 teaspoon Dijon mustard
1 teaspoon sea salt
black pepper

Blend all ingredients together in a blender or food processor. Adjust the seasoning. Use to replace ordinary egg-based mayonnaise in your diet.

Vary the mayonnaise by adding chopped fresh herbs, such as dill, tarragon or chives. Lemon juice can be used instead of the vinegar.

Fresh pepper coulis

🍷 ☕ 🥄 🍴 ❗ 🎉 ❌ Ⅴ ⊘ ◑ 📅

Calories:	101
Total fat:	6.1g
Saturated fat:	1g
Fibre:	2.6g
Protein:	low
Carbohydrate:	
medium	
Vitamins: B6, folate, A, carotenoids, C	

2 medium red peppers
1 tablespoon extra-virgin olive oil
1 teaspoon sea salt
black pepper

Simmer the peppers whole in water for 10 minutes, then drain, reserving the cooking water. When cool, peel off the skins. Deseed the peppers and chop the flesh.

Put the chopped peppers in a blender or food processor together with 2-3 tablespoons of the reserved cooking water, the oil and seasoning. Whiz for a few seconds until you have a smooth sauce, adding a little more cooking liquid if the sauce is to thick. Adjust the seasoning. Serve hot or cold.

Chilli sauce to taste can be added for a sauce with more bite.

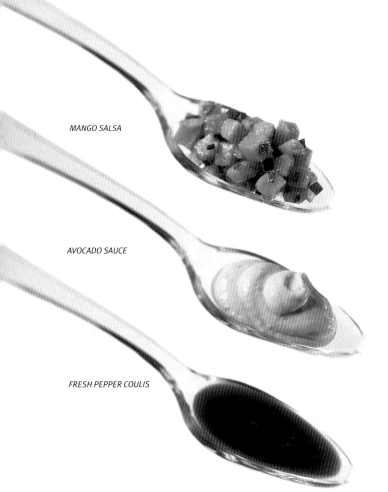

MANGO SALSA

AVOCADO SAUCE

FRESH PEPPER COULIS

Tomato and bean salsa

Calories: 194
Total fat: 6.5g
Saturated fat: 1g
Fibre: 6.9g
Protein: high
Carbohydrate: high
Vitamins: B1, nicotinic acid, B6, folate, A, carotenoids, C, E
Minerals: magnesium, potassium, iron, copper

2 large tomatoes, halved, deseeded and
    chopped
1 medium red onion, chopped
1 small yellow pepper, deseeded and
    chopped
5-cm (2-inch) piece of cucumber,
    deseeded and chopped
200-g (7-oz) can of mixed pulses, rinsed
    and drained
1 green chilli, deseeded and chopped
2 tablespoons chopped fresh coriander
1 tablespoon olive oil
1 tablespoon lime juice
1 teaspoon sea salt
black pepper

Combine all ingredients together in a bowl and leave to marinate for 30 minutes. Serve cold.

Sauce verde

Calories: 108
Total fat: 11g
Saturated fat: 1.6g
Fibre: 0.3g
Protein: low
Carbohydrate: low

1-2 garlic cloves, crushed
1 teaspoon sea salt
1 teaspoon Dijon mustard
2 tablespoons chopped fresh flat-leaved
    parsley
2 tablespoons chopped fresh mint or
    basil
juice of ½ lemon
2 tablespoons extra-virgin olive oil
black pepper

Blend together the garlic and sea salt. Then, using a blender or food processor on slow, blend in the mustard, herbs and lemon juice. With the machine still running, slowly add the olive oil, blending as you do, until you have a green sauce. Add black pepper and adjust the seasoning.

Tomato sauce

Calories: 126
Total fat: 5.9g
Saturated fat: 0.8g
Fibre: 2.7g
Protein: medium
Carbohydrate: medium
Vitamins: B1, B6, folate, carotenoids, C, E
Minerals: potassium, copper

1 tablespoon olive oil
1 medium onion, finely chopped
1 fresh juicy garlic clove, chopped
one 400-g (14-oz) can of chopped
    tomatoes (with their liquid)
2 teaspoons tomato paste
1 heaped teaspoon soft brown sugar
2 teaspoons lemon juice
1 teaspoon salt
black pepper

Heat the oil in a non-stick frying pan and sauté the onion until soft. Add the garlic and stir for a minute.

Add the remaining ingredients, bring to a simmer and cook, uncovered, for 30 minutes or more, until you have a rich sauce.

If too much liquid evaporates, add a little water or tomato juice.

Avocado sauce

Calories: 257
Total fat: 25g
Saturated fat: 7.3g
Fibre: 3.3g
Protein: low
Carbohydrate: low
Vitamins: B2, B6, E

1 large good-quality ripe avocado
juice of 1 small lemon
125 ml (4 fl oz) Greek-style yoghurt
black pepper
1 teaspoon sea salt

Peel and stone the avocado and chop the flesh. Put it immediately in a blender or food processor with the lemon juice and whiz for a few seconds until smooth.

Stir in the Greek yoghurt (by hand) and the seasoning. Serve cold.
Good with fish and seafood, chicken, gammon and eggs, or as a pasta sauce or dip.

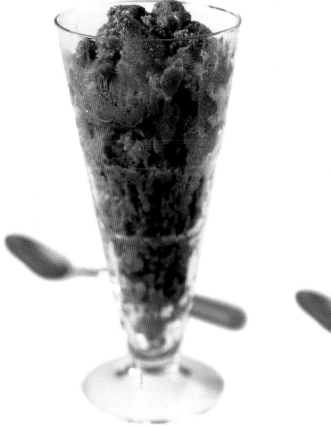
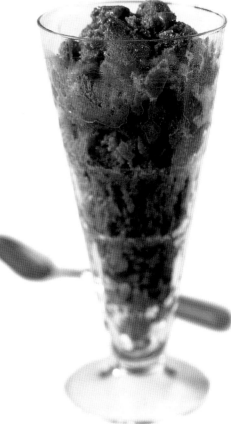

Blackberry ice sundaes

Calories: 193	
Total fat: 1.2g	
Saturated fat: 0.6g	
Fibre: 6.3g	
Protein: high	
Carbohydrate: high	
Vitamins: B2, folate, C, E	
Minerals: calcium, magnesium, potassium, iodine	

40 g (1½ oz) fructose
1 teaspoon agar-agar
100 ml (3½ fl oz) skimmed milk
275 g (10 oz) blackberries
200 g (7 oz) low-fat bio yoghurt
3 tablespoons orange juice

In a small pan, heat the fructose, agar-agar and milk with 3 tablespoons water until the fructose and agar-agar are dissolved. Stir well.

Purée the berries in a blender or food processor and pass through a sieve to remove the pips. Mix this well with the fructose syrup and the remaining ingredients and transfer to a freezable container or ice-cream maker.

If using an ice-cream maker, follow the manufacturer's instructions. If using a container, put the lid on and place in fast-freezer for a few hours or until half-frozen. Take out and stir well. Repeat this process twice more before the ice is totally frozen. Serve frozen.

Other berries can be used in place of the blackberries; if using strawberries or raspberries you don't really need to pass the purée through a sieve. If using ripe fruit at the height of their season, you could reduce the amount of added fructose.

Summer fruit compote

Calories:	54
Total fat:	0.3g
Saturated fat:	
negligible	
Fibre:	4.2g
Protein:	medium
Carbohydrate:	
high	
Vitamins:	folate, C
Minerals:	copper

200 g (7 oz) strawberries
100 g (3½ oz) raspberries
100 g (3½ oz) blackcurrants
40 g (1½ oz) fructose
1 cinnamon stick
dash of lemon juice
Greek-style yoghurt or ice-cream, to serve

Preheat the oven to 160°C/ 325°F/ gas 3. Prepare the fruit if necessary, halving any over-large strawberries and topping and tailing and rinsing the blackcurrants. (Don't rinse the raspberries, just pick over carefully.)

Place the fruit, fructose and cinnamon in a shallow baking dish with 2-3 tablespoons water. Cover and bake in the oven for 30 minutes, stirring gently once, or until the fruit is soft and there is a rich juice.

Remove the cinnamon stick, stir in the lemon juice and serve with Greek-style yoghurt or ice-cream.

Peach and banana fool

Calories:	174
Total fat:	neg
Saturated fat:	4g
Fibre:	1.4g
Protein:	medium
Carbohydrate:	
medium	
Vitamins:	C

1 ripe peach
1 medium just-ripe banana
2 teaspoons icing sugar
1 tablespoon orange juice
150 ml (¼ pint) Greek-style
    yoghurt

Peel and chop the peach and banana and place them in a blender or food processor with the icing sugar and orange juice.

Blend until fairly smooth.

Fold the fruit mixture into the yoghurt, divide between 2 glass dessert bowls or glasses and chill.

Citrus granita

Calories:	142
Total fat:	neg
Saturated fat:	
negligible	
Fibre:	0.2g
Protein:	low
Carbohydrate:	
high	
Vitamins:	C

150 ml (¼ pint) water
60 g (2 oz) fructose
125 ml (4 fl oz) each fresh orange juice
    and lemon juice
3 tablespoons lime juice

Heat the water and dissolve the fructose in it. Stir in all the remaining ingredients and transfer to a sorbet maker or into a freezable container. Follow the process as for Blackberry Ice Sundaes opposite.

Serve frozen — the granita won't be all that solid, even straight from freezer.

Raspberry gratin

Calories:	218
Total fat:	12g
Saturated fat:	
7.7g	
Fibre:	2.5g
Protein:	medium
Carbohydrate:	
low	
Vitamins:	folate, C
Minerals:	calcium

200 g (7 oz) fresh raspberries
7.5 g (¼ oz) fructose
100 ml (3½ fl oz) Greek yoghurt
100 ml (3½ fl oz) half-fat crème fraîche
1 teaspoon cornflour
2 teaspoons soft brown sugar

Preheat the grill. Divide the raspberries between two individual soufflé dishes and sprinkle the fructose on them.

Beat together the yoghurt, créme fraîche and cornflour and spoon evenly over the top of the raspberries. Sprinkle the brown sugar on top.

Put the soufflé dishes underneath the grill. Grill the gratins until the tops begin to bubble and brown. Serve at once.

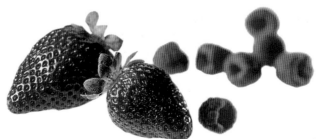

Stir-fried fruit salad

Calories: 214	
Total fat: 6.6g	
Saturated fat: 3.1g	
Fibre: 3.4g	
Protein: low	
Carbohydrate: high	
Vitamins: A, C, E	
Minerals: magnesium, potassium	

1 large barely ripe banana
1 teaspoon safflower oil
7.5 g (¼ oz) unsalted butter
2 slices of fresh pineapple, each halved
1 small ripe mango, peeled, stoned and
    quartered
2 teaspoons lime juice
1 tablespoon sweet dessert wine
Greek-style yoghurt, half-fat crème
    fraîche or half-fat single cream,
    to serve

Peel the banana and cut it into wedges. Heat the oil and butter in a non-stick frying pan and, when very hot, add the fruit. When it starts to brown, stir gently.

Add the lime juice, stir again and add the dessert wine. When the wine has bubbled for a few seconds, serve with some Greek-style yoghurt, half-fat crème fraîche or half-fat single cream.

Mango filo tarts

Calories: 232	
Total fat: 1.5g	
Saturated fat: negligible	
Fibre: 4.5g	
Protein: low	
Carbohydrate: high	
Vitamins: A, carotenoids, C	

3 oblong sheets of filo pastry
'Fry Light' spray
1 large ripe mango
2 teaspoons fructose
2 teaspoons lime juice
pinch each of ground cinnamon and
    ginger
1 tablespoon sultanas
yoghurt, ice-cream or raspberry coulis,
    to serve (optional)

Preheat the oven to 200°C/ 400°F/ gas 6. Cut the filo sheets in half to make six squares. Spraying each sheet with 'Fry Light' as you go, arrange three sheets at angles to each other to produce a decorative edge in 2 patty tins, or similar, to make 2 pastry shells. Bake for 10 minutes, or until just turning golden. Remove from the oven.

Meanwhile, peel, stone and chop the mango. Mix this with the remaining ingredients. Heat through in a small saucepan or microwave to combine the flavours.

When the pastry cases are ready, fill them with the mango mixture and serve immediately with yoghurt, ice-cream or a raspberry coulis if you like.

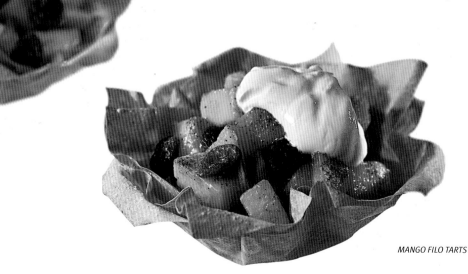

MANGO FILO TARTS

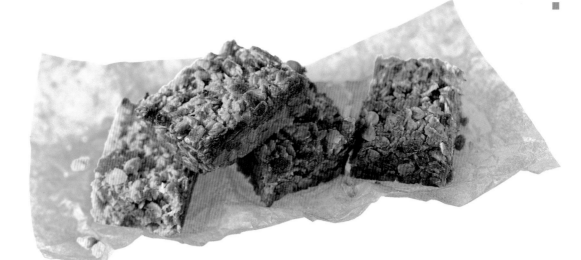

FLAPJACKS

Oat bread

♨ ▼ ∀ ◑ ♻

Makes two 450g (1 lb) loaves

Calories: 78 per slice

Total fat: 2g

Saturated fat: 0.4g

Fibre: 1.5g

Protein: medium

Carbohydrate: high

Vitamins: B, folate

Minerals: magnesium, iron, zinc, copper

475 g (1 lb / 1 oz) oat flour (see note)
40 g (1½ oz) soy flour
7.5 g (1¼ oz) sachet of quick-blend dried yeast
1 teaspoon sea salt
1 level tablespoon soft brown sugar
400 ml (14 fl oz) water, slightly warm
1 tablespoon sunflower oil

Put the flours into a mixing bowl with the yeast, salt and sugar. Add the oil and water and mix thoroughly. When a dough has begun to form, knead it thoroughly for 5-10 minutes.

Divide the dough between 2 lightly oiled 450-g (1-lb) loaf pans and leave in a warm place, covered with a tea towel, for 30 minutes until well risen. Preheat the oven to 180°C/350°F/gas 4. Bake the loaves for 50 minutes, or until they sound hollow when tapped on the base. Turn out on racks and leave to cool well before serving. The bread will keep for a day in an airtight container, or freeze.

NOTE: if your health-food store cannot sell you ready-made oat flour, simply process porridge oats in a blender or food processor until you have a flour, being careful not to over-process to dust. Soy flour can be found in most health-food stores.

Flapjacks

♨ ▼ ✗ ∀ ◑ ♻

Makes 10

Calories: 189 each

Total fat: 8.7g

Saturated fat: 1.8g

Fibre: 2g

Protein: low

Carbohydrate: high

Vitamins: B, D, E

140 g (4¾ oz) Flora Light or other low-fat margarine
150 ml (¼ pint) apple concentrate
225 g (8 oz) porridge oats
pinch of sea salt
25 g (¾ oz) sunflower seeds
50 g (1¾ oz) ready-to-eat dried apricots, chopped

Preheat the oven to 190°C/ 375°F/ gas 5.

In a saucepan, gently melt the margarine with the apple concentrate. Add the oats, salt, seeds and apricots and stir well to mix.

Spoon the mixture into a shallow 17.5 cm (7 inch) square cake pan. Press down well and smooth the top level. Bake for 20-25 minutes, until golden brown, then mark into 8 pieces before allowing to cool.

When cool, remove from the pan and cut through the marks to serve.

Vegetable cup

Calories:	48
Total fat:	0.6g
Saturated fat: 0.2g	
Fibre:	12g
Protein:	high
Carbohydrate: high	
Vitamins: nicotinic acid, folate, A, carotenoids, C, E	
Minerals: potassium	

225 g (8 oz) ripe tomatoes
1 medium carrot
1 celery stalk
handful of watercress
1 teaspoon yeast extract dissolved in a little boiling water
125 ml (4 fl oz) tomato juice
pinch of celery salt
black pepper

Skin, halve and deseed the tomatoes. Peel and finely chop the carrot and chop the celery.

Add everything to a blender or food processor and purée until smooth. Serve cold.

You can use a wide range of additional vegetables in this cup: try adding some sorrel or spinach leaves, cauliflower and/or broccoli florets and Swiss chard.

CLOCKWISE FROM THE TOP: STRAWBERRY COOLER, MANGO AND PEACH BOOSTER, BANANA AND STRAWBERRY SMOOTHIE, VEGETABLE CUP

Strawberry cooler

Calories: 68
Total fat: 0.9g
Saturated fat: 0.6g
Fibre: 0.9g
Protein: high
Carbohydrate: high
Vitamins: C

150 g (5 oz) strawberries
100 ml (3½ fl oz) skimmed milk
100 ml (3½ fl oz) WeightWatchers or
    other low-fat strawberry ice-cream or
    frozen yoghurt

Hull and halve the strawberries and place in blender or a food processor.
    Add the milk and ice-cream and blend until smooth and frothy. Serve immediately.

Mango and peach booster

Calories: 150
Total fat: 0.8g
Saturated fat: 0.4g
Fibre: 3.3g
Protein: medium
Carbohydrate: high
Vitamins: B2, A, carotenoids, C
Minerals: calcium, iodine

1 mango
1 peach
5 tablespoons orange juice
150 ml (¼ pint) low-fat bio yoghurt
2 teaspoons pouring honey

Peel, stone and chop the mango and the peach and place in a blender or food processor. Blend until smooth. Add the other ingredients and blend briefly to mix well. Serve chilled.

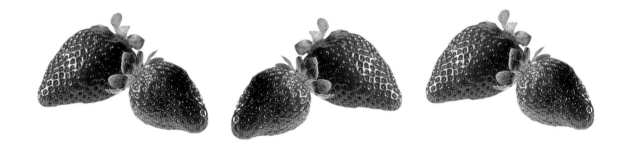

Banana and strawberry smoothie

Calories: 103
Total fat: 0g
Saturated fat: 0.2g
Fibre: 1.4g
Protein: high
Carbohydrate: high
Vitamins: B6, B12, C

1 medium banana
2 teaspoons lemon juice
75 g (2¾ oz) fresh strawberries, chopped
1 teaspoon wheatgerm
1 teaspoon fructose
175 ml (6 fl oz) skimmed milk

Peel and chop the banana and put in a blender or food processor with the lemon juice. Add the strawberries, wheatgerm, fructose and half the milk and blend until smooth.
    Add the rest of the milk and blend again. Serve chilled.

Watermelon refresher

Calories: 50
Total fat: 0.4g
Saturated fat: negligible
Fibre: 0.2g
Protein: low
Carbohydrate: high
Vitamins: C

400 g (14 oz) watermelon
1 teaspoon grated peeled fresh root ginger
2 teaspoons fructose
3 tablespoons mineral water or diet American ginger ale

Peel the watermelon and deseed. Chop the flesh into pieces and add to a blender or food processor with the ginger and fructose. Blend.
    Add the mineral water or ginger ale and blend again. Serve chilled.
Root ginger freezes well and can be grated from frozen.

Summer punch

Calories: 39
Total fat: negligible
Saturated fat: negligible
Fibre: 0.1g
Protein: low
Carbohydrate: high
Vitamins: C

dash of Angostura bitters
dash of Grenadine
100 ml (3½ fl oz) pineapple juice
100 ml (3½ fl oz) orange juice
2 tablespoons lemon juice
100 ml (3½ fl oz) sparkling mineral water

All the ingredients should be nice and cold. Mix together everything but the mineral water. Then stir in the mineral water and serve.

Orange and pineapple crush

Calories: 36
Total fat: negligible
Saturated fat: negligible
Fibre: 0.6g
Protein: low
Carbohydrate: high
Vitamins: C

2 rings of fresh pineapple
100 ml (3½ fl oz) orange juice
200 ml (7 fl oz) diet lemonade

Chop the pineapple and process in a blender or food processor for a few seconds until it is well crushed.

Mix together the orange juice and lemonade.

Divide the crushed pineapple between 2 glasses and top with the lemonade mixture. Serve chilled.

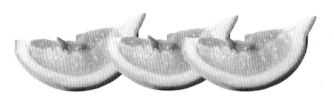

Apple and apricot shake

Calories: 169
Total fat: 2.6g
Saturated fat: 1.5g
Fibre: 3g
Protein: medium
Carbohydrate: high
Vitamins: B1, B12
Minerals: calcium, potassium, iodine

2 fresh and tasty eating apples
4 pieces ready-to-eat dried apricot
300 ml (½ pint) semi-skimmed milk
2 teaspoons pouring honey
pinch of ground cinnamon

Peel, core and chop the eating apples and put in a blender or food processor.

Chop the apricots and add to the blender with one-third of the milk, the honey and the cinnamon. Blend to a purée, then gradually add the rest of the milk. Serve chilled.

Sangria

Calories: 132
Total fat: negligible
Saturated fat: negligible
Fibre: 1.4g
Protein: low
Carbohydrate: low
Vitamins: C

1 organic orange
1 organic lemon
300 ml (½ pint) light and fruity red wine
100 ml (3½ fl oz) soda water

Wash the fruit and peel a few long strips of peel off each. Reserve. Peel the fruit, removing all the pith. Segment the fruit over a suitable jug so that you retain all the juices, again removing all pith and pips.

Halve the segments and add to the jug containing the retained juices, together with the peel. Pour the wine over, stir and chill for at least 30 minutes.

When ready to serve, stir in the soda water.

Lemon balm tea

Calories:
negligible

Total fat:
negligible

Saturated fat:
negligible

Fibre: negligible

Protein:
negligible

4 tablespoons fresh lemon balm leaf,
   finely chopped
1.25 litres (2 pints) boiling water
whole lemon balm leaves, to garnish
lemon slices, to garnish

Place the chopped lemon balm in a warmed teapot and pour on the boiling water. Leave to infuse for 5 minutes, then strain into mugs.

Serve hot or cold garnished with lemon balm leaves and lemon.

Lemon balm tea is calming and also anti-viral. Herbal infusions can also be made with various other fresh herbs such as mint (for indigestion), nettles (diuretic and detoxifying), parsley (diuretic and stimulating), rosemary (tonic and circulatory stimulant).

Dandelion and burdock tea

Calories:
negligible

Total fat:
negligible

Saturated fat:
negligible

Fibre: negligible

Protein:
negligible

25g (1 oz) finely chopped cleaned
   dandelion root
25g (1 oz) finely chopped cleaned
   burdock root

To make a tea out of plant roots, they must be simmered in boiling water for some time rather than simply steeped in boiling water – a decoction. Place the chopped roots in a pan, add 1 litre (1¾ pints) water, bring to simmer and simmer gently for 30 minutes until reduced by half. Strain and serve. The decoction can be kept in the fridge for a day or two.

Dandelion and burdock tea is a good detoxifier, aiding liver function. It is also diuretic and purifying, with a laxative effect due to the burdock.

*CLOCKWISE FROM TOP: ORANGE AND PINEAPPLE CRUSH,
SUMMER PUNCH, APRICOT AND APPLE SHAKE, SANGRIA*

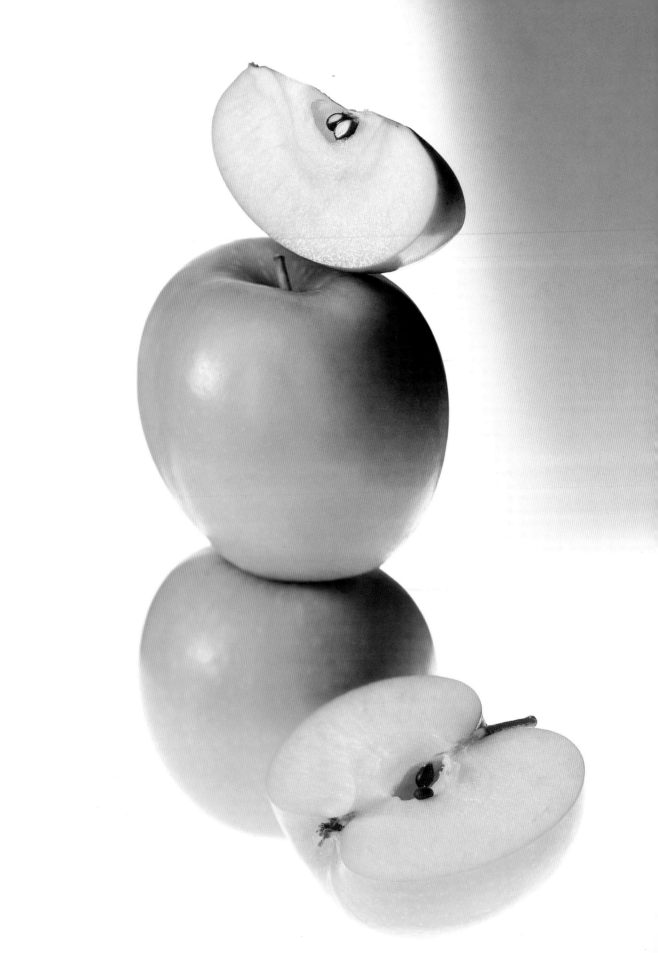

Food at a glance

The charts that follow list the nutrient breakdown of about 400 common and not-so-common foods. Whenever you want to know what is in the food that you eat, this is the section to which you should refer. Where appropriate, there are also interesting health notes for individual foods and food groups to give you extra information that the tables may not supply — for example, news about new micro-nutrients and their effect. The nutrient information is calculated from published analysis and manufacturers' data. However, individual foods vary in their precise nutrient content for various reasons — time of year (especially with fresh fruits and vegetables), method of storage (poor storage loses vitamins, for example), reformulation of manufactured products, and so on. There are also sometimes quite significant variations in nutritional content of some branded foods made by different manufacturers — e.g. different brands of beefburgers. However, the charts will still give you a very reasonable indication of nutrients.

The food charts

Name of food

Usually a general name (for staple foods) but when a food is familiarly known under a manufacturer's name, (e.g. Weetabix), that is given.

Food state

This column tells you whether or not the food has been analysed raw or cooked and, if the latter, how cooked.

Portion size
(sometimes given at start of section)

We have tried as far as possible to give portion sizes which are quantities of the food that will normally be eaten, including official UK Government medium portion sizes, and portions as indicated by manufacturers. All other nutrient information refers to this portion size. For example, most breakfast cereals are given as per 30 g average portion. Therefore the calorie, fat, protein, etc., content listed is what is in that 30 g portion. Bread is usually given per 100 g — equivalent to about three slices.

We have tried to use our common sense when offering portion sizes — obviously, for a more accurate breakdown of what nutrients you are getting in your own diet, you may want to weigh your own portions and then raise or lower the nutrient content accordingly.

KiloCalorie content (calories) and KiloJoules (joules)

A KiloCalorie is a measurement of energy and is popularly known as a 'calorie'. Calorie content is given per portion stated. A KiloJoule — popularly known as a 'joule' — is another way of measuring energy which is used alongside the KiloCalorie method in most countries. A KiloJoule is roughly 4.184 times each calorie, but as joules

are measured in a slightly different way from calories, values can often be less or greater than this. For more information on typical energy (calorie/joule) content of various diets, see Section One.

Total fat (g) and percentages of types of fat

Total fat content of each portion of food is given in grams. The next three columns then offer a percentage breakdown of the types of fat within the total fat content. These are: percentage of polyunsaturated fats, percentage of monounsaturated fats, and percentage of saturated fat. This total fat column also includes trans (hydrogenated) fats, which have a similar effect within the body.

You will probably notice that, in all but a few cases, the three percentage columns don't actually add up to 100. This is because the total fat content of most foods also includes the non-fatty acid fats, such as glycerol and other fatty compounds, as well as polyunsaturated, monounsaturated and saturated fatty acids, so that out of the total weight of fat in a particular food, the 'missing' percentage will be these other fats.

If you are keeping a close eye on your fat intake, it is easy to work out what percentage of total calories in a particular food are fat calories. Check the total fat (g) column. Each gram of fat contains 9 calories, so multiply this column by 9. For example, Cheddar cheese contains 17 g fat, which equals 153 calories. Total calories in the cheese are 206. So the percentage of calories from fat in the cheese (153 divided by 206) = 74.27%. From this you can see that Cheddar is a very high-fat food. You can also see that 63% of those fat calories are from saturated fat, making it also a food extremely high in saturated fat.

For more information on fat within your diet and how much we need of the different types, turn to Section One.

★ SUPERFOODS

Around fifty of the foods in the charts that follow have been picked out with a ❂ in the margin by their names.

These are foods that we have named 'superfoods' because of their special abilities to help fight illness and/or promote good health, and because generally they also have no drawbacks either. These are foods that we should all try to include in our diets regularly (the exception to this is if you are allergic to any of the superfoods, or have been told by your physician to avoid any of them for any other medical reason).

This list is, of course, subjective and most of the foods in the charts have their own plus-points, so don't take the superfood selections too literally – we all need as wide a variety of foods in our diet as possible.

The Health Notes will point out benefits and drawbacks to the foods, and further help in the selection of foods of particular benefit in your own diet appear throughout the book.

Protein (g)

Protein content of the food is given in grams. In a similar way to fat, you can also work out the percentage of protein calories in any particular food.

Each gram of protein contains 4 calories. So, say, Cheddar cheese contains (13 x 4) = 52 protein calories. This is (52 divided by 206) = 25.24% protein, making cheese a high-protein food (because we need no more than 10-15% of our total daily calories as protein).

For more information on protein within your diet and how much we need for health, turn to Section One.

Total carbohydrate (g)

Total carbohydrate content of the food is given in grams and then, in the next two columns, this is broken down into starches and sugars, both also given in grams. For an explanation of these different types of carbohydrate, turn to Section One.

If you would like to work out the percentage of calories from total carbohydrates, starch, or sugars, in any food, simply multiply the grams by 3.75 as each gram of carbohydrate contains 3.75 calories. (E.g. one crumpet contains 17 g of carbohydrate. That is (17 x 3.75) = 63.75 calories. The total calories in the crumpet are 80, so each crumpet contains (63.75 divided by 80) = 79.68% of its calories as carbohydrate, making crumpets a high-carbohydrate food. For more information on carbohydrates and how much we need in our diets for health, turn to Section One.
NOTE: Due to EU labelling regulations, a conversion factor of 4, not 3.75, is used for packeted foods, therefore if calculating from packet information, use 4 and not 3.75.

Total fibre (NSP) (g) and soluble fibre (g)

The fibre columns give fibre (non-starch polysaccharides) content of each food – total fibre, measured by the Englyst method (see page 14), and soluble fibre. For more information about the types of fibre and how much we should get in our diets for good health, turn to Section One.

Cholesterol (mg)

Cholesterol content of foods is listed in milligrams (mg). This column will be useful for anyone who has been asked to follow a diet low in cholesterol by their physician, for instance, people with high blood cholesterol levels or a history of heart disease.

For more information on cholesterol within foods and its importance in a healthy diet, turn to Section One.

Vitamins (useful source of)

This column lists all the vitamins that appear in this portion size of food in useful quantities. A 'useful quantity' in most instances is about 17% or more of the daily EU RDA (recommended daily amount) which has been laid down by the European regulators. Where there is no EU RDA for a nutrient, the UK Department of Health's RNI (reference nutrient intake) has been used.

The Health Notes will sometimes clarify this — for example, when content of a certain vitamin has come out at marginally below 17% and you eat a lot of it, that food will make a useful contribution to that vitamin content of your diet and this will usually be mentioned.

For more advice on vitamins and how much of them we need in our diets, turn to Section One, where you will also find charts listing the principal sources for all major vitamins and minerals.

Minerals (good source of)

Exactly the same criteria have been used for minerals as for vitamins (see above) and again, for more information on minerals in your diet, and charts listing the best sources of each, turn to Section One.

Sodium content has not been listed for each food but if a food is particularly high in sodium this is mentioned in the Health Notes. For a list of foods with high sodium content, see Section One.

Special health notes

Sometimes these are applicable to just one food in a group; at other times they run down several items as group notes.

Classification of the foods

To help you find your way about the charts, the foods are classified under the following headings in the order given:
Breads and other baked goods
Breakfast cereals
Dairy products and eggs
Condiments, sauces and other store-cupboard items
Drinks, alcoholic
Drinks, non-alcoholic
Fats and oils
Fish and seafood
Fruit
Meat, poultry and game
Nuts, seeds and savoury snacks
Puddings and desserts
Rice, grains and pasta
Spreads, dips and pâtés
Sweeteners and confectionery
Vegetables and pulses

VITAMIN ABBREVIATIONS

B1	also known as thiamine	folate	also known as folic acid
B2	also known as riboflavin	pant ac	pantothenic acid, B5
nic ac	nicotinic acid, also known as niacin, B3	b-carotene	beta-carotene (pro-vitamin A)
B6	also known as pyridoxine	C	also known as ascorbic acid

MINERAL ABBREVIATIONS

cal	calcium	manga	manganese
cop	copper	phos	phosphorous
iod	iodine	potas	potassium
magnes	magnesium	sel	selenium

Breads and other baked goods

	food state	portion size	calories	k joules	total fat (g)	% poly	% mono	% sat	protein (g)	carbo (g)	starch (g)	sugars (g)	
Brown		100g	218	927	2.0	30	15	20	9	44	41	3	
Ciabatta		100g	270	1,130	3.5	40	23	37	8.8	50	48	1.9	
Croissant		1 x 60g	216	903	12.2	24	40	32	5	23	22	0.6	
French		100g	270	1,149	2.7	22	19	26	9.6	55	54	1.9	
Granary		100g	235	999	2.7	26	22	19	9.3	46	44	2.2	
Malt		100g	268	1,139	2.4	42	13	13	8.3	57	31	26	
Pitta white		1 x 75g	195	827	0.8	46	n/k	46	7.1	40	37	1.7	
Rye dark		100g	219	931	1.7	n/k	n/k	n/k	8.3	45.8	n/k	n/k	
Wheatgerm		100g	232	937	2.5	n/k	n/k	n/k	9.2	43	40	2.4	
White		100g	235	1002	1.9	26	21	21	8.4	49	47	2.6	
Wholemeal		100g	215	914	2.5	28	20	20	9.2	42	40	1.8	
Cream cracker		3	92	390	3.4	1.3	40	39	2.0	14	14	tr	
Oatcake		2	115	482	4.8	29	44	21	2.6	16	16	0.8	

total fibre (g)	soluble fibre (g)	chol (mg)	useful source of vitamins	good source of minerals
4	1	0	B1, nic ac, folate	magnes, iron, cop, manga
2.6	n/k	0	nic ac	cal, iron, sel, manga
1.0	0.5	4.5	nic ac, folate	
1.5	0.9	0	nic ac	cal, iron, sel, manga
4.3	2.1	0	B1, nic ac, folate	magnes, phos
n/k	n/k	1	B1, nic ac	potas, phos, iron, cop, iod, manga
1.5	n/k	0		
4.4	n/k	0	B1, B2, nic ac, E	cal, iron, phos
3.3	1.3	n/k	B1, nic ac, folate	cal, magnes, iron, cop, iod, manga, potas, phos
1.5	0.9	0	B1, nic ac	cal, manga
5.8	1.6	0	B1, nic ac, folate	magnes, potas, phos, iron, sel, manga
0.5	0.3	n/k		
1.5	0.9	2	manga	

special health notes

Bread is a staple food and, for most people, a healthy one, as a source of carbohydrate and reasonable amounts of protein. Most breads are also low in fat, notable exceptions being croissants and some speciality breads.

Bread is usually made from wheat flour – wholemeal contains 100% of the milled grain, brown and granary 85-95%, and white bread up to 80% of the whole grain but none of the bran (outer layers) or wheat-germ (the centre). Because many of the vitamins and minerals are contained in these parts of the grain, white bread is naturally much lower in vitamins and minerals than wholemeal bread. In the UK, however, by law white bread flour is fortified with B1, nicotinic acid, iron and calcium. Folic acid, a vitamin especially important in pregnancy for the health of the foetus, is due to be added by law to white bread in the near future but not to wholemeal.

Salt content of bread can be high or fairly high, a point worth remembering if you eat a lot of bread and have been asked to follow a low-sodium diet.

Bread is high on the list of foods which can produce allergic reactions in some people – the main allergens being gluten (the constituent which gives dough its elasticity) or wheat or yeast (see Gluten Intolerance, Allergies). Several manufacturers now make wheat-and/or gluten-free loaves and some flat breads are made without added yeast (check labels carefully as many flat breads, such as commercial pittas, DO contain yeast). Soda bread is a yeast-free alternative, though with a short shelf-life. Note that even breads which appear to contain no wheat – e.g. rye bread or oat bread, usually do, in fact, have a proportion of wheat in the recipe to give a lighter loaf. Check the ingredients list.

Commercial, mass-produced budget loaves may contain several additives such as bleach, soya bean flour and caramel. Organic and traditionally made bread is now fairly widely available.

For people following a calorie-restricted diet, dark rye bread is a good choice as it has a medium glycaemic index, unlike wheat loaves which have a high glycaemic index, and so keeps hunger at bay for longer.

Savoury biscuits and crackers tend to be high in salt and fat. Cream crackers are particularly high in saturated and trans fats and salt, and low in fibre. Oatcakes are higher in unsaturated fats and contain much more fibre; as regular eating of oat foods is linked with lowering of blood cholesterol they could be a healthier alternative. Rye crisp-breads are a healthy wholefood, containing nothing but rye and a very little salt, and may be useful for people with wheat intolerance.

	food state	portion size	calories	k joules	total fat (g)	% poly	% mono	% sat	protein (g)	carbo (g)	starch (g)	sugars (g)	
Rice cake		3	77	322	0.6	33	17	17	1.7	17	17	0.3	
Rye crispbread		3	81	338	0.45	50	17	17	2.7	16.5	14.4	2.1	
Apple pie		average slice 110g	293	1,227	15	7	35	49	3.2	39	24	15	
Cereal chewy bar		1 x 33g bar	138	583	5.4	46	42	12	2.4	21	8	11	
Chocolate cake rich		50g	228	954	13	43	32	9	3.7	25	11	14	
Digestive biscuit		x 2	141	593	6.3	8	46	41	1.9	21	17	4	
Digestive biscuit chocolate-coated		2	177	746	8.7	7	37	51	2.4	24	14	10	
Doughnut jam		1	252	1,061	11	25	37	29	43	37	23	14	
Eclair chocolate	frozen	1 x 35g	139	576	11	6	33	52	2.0	9	6.8	2.3	
Fruit cake rich		50g	171	719	5.5	25	40	31	1.9	30	5.6	24	
Rich tea biscuit		2	64	270	2.3	7	35	48	0.9	11	7.3	3.1	
Scone plain		1	174	731	7.0	24	37	34	3.5	26	23	2.8	
Sponge Victoria		50g	151	640	2.5	12	36	32	2.1	32	8.3	24	
Filo pastry		25g	79	332	0.9	n/k	n/k	8	2.2	15	15	0.3	

total fibre (g)	soluble fibre (g)	chol (mg)	useful source of vitamins	good source of minerals	special health notes
0.8	n/k	0			Rice cakes are another low-fat, low-salt alternative to wheat crackers, though they are low in fibre.
3.6	1.2	0		manga	
1.9	1	n/k	C		Calorie content of an apple pie can be reduced by using fructose to sweeten the apples and by making a top pie crust only.
1.1	n/k	n/k		manga	Most bakery items are high in fat, particularly saturated fats. Mass-produced commercial baked goods are often high in trans fats, which are now thought to be equally as bad – or even worse – for health than the saturates.
n/k	n/k	76	A, D, E		A few baked goods are not high in fat – crumpets are particularly low in fat, for example – check labels. Most bakery produce is also low in fibre, vitamins and minerals, and high in sugars and (often) in cholesterol. Cake-lovers should consider all these factors before indulging too often. Most people view cereal bars as a healthier alternative to cakes and biscuits, but they are higher in sugars than many other sweet foods and fat content can also be high.
0.7	0.3	12			
0.8	0.4	18			Nutritional values given here are for guidance only, as recipes vary from manufacturer to manufacturer. Homemade cakes using unsaturated fats, natural ingredients, wholemeal flours and less sugar will produce a much healthier nutritional profile.
n/k	n/k	11			
0.3	0.1	53			
0.9	0.3	32	A, D, E*		(* Dependent upon type of fat used in recipe.)
0.2	0.2	4			
0.9	0.4	14			
0.9	n/k	76			
0.8	n/k	n/k			Filo comes with hardly any fat, so the cook controls the amount and type of fat added. If lightly brushed with olive oil this is the healthiest pastry you can get. Values here are for the pastry before adding oil.

	food state	portion size	calories	k joules	total fat (g)	% poly	% mono	% sat	protein (g)	carbo (g)	starch (g)	sugars (g)
Puff Pastry		25g	93	390	5.9	16	42	49	3	7.7	7.3	0.5
Shortcrust pastry		25g	110	459	7.1	18	41	36	1.1	11	11	0.2
Pizza cheese and tomato		200g slice	474	1,990	24	18	31	45	18	50	46	4
Pork pie individual		140g	526	2,190	38	10	46	38	14	35	34	0.7
Sausage roll		1 average 75g	358	1,489	27	15	43	37	5.3	24	23	0.9

Breakfast cereals

	food state	portion size	calories	k joules	total fat (g)	% poly	% mono	% sat	protein (g)	carbo (g)	starch (g)	sugars (g)
All Bran		30g	78	333	1.0	40	10	20	4.2	14	8.3	5.7
Bran Flakes		30g	95	406	0.6	50	17	17	3.1	21	15	5.6
Cornflakes		30g	108	461	0.2	50	0	0	2.4	26	23	2.5
Fruit 'n Fibre		30g	105	444	1.4	21	29	57	2.7	22	14	7.3
★ **Muesli** no added sugar		50g	183	776	3.9	31	46	21	5.3	34	26	7.8
★ **Porridge oats**	raw	30g	113	476	2.8	39	36	18	3.4	20	20	0.3
Porridge	made with water	200g	98	418	2.2	36	36	18	3.0	18	18	tr
Pop Tart		1	210	870	6.0	n/k	n/k	17	2.5	36	19	17

total fibre (g)	soluble fibre (g)	chol (mg)	useful source of vitamins	good source of minerals	special health notes
1.5	n/k	n/k			The fat content of these traditional pastries is quite high and saturates are high unless a polyunsaturated margarine which is low in hydrogenated fats is used (check labels).
0.5	0.2	9			
2.8	1.2	44	A, b-carotene, B1, B2, nic ac, E	cal, potas, phos, iod, manga	The tomato sauce is high in lycopene, which helps to protect against heart disease and cancer. Cheese and tomato pizza is also a very good source of calcium. Fibre content can be boosted with extra veg.
1.3	n/k	73	B1, nic ac, B12,	phos	High in calories and fat, but the meat content gives some B vitamins and minerals.
0.9	n/k	37	nic ac, B12		A high-fat food, as both pastry and sausagemeat are high in fats.
7.3	1.2	0	B1, B2, nic ac, B6, B12, folate, D	magnes, potas, phos, iod, iron, cal	Very high-fibre cereal, useful for helping regular bowel movement and good source of nutrients, but contains reasonably high amount of sugar.
3.9	0.9	0	B1, B2, nic ac, B6, B12, folate, D	iron	Wheat bran-based cereal; less fibre than All Bran but still higher than most commercial cereals; vitamin- and mineral-fortified.
0.3	0.1	0	B1, B2, nic ac, B6, B12, folate, D	iron	Wheat-free cereal, low in fibre but fortified with vitamins and minerals. Fairly high in sugar, but a better choice for people trying to limit their sugar intake than 'frosted' cereals such as Frosties.
2.1	0.8	0	B1, B2, nic ac, B6, B12, folate, D	iron	Wheat-based cereal, higher in saturated fats than other cereals because of the coconut content; vitamin- and mineral-fortified.
3.8	n/k	tr	nic ac, E	manga, cop	Muesli is a whole-grain cereal (usually containing a range of grains such as wheat, oat and rye flakes – check label if avoiding wheat; some brands don't include it) providing a good range of vitamins and minerals (though mostly not in sufficient quantities to appear on chart). Oats are rich in soluble fibre, which can help lower blood cholesterol, and with a low glycaemic index providing lasting energy and keeping hunger at bay. Muesli is high in natural sugars from the fruit, but low in salt and high in monounsaturated fats. Porridge is also a whole-grain oat cereal, high in unsaturated fats and soluble fibre, and with a medium glycaemic index.
2.1	1.2	0		manga	
1.6	1.0	0			
0.8	n/k	0	B1, B2, nic ac, B6, B12, folate		Wheat-based breakfast snack fortified with vitamins and minerals; rather high in fats and low in fibre.

	food state	portion size	calories	k joules	total fat (g)	% poly	% mono	% sat	protein (g)	carbo (g)	starch (g)	sugars (g)	
Puffed Wheat		30g	96	410	0.4	50	2.5	2.5	4.3	20	20	0.1	
Rice Crispies		30g	111	472	0.3	33	33	33	1.8	27	24	3.2	
Shredded Wheat		2 biscuits	146	623	1.4	43	14	14	4.8	31	30	0.4	
Special K		30g	113	481	0.3	33	33	33	4.6	25	19	5.2	
Weetabix		2 biscuits	127	540	1.0	46	18	18	4.4	25.2	28	1.8	

Dairy products and eggs

	food state	portion size	calories	k joules	total fat (g)	% poly	% mono	% sat	protein (g)	carbo (g)	starch (g)	sugars (g)	
Cows' Milk whole		100ml	66	275	3.9	3	28	62	3.2	4.8	0	4.8	
Cows' Milk semi-skimmed		100ml	46	195	1.6	tr	31	63	3.3	5	0	5	
Cows' Milk skimmed		100ml	33	140	0.1	0	0	100	3.3	5	0	5	
Goats' Milk		100ml	60	253	3.5	3	23	66	3.1	44	0	4.4	
Soya Milk		100ml	32	132	1.9	58	21	16	2.9	0.8	0	0.8	
Cream single		50ml	99	409	9.6	3	29	62	1.3	2	0	2	
Cream half-fat		50ml	74	307	6.7	3	29	62	1.5	2.2	0	2.2	
Cream double		50ml	225	925	24	3	29	62	0.9	1.4	0	1.4	

total fibre (g)	soluble fibre (g)	chol (mg)	useful source of vitamins	good source of minerals	special health notes
1.7	n/k	0	nic ac	cop	Whole-grain wheat cereal, high in polyunsaturates and low in salt and sugar.
0.2	0	0	B1, B2, nic ac, B6, B12, folate, D	iron	Rice-based cereal fortified with vitamins and minerals; low in fibre.
4.4	0.9	0	nic ac	magnes, cop	Wholewheat cereal high in polyunsaturates and fibre and low in sugar and salt.
0.6	0.2	0	B1, B2, nic ac, B6, B12, folate, D	iron	Rice- and wheat-based cereal, fortified with vitamins and minerals; low in fibre and fairly high in sugars and salt.
2.9	1.2	0	B1, B2, nic ac	iron, cop	Wholewheat cereal fortified with vitamins and iron; fairly low in salt and added sugars.
0	0	14	A, B2, B12	cal, iod, potas, phos	Skimmed and semi-skimmed milks are a good very low or low-fat source of protein and one of the Western world's most common sources of calcium, a low intake of which has been linked with heart disease, colon cancer and, of course, osteoporosis. It is also one of our few major sources of iodine. Whole milk contains, however, more than half of its calories as fat, two-thirds of which is saturated and so people following a diet low in saturates should use skimmed milk or soya milk.
0	0	7	B2, B12,	cal, iod, potas, phos	
0	0	2	B2, B12,	cal, iod, potas, phos	Some people are allergic to, or intolerant of, cows' milk, either because of lactose intolerance or an inability to digest the milk proteins, in which case goats' milk is often an acceptable alternative. See Allergies.
0	0	10	A, B2, B12,	cal, iod, potas, phos	Almost as high in fat and saturates as whole cows' milk, but may be tolerated by people allergic to cows'-milk products.
0	0	0	B2, E	cop	People who eat no dairy produce should probably buy calcium-fortified soya milk. Soya milk is made from the soya bean, one of few sources of complete plant protein. See Soya Beans on page 316.
0	0	28	A		Whatever type of dairy cream you buy, most of the calories it contains will be from fat, two-thirds of which is saturated. Cream should be used sparingly within a healthy diet.
0	0	20	A		
0	0	65	A		

	food state	portion size	calories	k joules	total fat (g)	% poly	% mono	% sat	protein (g)	carbo (g)	starch (g)	sugars (g)	
Cream whipping		50ml	187	770	20	3	29	62	1	1.5	0	2.5	
Crème fraîche full-fat		50ml	190	784	20	3	24	66	1.2	1.4	0	1.4	
Yoghurt Natural low-fat		100g	56	236	0.8	tr	25	63	5.1	7.5	0	7.5	
Yoghurt Natural whole-milk		100g	79	333	3	7	30	30	5.7	7.8	0	7.8	
Yoghurt Natural Greek		100g	106	442	7.5	5	25	64	4.4	5.6	0	5.6	
Yoghurt Low-fat fruit		125ml tub	90	382	0.7	tr	29	57	4.1	18	0	18	
Yoghurt Diet fruit		125ml pot	51	221	0.3	tr	33	33	5.4	7.5	0	7.5	
Fromage frais natural, 8% fat		100g	113	469	7.1	3	30	62	6.8	5.7	0	5.7	
Fromage frais natural, 0% fat		100g	58	247	0.2	tr	50	50	7.7	6.8	0	6.8	
Fromage frais fruit		100g	131	551	5.8	3	29	62	6.8	14	0	14	
Fromage frais diet fruit		100g	64	269	1.2	2	25	58	5.6	7	0.5	6.5	
Brie		50g	160	662	13	3	29	63	9.6	tr	0	tr	
Cheddar full-fat		50g	206	854	17	4	27	63	13	0.1	0	0.1	
Cheddar half-fat		50g	131	546	7.5	3	29	63	16	tr	0	tr	

total fibre (g)	soluble fibre (g)	chol (mg)	useful source of vitamins	good source of minerals	special health notes
0	0	53	A		
0	0	53	A		
0	0	4	B2, B12	cal, potas, phos, iod	Good low-fat source of calcium and protein. Bio yoghurt contains bacteria that may help the digestive system, IBS, etc.
0	0	11	B2, B12	cal, potas, phos, iod	Over one-third of its calories are fat, but still a good source of calcium.
0	0	14	B2, B12	cal, potas, phos, iod	Over 50% of its calories are fat and much of this is saturated fat.
0	0	4	B2, B12	cal, potas, phos, iod	Fruit yoghurts tend to contain a lot of sugar.
0	n/k	1	B1, B12	cal, potas, phos, iod	Similar to low-fat fruit yoghurt except that the sugar content is less; usually artificial sweeteners will be used to reduce the calorie content.
0	0	25	B2, B12, A		Eaten in reasonable quantities, can make a good contribution to calcium intake, at 86mg/100ml, but saturated fat content is quite high.
0	0	1	B2, B12		Calcium content same as 8% fromage frais above, but fat content much lower.
tr	tr	21	B2, B12		
0.1	n/k	n/k	B2, B12		
0	0	50	B2, A, B12	cal, phos	Cheese is perceived by many as a 'protein' food and yet, weight for weight, many cheeses contain more fat than protein – and, as a percentage of total calories, fat is by far the dominant nutrient in cheese unless specifically labelled otherwise. Even 'half-fat' cheeses may contain up to 50% of their calories as fat. For further guidance see Food Labelling, page 77.
0	0	50	B2, A, B12	cal, phos	Cheeses are particularly high in saturated fats and many are high in sodium. Hard cheeses are, however, an excellent source of calcium, which is important in helping to prevent osteoporosis, and cheese is one of few good sources of vitamin B2, and a good source of B12 for
0	0	22	B2, B12	cal, phos	people who don't eat meat. Hard cheeses also provide iodine in

	food state	portion size	calories	k joules	total fat (g)	% poly	% mono	% sat	protein (g)	carbo (g)	starch (g)	sugars (g)	
Cheese spread full-fat		50g	138	572	11	3	29	63	6.8	22	0	2.2	
Cheese spread half-fat		50g	94	392	5	3	24	66	8	3.2	0	3.2	
Cottage cheese standard		50g	49	207	2.0	5	30	60	6.9	1.0	0	1.0	
Cream cheese full-fat		50g	220	904	24	3	29	63	1.5	tr	0	tr	
Danish Blue		50g	174	719	15	3	29	63	10	tr	0	tr	
Edam		50g	167	691	13	2	29	62	13	tr	0	tr	
Feta Greek		50g	125	519	10	3	20	67	7.8	0.8	0	0.8	
Gruyère		50g	205	848	17	3	29	63	14	tr	0	tr	
Mascarpone		50g	225	926	23	3	24	66	1.4	2.4	0	2.4	
Mozzarella Italian		50g	145	602	11	3	29	63	13	tr	0	tr	
Parmesan		10g (l tbsp)	45	188	3.3	2	29	63	4	tr	0	tr	
Processed cheese slice		1	66	273	5	4	28	61	4.2	0.2	0	0.2	
Soft-cheese low-fat		50g	98	405	7.5	3	24	66	6.0	1.5	0	1.5	
Stilton		50g	206	851	18	3	29	62	11	0.1	0	0.1	

total fibre (g)	soluble fibre (g)	chol (mg)	useful source of vitamins	good source of minerals
0	0	33	A, B12	cal, phos
0	0	n/k	B12	cal, phos
0	0	7	B12	
0	0	48	A, B12	
0	0	38	A, B12	cal, phos
0	0	40	nic ac	cal, iod, phos
0	0	35	B12	cal, phos
0	0	50	A, B12	cal, phos
0	0	n/k	A, B12	unknown
0	0	33	A, B12	cal, phos
0	0	10	B2, B12	cal
0	0	17	B12	phos
0	0	n/k	B12	
0	0	53	A, B2, B12	cal, iod, phos

special health notes

reasonable amounts. Vegetarians who want to avoid eating animal products should buy rennet-free cheeses, which are now becoming more widely available.

Official guidelines recommend that unpasteurized soft cheeses, such as Brie, should be avoided during pregnancy and by the elderly as they may contain the listeria bacterium which can cause food poisoning.

People with a cow's-milk intolerance can choose all kinds of cheeses – including Cheddar-types and blue cheeses – made from goats' or ewes' milk. These are now widely available in supermarkets as well as at specialist cheese shops and delicatessens (see Allergies).

Cheese is said to be a trigger for migraine in some susceptible people. Migraine sufferers may find they can eat soft cheeses but may have to avoid mature hard cheeses, which contain an enzyme called tyramine that may be the key to an attack.

There is some research to show that eating cheese at the end of a meal may help to reduce the formation of plaque and thus help prevent gum disease.

	food state	portion size	calories	k joules	total fat (g)	% poly	% mono	% sat	protein (g)	carbo (g)	starch (g)	sugars (g)
Eggs Small		1	69	288	5	12	44	30	6	tr	0	tr
Eggs Medium		1	84	349	6.1	12	43	30	7.2	tr	0	tr
Eggs Large		1	98	410	7.2	11	43	29	8.5	tr	0	tr
Medium egg	fried in vegetable oil	1	102	447	7.9	11	43	29	7.8	tr	0	tr

Condiments, sauces and other store-cupboard items

	food state	portion size	calories	k joules	total fat (g)	% poly	% mono	% sat	protein (g)	carbo (g)	starch (g)	sugars (g)
Apple sauce		1 tbsp (15ml)	10	41	tr	0	0	0	0	2.5	0	2.5
Brown sauce		1 tbsp (15ml)	15	63	0	0	0	0	0.2	3.8	0.3	3.5
Burger relish		1 tbsp (15ml)	14	59	tr	0	0	0	0.2	3.3	n/k	n/k
French dressing (vinaigrette)		1 tbsp (15ml)	69	285	7.4	25	61	9	0	0.7	0	0.7
Mayonnaise		1 tbsp (15ml)	104	426	11	60	23	15	0.2	0.3	0.1	0.2
Mayonnaise light		1 tbsp (15ml)	43	178	4.2	n/k	n/k	16	0.2	1.2	0.5	0.7
Pesto		1 tbsp (15ml)	78	321	7.1	21	47	27	3.1	0.3	0.1	0.2
Plum sauce		1 tbsp (15ml)	37	155	0	0	0	0	n/k	9.8	n/k	n/k
Salad cream		1 tbsp (15ml)	52	216	4.7	62	15	13	0.2	2.5	tr	2.5

total fibre (g)	soluble fibre (g)	chol (mg)	useful source of vitamins	good source of minerals	special health notes
0	0	179	B12, folate, A, D	iod	Eggs can also significantly contribute towards intake of B2, E, Nicotinic Acid. Iron is present but not well absorbed. High in cholesterol, but a recent review finds they have no significant impact on heart disease or blood cholesterol levels. The WHO suggests an upper limit of 10 eggs a week, including those eaten in cakes, dressings, desserts, etc. Raw and lightly cooked eggs should be avoided by the young, elderly, pregnant and invalids, because of the risk of salmonella, but risks can be reduced by purchasing Lion-stamped UK eggs. Organic eggs are likely to contain higher levels of omega-3 fats than caged hen eggs.
0	0	217	B12, folate, A, D	iod	
0	0	255	B12, folate, A, D	iod	
0	0	217	B12, folate, A, D	iod	Make fried eggs as healthy as possible by using a non-stick griddle or pan just brushed with a good-quality pure vegetable oil. If shallow-frying, drain thoroughly before serving.
0.2	n/k	0			Fruit- and vegetable-based sauces, such as apple sauce, tomato sauce, pickles and relishes, are normally eaten in fairly small quantities and therefore don't make a great contribution to the nutritional content of our diets. However, some contain reasonable amounts of sugar and salt, and if tomato ketchup and tomato sauces are eaten regularly they may make a useful contribution to carotenoid intake.
0.1	n/k	0			
n/k	n/k	0			Condiments based on oil, such as French dressing, mayonnaise, pesto and salad cream, are much higher in calories and fat. They can make a surprising contribution to the calorie and fat content of a meal and should be treated with caution if following a reduced-calorie diet. However the fats they contain are mostly unsaturated.
0	0	0	E		
0	0	11	E		
0	0	3	E		
n/k	n/k	6			
n/k	n/k	0			
0	0	6	B12, E		

	food state	portion size	calories	k joules	total fat (g)	% poly	% mono	% sat	protein (g)	carbo (g)	starch (g)	sugars (g)	
Soy sauce		1 tbsp (15ml)	10	40	0	0	0	0	1.3	1.2	n/k	n/k	
Sweet pickle		1 tbsp (15ml)	21	91	0	0	0	0	0.1	5.4	0.3	5.1	
Tomato ketchup		1 tbsp (15ml)	17	73	0	0	0	0	0.2	4.3	0.2	4.1	
Tomato sauce Italian (jar)		1 tbsp (15ml)	7	30	0.2	50	0	0	0.3	1.0	0.2	0.9	
Tomato purée		20g (1 level tbsp)	15	65	0.1	tr	tr	tr	1	2.8	0	2.8	
Worcestershire sauce		1 tbsp (15ml)	10	41	0	0	0	0	0.2	2.3	0.1	2.2	
Coconut creamed, block		25g	167	690	17	2	6	86	1.5	1.8	0	1.8	
Coconut milk canned		100ml	22	95	0.3	tr	tr	67	0.3	4.9	0	4.9	
Vinegar		1 tbsp	3	13	0	0	0	0	0.1	0.1	0	0.1	

Drinks, alcoholic

	food state	portion size	calories	k joules	total fat (g)	% poly	% mono	% sat	protein (g)	carbo (g)	starch (g)	sugars (g)	
Beer standard		275ml	88	363	0	0	0	0	0.8	6.3	0	6.3	
Beer low-alcohol		275ml	36	149	0	0	0	0	0.6	5.8	0	3.3	
Cider dry		275ml	99	418	0	0	0	0	tr	7.1	0	7.1	
Cider sweet		275ml	116	484	0	0	0	0	0	11.8	0	11.8	

total fibre (g)	soluble fibre (g)	chol (mg)	useful source of vitamins	good source of minerals	special health notes
0	0	0			Some sauces, particularly soy, teriyaki and Worcestershire, are high in salt (though reduced-salt soy sauce is now available) and should be limited for those following a low-sodium diet.
0.2	n/k	0			
0.1	n/k	0			
n/k	n/k	0			
0.6	n/k	0	b-carotene, E	potas, cop	High in lycopene, the pigment that helps prevent cancer and heart disease.
0	0	0			
n/k	n/k	0		manga	Coconut is one of the few plant foods to contain a large proportion of its fats as saturated fat. However there is some evidence that the saturated fat in coconut doesn't act like the saturated fat in animal and dairy produce and it may be therefore that coconut fat isn't such a risk factor for heart disease.
tr	tr	0		manga	
0	0	0			Often used as an anti-inflammatory by arthritis sufferers, though there is no real proof that this works. Should be avoided by people with a yeast allergy.
0	0	0	B12	cop, iod	Beer contains phytochemicals which have been shown to help protect against heart disease (See also Spirits and Wine overleaf). It aids digestion by encouraging acid production in the stomach.
0	0	0	nic ac		May not have the same protective effect as alcoholic beers.
0	0	0			
0	0	0			

	food state	portion size	calories	k joules	total fat (g)	% poly	% mono	% sat	protein (g)	carbo (g)	starch (g)	sugars (g)
Cider low-alcohol		275ml	47	204	0	0	0	0	0	9.9	0	9.9
Lager standard		275ml	80	333	0	0	0	0	0.8	tr	0	tr
Lager low-alcohol		275ml	28	113	0	0	0	0	0.6	4.1	0	2.8
Port		50ml	79	328	0	0	0	0	0.1	6.0	0	6.0
Sherry medium		50ml	58	241	0	0	0	0	0.1	3.0	0	3.0
Spirits all kinds		1 pub measure (25ml)	48	197	0	0	0	0	tr	tr	0	tr
Stouts (Guinness)		275ml	83	347	0	0	0	0	1.1	4.1	0	4.1
Wine white, dry		140ml	92	385	0	0	0	0	0.1	0.8	0	0.8
Wine white, sweet		140ml	132	552	0	0	0	0	0.3	8.3	0	8.3
Wine red		140ml	95	396	0	0	0	0	0.1	0.3	0	0.3

Drinks, non-alcoholic

	food state	portion size	calories	k joules	total fat (g)	% poly	% mono	% sat	protein (g)	carbo (g)	starch (g)	sugars (g)
Coffee instant		1 tea-spoon	2	6	tr	tr	tr	tr	0.3	0.1	0.1	0
Coffee freshly ground	black	1 cup (190ml)	4	15	tr	tr	tr	tr	0.4	0.4	0	0
Hot chocolate	made with whole milk	1 cup (190ml)	171	716	7.8	2.6	30	62	6.5	20	0.6	20

total fibre (g)	soluble fibre (g)	chol (mg)	useful source of vitamins	good source of minerals	special health notes
o	o	o			
tr	n/k	o	nic ac, folate		
tr	n/k	o	nic ac		
o	o	o			High levels of congeners, so more likely to produce hangover than 'pale' alcoholic drinks, like vodka and white wine. Also more likely to trigger migraine. May contain same flavonoids as Red wine (below).
o	o	o			
o	o	o			Taken in moderate amounts – 1-2 measures, 5-6 times a week – these offer protection against heart disease. The ethanols in aged whisky and brandy contain antioxidants. (See also Beer and Wine).
o	o	o	nic ac		Stouts and dark beers contain more of the protective flavonoids than light beers.
o	o	o			Red wines contain higher levels of flavonoids than any other alcoholic drink, offering protection against heart and arterial disease, probably because their antioxidant effect helps keep arteries free from 'furring'. Red wines also help prevent blood clotting and help increase 'good' HDL blood cholesterol. Optimum level appears to be a minimum of 1 drink and a maximum of 4 for men, and a minimum of 1 drink and a maximum of 2 for women, on 5-6 days a week. Also appears to protect against Alzheimer's disease in older people and may help protect against peptic ulcers. White wines contain lower levels of flavonoids and polyphenols, providing moderate protection against heart disease.
o	o	o			
o	o	o		iron	
o	o	o			Recent studies on coffee drinkers have shown that 1–2 cups a day can protect against liver and colon cancer, gallstones and kidney stones, type-2 diabetes and Parkinson's disease. All coffee contains high levels of antioxidants and tannins which are good for the heart and arteries. Caffeine is a stimulant which can improve concentration and alertness and help fat-burning, and is a mild laxative and diuretic. High intake (many cups a day) can rob body of minerals such as calcium and may have other negative side-effects.
o	o	o			
tr	o	23	B2, B12	cal, potas, phos, iod	Cocoa powder contains antioxidant flavonoids; an average cup of hot chocolate will have almost the same antioxidant strength as a glass of red wine.

	food state	portion size	calories	k joules	total fat (g)	% poly	% mono	% sat	protein (g)	carbo (g)	starch (g)	sugars (g)	
Instant low-calorie hot chocolate		1 sachet	38	161	1.5	n/k	n/k	87	2.0	4.2	n/k	2.5	
Tea	black	1 cup (190ml)	1	5	tr	tr	tr	tr	0.2	tr	0	tr	
Cola		330ml	142	574	0	0	0	0	tr	36	0	36	
Diet cola		330ml	1.3	5	0	0	0	0	tr	tr	0	tr	
Lemonade		330ml	75	319	0	0	0	0	tr	20	0	20	
Orange squash		275ml	54	229	0	0	0	0	tr	14	0	14	
Apple juice		100ml	38	164	0.1	100	0	0	0.1	10	0	10	
Cranberry juice		100ml	57	238	0	0	0	0	0	14	0	14	
Grape juice		100ml	46	196	0.1	tr	tr	tr	0.3	12	0	12	
Grapefruit juice		100ml	33	140	0.1	tr	tr	tr	0.4	8.3	0	8.3	
Orange juice		100ml	36	153	0.1	tr	tr	tr	0.5	8.8	0	8.8	
Pineapple juice		100ml	41	177	0.1	tr	tr	tr	0.3	11	0	11	
Tomato juice		100ml	14	62	tr	tr	tr	tr	0.8	3	tr	3	
Vegetable juice		100ml	21	88	0.5	n/k	n/k	n/k	0.8	3.3	0.4	2.9	

total fibre (g)	soluble fibre (g)	chol (mg)	useful source of vitamins	good source of minerals	special health notes
0.7	n/k	n/k		manga	See Hot chocolate on previous page.
0	0	0			Black and green tea contain powerful antioxidants, flavonols called quercetin, which may reduce risk of stroke, some cancers and heart disease. Tea has less caffeine than coffee but still is a mild stimulant.
0	0	0			Cola contains caffeine, a stimulant (see Coffee). Apart from that, it contains little except a lot of sugar and various flavourings, and has been linked with bone loss.
0	0	0			Diet drinks are high in artificial sweeteners; it is wise to limit intake of these to 1 a day particularly if following a slimming diet containing several other reduced-sugar products.
0	0	0			Carbonated drinks can contribute to tooth decay due to their acids, and have been linked with calcium loss in bones, due to phosphorous content. Artificial flavourings, etc, are linked to ADHD and allergies.
0	0	0			Most commercial squashes contain little real fruit juice but consist mainly of sugar and/or sweeteners, flavourings and colourings. Check label for juice content.
tr	tr	0	C		Some commercial brands contain added vitamin C because apples are not one of the better fruit sources of C. Cloudy varieties may be preferable to clear.
n/k	n/k	0	C		Compounds in cranberry juice are said to help prevent, and relieve, attacks of cystitis by preventing bacteria adhering to cells in bladder walls and urinary tract.
0	0	0	C		Red grape juice contains antioxidant compounds on a similar level to red wine, as well as vitamin C, another antioxidant.
tr	tr	0	C		Good source of vitamin C. If taken with some medicines, it can lead to toxicity from inhibition of liver mechanism – check with doctor if taking any medications for blood pressure, Aids, anxiety or hay fever.
0.1	0.1	0	C		Rich in vitamin C. Freshly squeezed is preferable to the long-life commercial brands as fresh juice contains bioflavonoids which act together with vitamin C as antioxidants.
tr	tr	0	C	manga	Contains the enzyme bromelain which helps to break down protein in the diet.
0.6	n/k	0	C, E, carotenoids	potas	Tomato juice is rich in lycopene, shown to be a powerful protectant against some cancers. Research shows a 50% reduction in heart attacks in men who eat tomato-rich diet. Also rich in beta-carotene, an antioxidant thought to help combat heart disease. There is evidence that tomatoes exacerbate rheumatoid arthritis. For other vegetable juices, see individual vegetables, but remember juicing removes most of the fibre.
1	n/k	0	C, carotenoids	potas	

Fats and oils

	food state	portion size	calories	k joules	total fat (g)	% poly	% mono	% sat	protein (g)	carbo (g)	starch (g)	sugars (g)	
Butter		25g	184	758	20	3.4	25	67	0.1	tr	0	tr	
Lard		25g	223	916	25	10	44	41	tr	0	0	0	
Low-fat spread		25g	98	401	10	25	44	28	1.5	0.1	0	0.1	
Very-low-fat spread		25g	62	255	5.9	20	50	26	1.5	0.6	tr	0.3	
Margarine hard, vegetable fat		25g	185	760	20	11	41	44	0.1	0.3	0	0.3	
Margarine sunflower		25g	187	767	21	44	32	21	tr	0.1	0	0.1	
Margarine olive oil, 60% fat		25g	137	571	15	18	54	21	0.1	0.3	0	0.3	
Suet vegetable		25g	209	861	22	15	30	51	0.3	2.5	2.5	0	
Suet animal		25g	224	936	25	1	37	56	0.2	0	0	0	
Corn oil		25g	225	924	25	51	30	14	tr	0	0	0	
Groundnut (peanut) oil		25g	225	924	25	31	44	20	tr	0	0	0	
Olive oil		25g	225	924	25	10	73	14	tr	0	0	0	
Rapeseed oil		25g	225	924	25	29	59	6	tr	0	0	0	

total fibre (g)	soluble fibre (g)	chol (mg)	useful source of vitamins	good source of minerals	special health notes
0	0	58	A, D		High in saturated fat, which is linked with heart disease.
0	0	23			High in saturated fat.
0	0	2	A, D, E		Lower in calories and fat than butter or margarine. Usually made from water blended with vegetable fats or butter. May contain trans fats, now believed by some to be linked with heart disease even more than saturated fat, though some formulations have now reduced trans fats to a minimum and will therefore contain a lower percentage than the averages given. Very-low-fat spreads are about 60% or more water.
0	0	2	A, D, E		
0	0	4	A, D, E		Contains a high proportion of trans fats (see above). May also contain fish by-products and so unsuitable for vegetarians.
0	0	1	A, D, E		High in polyunsaturated fats and vitamin E. Other soft margarines include Benecol, which contains sterol esters that help to lower blood cholesterol.
0	0	tr	A, D, E		The only spread to be high in monounsaturates; many experts now believe that these are the healthiest of all the types of fat, as they can lower blood cholesterol levels. For more information see pages 15-19.
0	0	0	E		Contains high levels of trans fats, despite being low in saturated fat.
0	0	15			High in saturated fat.
0	0	0	E		All plant oils are a good source of unsaturated fats and vitamin E, although all do still contain some saturated fat. Corn, safflower, sesame, sunflower, walnut and blended vegetable oils are highest in polyunsaturated fats. Olive, rapeseed and groundnut (peanut) oils are highest in monounsaturated fats. All oils are extremely high in calories and intake should be moderate in people attempting to lose weight or keep weight off — but should not be banned, as unsaturated oils are now known to have health benefits, including lowering of blood cholesterol and possible cancer prevention, and are a good source of the antioxidant vitamin E. However, the right balance of polyunsaturates is important – most of us eat too many omega-6s and not enough omega-3s (see pages 15-19).
0	0	0	E		
0	0	0	E		
0	0	0	E		

	food state	portion size	calories	k joules	total fat (g)	% poly	% mono	% sat	protein (g)	carbo (g)	starch (g)	sugars (g)
Safflower oil		25g	225	924	25	74	12	10	tr	0	0	0
Sesame oil		25g	225	924	25	44	38	15	0.1	0	0	0
Sunflower oil		25g	225	924	25	63	20	12	tr	0	0	0
Walnut oil		25g	225	924	25	70	16	9	tr	0	0	0
Vegetable oil blended		25g	225	924	25	48	36	10	tr	0	0	0

Fish and seafood

	food state	portion size	calories	k joules	total fat (g)	% poly	% mono	% sat	protein (g)	carbo (g)	starch (g)	sugars (g)
Cod		100g	80	337	0.7	43	14	14	18	0	0	0
Cod	deep-fried in batter	100g	247	1,031	15	24	45	27	16	12	12	tr
Fish fillet in crumbs	baked	100g	188	786	11	15	15	50	11	13	13	0.1
Fish fingers		4	200	838	8.9	26	38	32	14	17	17	tr
Haddock smoked fillet		100g	81	345	0.6	33	17	17	19	0	0	0
★ **Herring fillet**		100g	190	791	13	21	42	25	18	0	0	0
Kipper fillet	grilled	100g	255	1,060	19	22	53	16	20	0	0	0
★ **Mackerel fillet**	fresh	100g	220	914	16	21	49	21	19	0	0	0

total fibre (g)	soluble fibre (g)	chol (mg)	useful source of vitamins	good source of minerals	special health notes
0	0	0	E		
0	0	0	E		
0	0	0	E		
0	0	0	E		
0	0	0	E		
0	0	46	nic ac, B12	phos, iod, sel, potas	Plain-cooked white fish, such as cod, haddock, brill, coley, is a good low-fat, low-calorie source of protein, vitamins and minerals, and ideal for slimmers. (Any plain white fish not in the list has a similar nutrient value to cod.)
0.5	n/k	n/k	nic ac, B12	phos, iod, sel, potas	Oily fish, such as herring, kipper, mackerel, salmon and sardines, are one of the few nutritional sources of the Omega-3 polyunsaturated fatty acids, which help to prevent heart disease and strokes and may help to prevent some cancers and help minimize the symptoms of
0.1	0.5	n/k	nic ac, B12	phos, iod, sel, potas	arthritis. Latest research shows that just one portion of fish per week can help prevent heart attacks. Some research indicates a link between a lack of Omega-3 fatty acids and depression. Most fishes are also a good source of the antioxidant mineral, selenium. For more detail about Omega-3 fats and a chart showing the amount in each
0.7	n/k	35	nic ac, B12	phos, iod, sel, potas	fish, turn to Section One, page 16. Smoked fish, such as kippers, may be carcinogenic due to the smoking process, and is high in salt. Salmon is best bought organic or with the Freedom Food label.
0	0	36	nic ac, B6, B12	phos, iod, sel, potas	While regular fish intake is to be encouraged, the UK Food Standards Agency has issued guidelines on minimum and maximum intakes – as, particularly with oily fish, a high intake may pose a health threat due to pollutant contamination. As follows:
0	0	50	nic ac, B6, B12, D	phos, iod, sel, potas	– Women intending to become pregnant or who are pregnant or breastfeeding, and girls under 16, should limit oily fish intake to 2 portions a week, while everyone else should limit it to 4 portions a week. – Nevertheless, everyone should have at least one portion of oily fish a week.
0	0	0	nic ac, B6, B12, D	phos, iod, sel, potas	– Children under 16 and women intending to become pregnant or who are pregnant or breastfeeding should avoid shark, marlin and swordfish, due to the high levels of mercury that they may contain. Everyone else should limit themselves to one portion a week of these fish.
0	0	54	nic ac, B6, B12, D	phos, iod, sel, potas	– Apart from these three white fish, everyone should eat at least one portion of white fish a week and there is no maximum level set.

	food state	portion size	calories	k joules	total fat (g)	% poly	% mono	% sat	protein (g)	carbo (g)	starch (g)	sugars (g)	
Mullet, red		100g	109	459	3.8	n/k	n/k	n/k	19	0	0	0	
★ **Salmon** fresh fillet		100g	180	750	11	28	40	9	20	0	0	0	
Salmon canned		100g	153	644	6.6	29	36	20	24	0	0	0	
Salmon smoked		50g (average serving)	71	299	2.3	26	39	17	13	0	0	0	
★ **Sardines** fresh	whole	3	281	1,176	16	29	36	20	21	0	0	0	
Sardines canned in oil	drained	100g	220	918	14	36	34	21	23	0	0	0	
Swordfish fillet		100g	109	458	4.1	27	39	22	18	0	0	0	
Trout fresh		1 medium (225g)	281	1,184	12	33	34	9	44	0	0	0	
Tuna fresh		100g	136	573	4.6	35	22	22	24	0	0	0	
Tuna canned in brine	drained	100g	99	422	0.6	33	17	33	24	0	0	0	
Tuna canned in oil	drained	100g	189	794	9	53	26	17	27	0	0	0	
Whitebait	deep-fried	100g	525	2,174	48	n/k	n/k	n/k	20	5.3	5.2	0.1	
Crabmeat	dressed	100g	128	535	5.5	29	27	13	20	tr	tr	tr	
Lobster		1/2 average (250g)	93	393	1.5	33	20	20	20	tr	tr	tr	

total fibre (g)	soluble fibre (g)	chol (mg)	useful source of vitamins	good source of minerals	special health notes
0	0	n/k	nic ac, B6, B12	phos, sel, potas	
0	0	50	B1, nic ac, B6, B12, D, E	phos, potas, sel, iod	
0	0	20	nic ac, B12, D, E	cal, phos, potas, sel, iod	
0	0	18	nic ac, B6, B12	phos, sel, potas	
0	0	92	B2, nic ac, B6, B12, D, pant ac	cal, phos, potas, sel, iod, iron, magnes	
0	0	65	B2, nic ac, B12, D, pant ac	cal, phos, potas, iron, sel, iod, zn	
0	0	41	nic ac, B6, B12	phos, potas, sel	
0	0	151	B1, B2, nic ac, B6, B12, D, E, pant	potas, phos, sel, iod	
0	0	28	nic ac, B6, B12, D	potas, phos, cop, sel, iod	
0	0	51	nic ac, B6, B12, D	phos, potas, sel	
0	0	50	nic ac, B6, B12, D, E	phos, potas, sel	
0.2	n/k	n/k		cal, phos, cop, sel, iod	
0	0	72	B2, nic ac	potas, phos, zn, cop, magnes	Plainly cooked shellfish is a low-fat, low-calorie source of protein, many minerals including the antioxidant selenium, zinc (which is not easy to come by in the average diet) and magnesium, as well as some B group vitamins. The prawn family are high in cholesterol and sodium. Only crabmeat and mussels contain significant amounts of Omega-3 fatty acids.
0	0	100	nic ac, B12, E	phos, zn, cop, sel, iod, potas	

	food state	portion size	calories	k joules	total fat (g)	% poly	% mono	% sat	protein (g)	carbo (g)	starch (g)	sugars (g)	
⭐ **Mussels**	shelled	100g	104	440	2.7	3.7	15	19	17	3.5	tr	tr	
Oysters	shelled	100g	65	275	1.3	31	15	15	11	2.7	tr	tr	
Prawns	shelled	100g	99	418	0.9	22	22	22	23	0	0	0	
Scallops	shelled	100g	118	501	1.4	29	7	29	23	3.4	tr	tr	
Scampi	deep-fried in breadcrumbs	100g	237	991	14	47	38	10	9.4	21	21	tr	
Squid		100g	81	344	1.7	35	12	24	15	1.2	tr	tr	

Fruit

	food state	portion size	calories	k joules	total fat (g)	% poly	% mono	% sat	protein (g)	carbo (g)	starch (g)	sugars (g)	
⭐ **Apple** dessert		1	47	199	0.1	100	0	0	0.4	12	tr	12	
Apple cooking		1	60	257	0.2	100	0	0	0.5	15	tr	15	
Apricot fresh		100g	29	123	0.1	tr	tr	tr	0.8	6.6	0	6.6	
⭐ **Apricot** dried ready-to-eat		50g	79	337	0.3	n/k	n/k	n/k	2.0	18.2	0	18.2	
Banana		1 medium	95	403	0.3	33	tr	33	1.2	23	2.3	21	
Blackberries		100g	25	104	0.2	50	50	tr	0.9	5.1	0	5.1	
⭐ **Blackcurrants**		100g	28	121	tr	tr	tr	0.4	0.9	6.6	0	6.6	

total fibre (g)	soluble fibre (g)	chol (mg)	useful source of vitamins	good source of minerals	special health notes
0	0	58	B2, nic ac, B12, folate	iron, zn, cop, sel, iod, phos, manga	
0	0	57	nic ac, B12, D	cal, magnes, phos, potas, zn, cop, sel, iod, manga	
0	0	280	nic ac, B12, E	potas, phos, magnes, zn, sel, iod	
0	0	47	nic ac, B12,	potas, phos, zn, sel, iod	
n/k	n/k	110	nic ac, B12	cal, phos, cop, sel, iod manga	
0	0	225	nic ac, B6, B12, E	potas, phos, sel, iod	
1.8	0.7	0	C	potas	Vitamin C content varies considerably with variety of apple and freshness. Levels of polyphenol antioxidants vary depending on the variety and colour – red-skinned varieties generally contain the most, while less sweet varieties, such as Cox, are higher in cancer-fighting salvestrols. The flavonoid quercetin in apples can help lower blood cholesterol and improve lung function. Useful for slimmers as apples have a low Glycaemic Index and keep hunger pangs at bay for longer than many other fruits.
2.7	1	0	C	potas	
1.6	0.9	0	b-carotene		Food with a low Glycaemic Index and very high in the antioxidant beta-carotene. Non-organic varieties of dried fruits may be high in preservatives such as sulphur.
3.1	2.0	0	b-carotene	potas, iron, manga	
1.1	0.7	0	B6, C	potas, manga	
3.1	1	0	C, folate, E	manga	One of few fruits to contain significant amounts of the antioxidant vitamin E and contains the flavonoid ellagic acid, which may block cancer cells.
3.6	1.6	0	C, b-carotene	potas	One of the richest sources of vitamin C, containing around 200mg per 100g fruit – that is, five times the daily RNI for adults. Also contains the anti-cancer carotenoid lutein.

	food state	portion size	calories	k joules	total fat (g)	% poly	% mono	% sat	protein (g)	carbo (g)	starch (g)	sugars (g)
Blueberries		100g	30	128	0.2	50	50	tr	0.6	6.9	0	6.9
Cranberries		100g	15	65	0.1	tr	tr	tr	0.4	3.4	0	3.4
★ **Cherries**		100g	39	168	0.1	tr	tr	tr	0.7	9.5	0	9.5
Coconut	flesh only	100g	351	1,446	36	2	6	86	3.2	3.7	0	3.7
Currants dried		50g	134	570	0.2	n/k	n/k	n/k	1.1	34	0	3.4
Dates fresh		100g	107	456	0.1	tr	tr	tr	1.3	27	0	27
Dates dried		50g	135	576	0.1	0	50	50	1.6	34	0	34
Fig fresh		100g	43	185	0.3	33	33	33	1.3	9.5	0	9.5
Fig dried		50g	114	484	0.8	n/k	n/k	n/k	1.8	27	0	27
Grapefruit		1/2	24	101	0.1	tr	tr	tr	0.6	5.4	0	5.4
★ **Grapes**		100g	60	257	0.1	tr	tr	tr	0.4	15	0	15
★ **Kiwi fruit**		1 average	29	124	0.3	n/k	n/k	n/k	0.7	0.4	0.2	6.2
Lemon		juice of 1	1	6	tr	tr	tr	tr	0.1	0.3	0	0.3
Lime		juice of 1	1	4	tr	tr	tr	tr	0	0.2	0	0.2

total fibre (g)	soluble fibre (g)	chol (mg)	useful source of vitamins	good source of minerals	special health notes
1.8	0.5	0	C	manga	Tests show that blueberries contain the highest levels of antioxidants of all commonly eaten fruits.
3	1.1	0	C	manga	Often used to prevent or treat cystitis and urinary tract infections (see Cranberry juice)
0.7	0.4	0	C		Contain ellagic acid, a phytochemical that may fight cancer, and anthocyanins which relieve pain.
7.3	1	0		potas	One of the few fruits which is high in saturated fats, though some research indicates that the saturated fat it contains is not the 'harmful' type founds in animal and dairy fats.
0.9	0.5	0		potas, cop, manga	
1.5	0.4	0	C	potas	
2	0.6	0		potas	
1.5	0.9	0	b-carotene		
3.8	2	0		potas, iron, manga	
1	0.7	0	C		Pink grapefruit contains beta-carotene.
0.7	0.4	0		potas	Red grape varieties contain powerful polyphenols, the same as those in red wine. These are antioxidants and have a positive effect in reducing heart disease. Also contain ellagic acid (see Cherries).
1.1	0.5	0	C	potas	Richer in vitamin C than oranges, an average fruit containing about 40mg which is a day's RNI for adults.
0	0	0	C		As with all citrus fruit, good source of vitamin C. Contains linolene, which helps ward off cancer.
0	0	0	C		

	food state	portion size	calories	k joules	total fat (g)	% poly	% mono	% sat	protein (g)	carbo (g)	starch (g)	sugars (g)	
★ Mango		1	107	457	0.3	n/k	n/k	n/k	1.4	26	0.6	25	
★ Melon cantaloupe		1 200g slice	26	110	0.2	tr	tr	tr	0.8	5.6	0	5.6	
Nectarine		1	60	257	0.2	tr	tr	tr	2.1	14	0	14	
★ Orange		1	60	253	0.2	tr	tr	tr	1.8	14	0	14	
★ Papaya		1	74	319	0.3	tr	tr	tr	1.1	18	0	18	
Passion fruit		1	5	23	0.1	33	33	33	0.4	0.9	0	0.9	
Peach		1	36	155	0.1	tr	tr	tr	1.1	8.2	0	8.2	
Pear		1	64	270	0.2	tr	tr	tr	0.5	16	0	16	
Pineapple	fresh	2 rings (100g)	41	178	0.2	50	50	tr	0.4	10	0	10	
Plums red dessert		2	34	145	0.1	tr	tr	tr	0.5	8.3	0	8.3	
Prunes	stoned	50g	71	301	0.2	tr	50	50	1.3	17	0	17	
Raisins		50g	136	580	0.2	n/k	n/k	n/k	1	35	0	35	
★ Raspberries		100g	25	109	0.3	33	33	33	1.4	4.6	0	4.6	
Rhubarb		100g	7	32	0.1	tr	tr	tr	0.9	0.8	0	0.8	

total fibre (g)	soluble fibre (g)	chol (mg)	useful source of vitamins	good source of minerals	special health notes
4.9	3	0	b-carotene, nic ac, C, E	manga, potas	Very best fruit source of antioxidant carotenoids. Extremely rich in fibre, particularly soluble fibre, important in keeping blood cholesterol low. Also one of the few good fruit sources of vitamin E.
1.4	0.4	0	b-carotene, C	potas	Orange- and red-fleshed melons, such as cantaloupe and watermelon, contain good amounts of beta-carotene, but pale-fleshed varieties do not.
1.8	0.9	0	C	potas	
2.7	1.8	0	folate, C	potas	One of the least expensive fruit sources of vitamin C, providing more than the daily RNI for adults in one average fruit (about 60mg per fruit). Rich in flavonoids such as rutin that have an antioxidant effect.
4.7	2.8	0	carotenoids, C	potas	Rich in beta-carotene and fibres. Particularly good source of soluble fibre (see Mango) and contains enzymes which aid digestion.
0.5	0.1	0	C, carotenoids		
1.6	0.8	0	C		
3.5	1.1	0	C	potas	Pears are a good fruit for children and others with a tendency to be allergic to fruits, as they have a low allergy rating. They contain an antioxidant (hydroxycinnamic acid) which has an antibacterial action.
1.2	0.1	0	C	manga	Contains the enzyme bromelain, which helps the digestion by aiding the breakdown of protein.
1.5	1	0	b-carotene	potas	Good source of fibres, and red-skinned varieties contain useful amounts of beta-carotene.
2.8	2	0		potas, iron	Laxative effect due to compounds which stimulate the bowel. Regular intake has been shown to reduce LDL cholesterol in the blood. May also protect against colon cancer. Good source of fibres and iron.
1	0.5	0		potas, iron	
2.5	0.7	0	folate, C	manga	One of the best fresh fruit sources of fibre.
1.4	0.5	0		cal, potas	Contains good amounts of calcium, but the oxalic acid content of rhubarb hinders its absorption, and also hinders absorption of iron. Excellent laxative.

	food state	portion size	calories	k joules	total fat (g)	% poly	% mono	% sat	protein (g)	carbo (g)	starch (g)	sugars (g)	
Satsuma		1	23	99	0.1	tr	tr	tr	0.5	5.4	0	5.4	
Strawberries		100g	27	113	0.1	tr	tr	tr	0.8	6	0	6	
Sultanas		50g	138	586	0.2	tr	tr	tr	1.4	35	0	35	

Meat, poultry and game

	food state	portion size	calories	k joules	total fat (g)	% poly	% mono	% sat	protein (g)	carbo (g)	starch (g)	sugars (g)	
Bacon lean back	raw	100g	136	568	6.7	13	42	37	19	0	0	0	
Bacon back, standard	raw	100g	120	500	6.9	13	42	37	14	0	0	0	
Bacon back, lean and fat	fried in blended vegetable oil	100g	465	1,926	41	11	45	39	25	0	0	0	
Bacon streaky	raw	100g	276	1,142	24	15	43	35	16	0	0	0	
Beef minced, average	raw	100g	225	934	16	3	44	44	20	0	0	0	
Beef minced, extra-lean	raw	100g	174	728	9.6	4	43	44	22	0	0	0	
Beef topside, sirloin	roast, lean meat only	100g	175	736	5.1	4	45	41	32	0	0	0	
Beef steak, rump	raw, lean only	100g	125	526	4.1	7	42	42	22	0	0	0	
Beefburger	grilled	1 quarter-pounder	254	1,057	19	3	46	45	21	0.1	0	0.1	
Beef corned		100g	217	905	12	3	40	52	27	0	0	0	

total fibre (g)	soluble fibre (g)	chol (mg)	useful source of vitamins	good source of minerals	special health notes
0.8	0.5	0			As with all citrus fruits, good source of vitamin C, containing approximately 20mg per average fruit, or half a day's RNI for adults.
1.1	0.5	0	C		Excellent source of vitamin C, approximately twice a day's RNI for adults (77mg) in 100g of fruit. Also contains ellagic acid (see Cherries).
1	0.4	0	potas, iron		
0	0	18	B1, nic ac, B6, B12, pant ac	potas, zn, phos	Bacon, like most meats, is a good source of B vitamins and an important source of zinc, which helps to boost the immune system. Surprisingly, bacon contains more monounsaturated fat than saturated. Bacon can be an extremely high-fat food, especially if fried, but if well trimmed and grilled, is a good source of protein. Don't grill bacon to the point where it is burnt, as the burnt bits are carcinogenic. Smoked bacon has also been linked with cancer; better to choose unsmoked as often as you can.
0	0	101	B1, nic ac, B6, B12, pant ac	potas, phos	
0	0	143	B1, nic ac, B6, B12, pant ac	potas, phos	All bacon is high in sodium, even the kinds labelled 'reduced-salt' and should be avoided by people with high blood pressure or who have been asked to follow a low-salt diet by their doctor.
0	0	97	B1, nic ac, B6, B12, pant ac	potas, zn, phos	
0	0	66	nic ac, B6, B12	potas, phos, zn, iron	Beef, like most meats, is a good source of B vitamins, zinc and iron. Lean cuts are not all that high in fat – just over one-quarter of lean beef's calories are fat calories. Of that, less than half is saturated. Consumption has declined in the UK slightly due to the possible link between the new strain of Creutzfeldt-Jakob disease and BSE in cattle. If this worries you, organic beef is BSE-free (and also free from antibiotics and growth hormones). The World Cancer Research Fund says that red meat intake should be limited to 80g a day. A recent International consensus study has suggested a strong link between meat eating and heart disease. The last UK COMA panel report recommended people who eat above average amounts of meat should cut down. USA studies link barbecued and grilled red meat with stomach cancer and UK studies have shown increased production of carcinogenic nitro-samines in the intestines of people who eat large amounts of meat. Minced beef, including burgers, should be well cooked so that no pink meat remains to prevent food poisoning such as E-coli, but don't cook meat until charred as charred portion is carcinogenic. For further detail on red meat and your health, see pages 71-72 and 80-81.
0	0	56	nic ac, B6, B12	potas, phos, zn, iron	
0	0	82	B2, nic ac, B6, B12	potas, phos, zn, iron	
0	0	59	B2, nic ac, B6, B12	potas, phos, zn, iron	
0	0	59	nic ac, B6, B12	potas, phos, zn, iron	
0	0	93	nic ac, B12	zn, iron	High in sodium and so should be limited by anyone following a low-sodium diet.

	food state	portion size	calories	k joules	total fat (g)	% poly	% mono	% sat	protein (g)	carbo (g)	starch (g)	sugars (g)	
Crocodile fillet	cooked	100g	160	674	4	23	48	30	31	0	0	0	
Gammon steak fat removed	grilled	100g	172	726	5.2	10	42	37	31	0	0	0	
Ham extra-lean		100g	107	451	3.3	15	46	33	18	1	0	1	
Ham Parma		50g	111	466	6.5	n/k	n/k	33	13.5	tr	0	tr	
Lamb loin chop, trimmed	grilled	1	150	624	7.5	6	37	46	29	0	0	0	
Lamb leg	roast, lean only	100g	203	853	9.4	6	42	40	30	0	0	0	
Lamb shoulder	roast	100g	235	982	14	4	39	46	28	0	0	0	
Kidney lambs'	fat removed	1	91	385	2.6	19	23	35	17	0	0	0	
Liver lamb's		100g	137	575	6.2	15	29	27	20	0	0	0	
Ostrich	cooked	100g	188	794	3.4	32	35	32	39	0	0	0	
Pork fillet	raw	100g	122	514	4	8	45	40	22	0	0	0	
Pork leg	roast, lean only	100g	185	779	5.1	14	41	35	35	0	0	0	
Pork crackling	roast	100g	550	2,280	45	18	44	34	36	0	0	0	
Pork chop, loin, lean	grilled	1	220	929	7.7	16	16	34	38	0	0	0	

total fibre (g)	soluble fibre (g)	chol (mg)	useful source of vitamins	good source of minerals	special health notes
0	0	n/k	n/k	n/k	Very low in fat and high in protein, a good alternative to higher-fat meats.
0	0	19	B1, B2, nic ac, B6	potas, phos, zn, cop	See Bacon.
0	0	58	B1, nic ac, B6, B12,	potas	Extra-lean ham is a good source of fairly low-fat protein. All ham contains reasonably high amounts of sodium, due to the curing process.
tr	n/k	n/k	n/k	n/k	
0	0	96	B2, nic ac, B6, B12, pant ac	potas, phos, iron, zn	Lamb contains similar levels of saturated fat to beef and pork, but contains around twice as much total fat as either. Even the lean cuts of lamb, such as leg, are comparatively high in fat. Like most meat, however, lamb is a good source of B vitamins and iron and zinc. See health notes for Beef for general notes on red meat and see also Heart Disease and Cancer in Section Two.
0	0	110	B2, nic ac, B6, B12, pant ac	potas, phos, iron, zn	
0	0	107	B2, nic ac, B6, B12, pant ac	potas, phos, iron, zn	
0	0	315	B1, B2, nic ac, B6, B12, pant ac, biotin	potas, phos, iron, zn, cop, sel	All offal is very high in nutrients. Kidneys are a good low-fat, low-calorie source of protein. Liver is one of the best dietary sources of iron and complete protein. However, it is high in cholesterol and should be avoided or limited by those on a low-cholesterol diet. Its very high content of vitamin A (which can be toxic) means it should be avoided by women in the first few months of pregnancy.
0	0	430	A, B1, B2, nic ac, B6, B12, folate, pant ac, biotin	potas, phos, iron, zn, cop, sel	
0	0	n/k	n/k	n/k	A low-fat source of protein.
0	0	89	B1, B2, nic ac, B6, B12 pant ac	potas, phos, zn, sel	Pork is one of the best sources of the range of B vitamins, and the lean meat contains only a little more total fat than beef. Good source of zinc and a useful source of selenium which, many experts now believe, may be lacking in many of our diets. Roast pork crackling is very high in fat. See health notes for Beef for general notes on red meat and see also entries for Heart Disease and Cancer in Section One.
0	0	110	B1, B2, nic ac, B6, B12, pant ac	potas, phos, zn, sel	
0	0	105			
0	0	110	B1, nic ac, B6, B12, pant ac	potas, phos, zn, sel	

	food state	portion size	calories	k joules	total fat (g)	% poly	% mono	% sat	protein (g)	carbo (g)	starch (g)	sugars (g)	
Salami		25g	109	453	10	11	45	37	5	0.5	0	0.5	
Sausage chorizo		100g	291	1,208	23	10	48	42	18	3.2	0.4	2.8	
Sausage pepperoni		100g	551	2,279	51	10	45	38	22	0.6	tr	0.6	
Sausage pork	grilled	2 large	254	1,056	20	11	45	39	11	9.2	7.8	1.4	
Sausage chipolata, low-fat	grilled	2	92	384	5.5	16	44	36	6.5	4.3	4	0.4	
Veal fillet		100g	109	459	2.7	15	44	33	21	0	0	0	
Venison fillet		100g	103	437	1.6	25	25	50	22	0	0	0	
Chicken fillet	no skin	100g	116	480	3.2	18	46	27	22	0	0	0	
Chicken breast	grilled, skin removed	1 breast	192	814	2.9	18	46	27	42	0	0	0	
Chicken leg quarter	casseroled	1	257	1,075	12	19	46	27	37	0	0	0	
Chicken roast	meat/skin only (no bone), avge	100g	177	742	7.5	20	45	28	27	0	0	0	
Duck farmed	roast, meat plus skin	100g	337	1,410	28	12.5	46	36	19	0	0	0	
Duck wild	breast, roast, meat only	100g	123	515	4.25	14	28	30	20	0	0	0	
Guinea fowl meat	raw	100g	148	622	6.2	23	37	33	23	0	0	0	

total fibre (g)	soluble fibre (g)	chol (mg)	useful source of vitamins	good source of minerals	special health notes
0.1	n/k	20	B1, nic ac, B6, B12, pant ac	potas, phos	Delicatessen cooked sausages are high in fat, saturated fat and sodium. Because of the smoking process, smoked sausages have been linked with some cancers.
tr	n/k	n/k	n/k	n/k	
tr	n/k	n/k	n/k	n/k	
0.6	n/k	53	nic ac, B12	cop	Over 70% of the calories in an average pork sausage are fat calories. Even well grilled, the proportion remains high. Low-fat sausages are less fatty but still contain over half their calories as fat.
0.6	n/k	22	nic ac, B12	cop	
0	0	84	B2, nic ac, B6, B12	potas, phos, zn	A low-fat, high-protein meat.
0	0	50	B2, nic ac, B6, B12	potas, phos, iron, zn, cop	A low-fat, high-protein meat, rich in vitamins and minerals. Good source of iron. The iron in all meats is more easily absorbed by the body than that in plant foods.
0	0	43	nic ac, B6, pant ac	potas, phos, sel	Chicken is only a low-fat source of protein if the skin is removed, preferably before cooking. If you eat the meat and skin, the fat content of chicken is much higher than beef and other red meats. Chicken is a good source of selenium, an antioxidant mineral which may be lacking in our diets.
0	0	122	nic ac, B6, pant ac	potas, phos, sel	Chicken should be cooked right through to avoid food poisoning and stored and re-heated carefully.
0	0	168	nic ac, B6, pant ac	potas, phos, zn, sel	
0	0	105	nic ac, B6, pant ac	potas, phos, zn, sel	
0	0	84	B1, B2, nic ac, B6, B12	potas, phos, iron, zn, cop, sel	Lean duck meat isn't as high in fat as many people believe, containing no more fat than lamb. But duck eaten with the skin – even crispy skin – becomes much higher in fat, although these fats are mostly the unsaturated type, unlike red meat. The lean meat is a good source of B vitamins and the important minerals iron, zinc and selenium. Wild duck is a healthy low-fat food.
0	0	77	B1, B2, nic ac, B6, B12, pant ac	potas, phos, iron, zn, cop, sel	
0	0	n/k	n/k	n/k	A low-fat source of protein.

	food state	portion size	calories	k joules	total fat (g)	% poly	% mono	% sat	protein (g)	carbo (g)	starch (g)	sugars (g)	
Pheasant	roast, meat no bone	100g	220	918	12	13	47	34	28	0	0	0	
Rabbit fillet	raw (no bone)	100g	137	576	5.5	33	24	38	22	0	0	0	
Turkey light meat, fillet	raw	100g	103	430	1.1	25	38	38	24	0	0	0	
Turkey dark meat, fillet	raw	100g	114	480	3.6	24	40	32	20	0	0	0	
Turkey light meat	roast	100g	153	648	1.4	25	35	35	34	0	0	0	

Nuts, seeds and savoury snacks

	food state	portion size	calories	k joules	total fat (g)	% poly	% mono	% sat	protein (g)	carbo (g)	starch (g)	sugars (g)	
★ **Almonds**		50g shelled weight	306	1267	28	25	62	8	11	3.5	1.4	2.1	
★ **Brazil nuts**		50g shelled weight	341	1407	34	34	38	24	7.1	1.5	0.3	1.2	
★ **Cashew nuts**		50g shelled weight	287	1187	24	18	58	20	8.9	9.1	6.8	2.3	
Chestnuts		50g shelled weight	85	360	1.4	41	37	19	1	18	15	3.5	
★ **Hazelnuts**		50g shelled weight	325	1343	32	10	79	7.5	7.1	3	1	2	
Macadamia nuts		50g shelled weight	374	1541	39	2	78	14	4	2.4	0.4	2	
Nuts mixed, chopped		50g	304	1258	27	27	52	16	11	4	2	2	
Peanuts	raw	50g shelled weight	282	1171	23	31	46	18	13	6.3	3.2	3.1	

total fibre (g)	soluble fibre (g)	chol (mg)	useful source of vitamins	good source of minerals	special health notes
0	0	220	B2, nic ac, B6, B12, potas	phos, iron	Higher in fat than some other game birds.
0	0	71	nic ac, B6, B12	potas, phos, sel	Very low-fat source of protein.
0	0	49	nic ac, B6, B12	potas, phos	Turkey is an extremely low-fat meat and a good choice for slimmers, being high in protein, B vitamins and selenium. The dark leg meat contains twice as much iron as the light breast meat and three times as much zinc, which is important for a healthy immune system.
0	0	81	B2, nic ac, B6, B12,	potas, phos, sel	
0	0	62	nic ac, B6, B12	potas, phos, sel	
3.7	0.6	0	B2, nic ac, E	cal, magnes, potas, phos, cop, manga	All nuts contribute significant amounts of iron, zinc and magnesium as a regular part of the diet. Nuts are quite high in protein, but the reason that their calorie content is so high is their high fat content. The fat in nuts is, however, mostly unsaturated. People who regularly eat nuts are up to half as likely to suffer a heart attack as people who never eat them. Most nuts, especially hazelnuts and macadamias, have a high monounsaturated fat content, but pine nuts and walnuts are higher in polyunsaturates. Chestnuts are the only low-fat nuts.
2.2	0.6	0	B1, E	magnes, potas, phos, zn, cop, sel, manga	
1.6	0.8	0	B1, nic ac, folate	magnes, potas, phos, iron, zn, cop, sel, manga	Brazil nuts are exceptionally high in magnesium and selenium, the antioxidant mineral which helps to protect against heart disease, cancer and ageing. Pecans are a good source of zinc, which helps to strengthen the immune system.
2	0.6	0		potas	Some people are allergic to peanuts and to a lesser extent, other nuts. A peanut allergy can produce an extremely serious reaction if even a minute amount of peanut is eaten, and can even cause death.
3.3	1.3	0	B1, nic ac, B6, folate, E	potas, phos, cop, magnes, manga	All fresh nuts should be eaten quickly as stale nuts can build up dangerous levels of contaminants that can cause illness. Young children under five should not have nuts as they can choke on them.
2.7	0.9	0		magnes, cop, manga	Peanuts, pistachio nuts, and diets containing 30% nut oils have been shown in several trials to reduce harmful LDL cholesterol levels in the blood as much as Mediterranean-type diets rich in olive oil.
3	0.9	0	nic ac, E	magnes, potas, phos, cop, manga	
3.1	0.9	0	B1, nic ac, B6, folate, E	magnes, potas, phos, cop, manga	

	food state	portion size	calories	k joules	total fat (g)	% poly	% mono	% sat	protein (g)	carbo (g)	starch (g)	sugars (g)
Pine nuts		50g shelled weight	344	1420	34	60	20	7	7	2	0.1	2
Pistachios		50g shelled weight	301	1243	28	32	50	13	8.9	4.1	1.3	2.8
Walnuts		50g shelled weight	344	1419	34	69	18	8	7.3	1.6	0.3	1.3
Pumpkin seeds		1tbsp (10g)	57	238	4.5	40	25	15	2.4	1.5	2.3	0.2
★ **Sunflower seeds**		1tbsp (10g)	57	238	4.5	65	21	10	3.2	3	2.6	0.3
Popcorn	plain	25g	148	617	11	46	34	10	1.5	12	12	0.3
Potato crisps salted		30g bag	159	665	10	15	40	41	1.7	16	16	0.2
Potato crisps salted, reduced fat		30g bag	137	577	6.4	12	41	43	2	19	19	0.4
Prawn crackers		40g	205	857	12	10	79	11	n/k	24	n/k	2.4
Tortilla chips		30g	138	578	6.9	30	47	18	2.3	18	17.7	0.3

Puddings and desserts

	food state	portion size	calories	k joules	total fat (g)	% poly	% mono	% sat	protein (g)	carbo (g)	starch (g)	sugars (g)
Custard ready-made		100ml serving	95	401	3	3	30	57	2.6	15	3.1	12
Ice-cream dairy, vanilla		100g serving	194	814	9.8	3	25	65	3.6	24	tr	22
Mousse, chocolate		100g serving	139	586	5.4	3	30	61	4	20	2.4	18

total fibre (g)	soluble fibre (g)	chol (mg)	useful source of vitamins	good source of minerals	special health notes
0.9	n/k	0	nic ac, E	magnes, potas, phos, iron, zn, cop, manga	
3	1.4	0	B1, nic ac, E	potas, magnes, potas, phos, cop, manga	
1.8	0.8	0	B1, B6, folate, E	magnes, potas, phos, cop, manga	
0.5	0.3	0		potas, phos, magnes, iron, zn, cop	Edible seeds are almost all a good source of many minerals and poly-unsaturated fats. They are high in calories because of their high fat content, but they weigh very light and so can be sprinkled on cereals, breads, soups, etc., without too much damage to a diet.
1	0.3	0	B1, E	magnes, iron, cop, manga	
n/k	n/k	0	E		Most snack products are very high in fat and salt without offering much nutritional benefit, and are best kept for occasional use. Many savoury snack foods are also high in artificial colourings and flavourings, and may be linked to allergic reactions.
1.6	0.8	0	E	potas	
1.8	1	0	E	potas	
0.6	n/k	0			
1.8	n/k	0	E	potas, manga	
0.1	n/k	11	A, B2	cal, potas, phos, iod	Most commercial desserts are high in sugar and fat unless specifically labelled otherwise. Puddings based on milk, such as custard and rice puddings, are a fairly good choice as they contain good amounts of calcium and sugar and fat content is not too high. Many ready-to-eat desserts, particularly those with a long shelf-life stored on shop shelves at room temperature, are high in preservatives and other additives. If you are trying to cut down on 'E numbers', give them a miss.
tr	0	31	A	cal	
n/k	tr	n/k		cal	

Rice, grains and pasta

	food state	portion size	calories	k joules	total fat (g)	% poly	% mono	% sat	protein (g)	carbo (g)	starch (g)	sugars (g)
Bulgar		50g dry weight	177	739	0.9	n/k	n/k	n/k	4.8	38	n/k	n/k
★ **Barley** pot		50g dry weight	151	641	1	n/k	n/k	15	5.3	32	31	0.9
Barley pearl		50g dry weight	180	768	0.9	n/k	n/k	15	4	42	42	0
Couscous instant		50g dry weight	175	745	0.9	n/k	n/k	n/k	5.3	39	39	0
Flour white		50g dry weight	171	725	0.6	50	17	17	4.7	39	38	0.8
★ **Flour** wholemeal		50g dry weight	155	659	1.1	45	14	14	6.3	32	31	1
Pasta white		50g dry weight	171	728	0.9	44	11	11	6	37	35	1.6
★ **Pasta** wholemeal		50g dry weight	162	690	1.3	44	12	16	6.7	33	31	1.9
Polenta		50g dry weight	172	720	0.8	n/k	n/k	33	4.3	37	36	1
★ **Rice** brown		50g dry weight	179	759	1.4	36	25	25	3.3	41	40	0.6
Rice white		50g dry weight	192	815	1.8	36	25	25	3.7	43	43	tr
Spaghetti in tomato sauce		215g can	138	587	0.9	50	25	25	4.1	31	19	12
Wheatgerm		2 tbsp	36	150	0.9	46	12	14	0.1	4	2.9	1.6

total fibre (g)	soluble fibre (g)	chol (mg)	useful source of vitamins	good source of minerals	special health notes
n/k	n/k	0	B1, nic ac	phos, iron, cop	A cracked wheat grain unsuitable for people with wheat or gluten intolerance or allergy. Good source of complex carbohydrate.
7.4	2	0	nic ac, B6	potas, iron, manga, phos	Pot barley contains the complete barley grain, which is rich in insoluble fibre and therefore good for helping constipation, and a good source of soluble fibre, which lowers blood cholesterol. Rich in minerals, good source of iron and a useful source of protein. Contains gluten. In pearl barley the outer husk of the barley, containing most of the nutrients, has been removed. A high-cereal diet helps to protect against bowel cancer and possibly diverticulitis and breast cancer.
3	n/k	0		manga	
1	0.5	0			Pre-cooked wheat semolina which, although a low-fat carbohydrate, contains few nutrients. Traditional couscous, available at health-food stores, contains more fibre, B vitamins and iron, but takes longer to cook.
1.5	0.8	0		cal	White flour has been milled until most of the outer wheat husk has been removed, therefore contains few nutrients in good quantities, except calcium.
4.5	1	0	B1, nic ac, B6	magnes, phos, cop, sel, manga	Good source of complex carbohydrate, containing all the goodness of the complete wheat husk and wheatgerm, plenty of fibre and useful amounts of protein.
1.5	0.8	0	nic ac	manga, cop	Wholewheat pasta is rich in nicotinic acid and fibre, with a low glycaemic index. With twice as much iron (2mg per 50g raw) as white, it is a helpful source of iron for vegetarians (even though iron does not appear in the chart as it is just under 17%, see page 30). White pasta contains less fibre, vitamins and minerals, but is still a good source of low-fat complex carbohydrates, with a medium glycaemic index.
4.2	1	0	B2, nic ac	manga, cop, magnes	
0.5	n/k	0		iron	Cornmeal, which is usually cooked with a lot of added butter and cheese, rendering the finished dish very high in fat and saturates. Suitable for those with a gluten or wheat intolerance.
0.9	tr	0	B1, nic ac	magnes, phos, cop, manga	Good source of B vitamins, with some fibre and low in fat, making it an ideal complex carbohydrate, particularly for those with a gluten or wheat intolerance, but also with a medium glycaemic index.
0.2	tr	0		manga	Contains less vitamins, minerals and fibre than brown rice but still a good low-fat carbohydrate food, suitable for those with a gluten or wheat intolerance.
1.5	n/k	0		potas	Canned spaghetti is a fairly useful low-fat food, but it is high in salt and sugar. Contains useful amounts of lycopene and beta-carotene in the tomato sauce.
1.6	0.3	0	B1, B6, folate, E		You need at least 2 tablespoons a day to make a significant contribution towards your daily intake of B vitamins, vitamin E or fibre (see note re vitamins and minerals on pages 22-33).

	food state	portion size	calories	k joules	total fat (g)	% poly	% mono	% sat	protein (g)	carbo (g)	starch (g)	sugars (g)	

Spreads, dips and pâtés

	food state	portion size	calories	k joules	total fat (g)	% poly	% mono	% sat	protein (g)	carbo (g)	starch (g)	sugars (g)	
Fruit conserve (jam)		25g	65	279	0	0	0	0	0.2	17	0	17	
Pure fruit spread		25g	30	130	0	0	0	0	0.2	7.8	0.2	7.8	
Peanut butter		25g	156	645	13	34	40	22	5.7	3.3	1.6	1.7	
Yeast extract		1tsp	16	69	0	0	0	0	3.7	0.3	0.2	0.1	
Hummus		25g	83	347	7.3	25	63	12	1.9	2.3	0.1	2.2	
Taramasalata		25g	126	519	13	32	55	8	0.8	1	1	0	
Liver pâté		25g	79	327	7.2	9	35	29	3.3	0.3	0.2	0.1	

Sweeteners and confectionery

	food state	portion size	calories	k joules	total fat (g)	% poly	% mono	% sat	protein (g)	carbo (g)	starch (g)	sugars (g)	
Honey		25g	72	307	0	0	0	0	0.1	19	0	19	
Fructose		25g	96	401	0	0	0	0	0	25	0	25	
Sugar white		25g	99	420	0	0	0	0	0	26	0	26	
Sugar brown		25g	91	387	0	0	0	0	0	25	0	25	
Syrup		25g	75	317	0	0	0	0	0.1	20	0	20	

total fibre (g)	soluble fibre (g)	chol (mg)	useful source of vitamins	good source of minerals	special health notes
n/k	n/k	0			High in sugar but with small amounts of vitamin C, depending upon variety.
n/k	n/k	0			Less sugar than jam, sweetness usually comes from fruit sugars.
1.4	0.4	0	nic ac, E	magnes	Peanuts are high in fat and calories, and so is peanut butter, but the fat is mostly unsaturated. Fairly good source of protein and useful for vegetarians. If eaten regularly, contributes valuable amounts of iron.
0	0	0	B1, B2, nic ac, folate		Yeast extracts, such as Marmite, are rich in B vitamins but as usually eaten in small quantities that has to be taken into account. Also very high in salt. Make good alternative to meat stocks for vegetarians.
3	n/k	0			Ready-made chickpea purée doesn't contain enough chickpeas to make a significant contribution to nutrients unless you eat lots. Homemade provides more, particularly magnes, iron, cop, manga and nic ac.
tr	n/k	06	B12		Extremely high in fat and salt.
tr	n/k	42	A, B12		Rich in vitamin A and best avoided in pregnancy. Very high in fats, but if eaten in reasonable amounts will contribute good amounts of iron and some B vitamins.
0	0	0			Honey (particularly the Manuka variety) is an antiseptic, reduces inflammation, and may help digestive problems. Organic, pure single-source honeys have more potent health properties.
0	0	0			Fructose (fruit sugar) has roughly the same calories as ordinary sugar (sucrose) but is twice as sweet and so offers a means of cutting calories. It is absorbed more slowly into the blood than sugar and so is less likely to produce fluctuations in blood sugar. It has also been shown to help disperse LDL cholesterols from the blood. However, an excess of fructose (around 25g plus/day) can cause diarrhoea and may raise triglyceride levels. Ordinary white sugar is the highly refined by-product of the sugar cane, containing no nutrients, fats, fibre, or anything except simple carbohydrate. Brown sugar is similar, though the darkest contain very small amounts of vitamins and minerals. Syrup is just processed sugar. High sugar intake has been linked with increased risk of various ailments, such as heart disease, but scientific evidence is scant and a new World Health Organization report says that sugary foods can be eaten up to four times a day as part of a healthy diet. See page 12.
0	0	0			
0	0	0			
0	0	0			

	food state	portion size	calories	k joules	total fat (g)	% poly	% mono	% sat	protein (g)	carbo (g)	starch (g)	sugars (g)	
Molasses blackstrap		25g	67	279	0	0	0	0	0	17	0	15	
Chocolate milk		25g	130	544	7.7	4	32	60	1.9	14	0	14	
Chocolate dark		25g	128	534	7	4	33	60	1.3	16	0.2	16	
Carob bar		25g	139	581	9.3	n/k	n/k	n/k	2.5	12	n/k	n/k	
Liquorice		25g	70	296	0.3	n/k	n/k	n/k	1.4	16	5.1	10	
Boiled sweets		25g	82	349	tr	0	0	0	tr	22	0.1	22	
Toffee		25g	107	448	4.7	4	40	51	0.6	17	tr	11	

Vegetables and pulses

	food state	portion size	calories	k joules	total fat (g)	% poly	% mono	% sat	protein (g)	carbo (g)	starch (g)	sugars (g)	
Artichoke globe		1 whole	9	39	0.1	100	0	0	1.4	1.4	tr	0.6	
Artichoke Jerusalem	boiled	100g	41	207	0.1	tr	tr	tr	1.6	11	tr	1.6	
⭐ **Asparagus**		100g	25	103	0.6	50	25	25	2.9	2	0.1	0.9	
Aubergine		100g	15	64	0.4	50	tr	25	0.9	2.2	0.2	2	
⭐ **Avocado**		1/2 medium	145	588	15	11	62	21	1.4	1.4	tr	0.4	
Bamboo shoots canned, drained		100g	11	45	0.2	50	0	50	1.5	0.7	tr	0.7	

total fibre (g)	soluble fibre (g)	chol (mg)	useful source of vitamins	good source of minerals	special health notes
tr	n/k	0		potas, magnes, manga	Molasses provides more nutrients than any other type of sweetener. In larger quantities, supplies good amounts of iron and calcium.
0.2	n/k	6			Chocolate is made from antioxidant cocoa beans, but milk chocolate doesn't contain a great deal of cocoa solids. Plain chocolate contains more cocoa solids — up to 70% — and therefore has a greater anti-oxidant potential. It also contains more caffeine and theobromine, two stimulants, and twice the magnesium of milk chocolate and more iron, but very little calcium.
0.6	n/k	2			
n/k	n/k	0			Often eaten as a 'healthier' alternative to chocolate, carob bars however still contain a lot of fat and sugars, and therefore calories, but they are free from caffeine and other stimulants.
0.5	n/k	0		potas, cal, magnes, iron, manga	Natural laxative, also contains useful amounts of several minerals. Virtually fat-free and if you must eat sweets a good choice, especially as evidence that a compound in liquorice may inhibit tooth decay.
0	0	0			Basically just sugar and additives, usually artificial flavourings and colourings. Frequent sucking and chewing of sweets can contribute to tooth decay.
0	0	4			High in sugar and fat, and very little else. Chewing toffee can contribute to tooth decay.
n/k	n/k	0	folate	potas	Compound in artichokes called cynarin said to boost liver function and help regulate blood cholesterol; it may also help with irritable bowel syndrome.
3.5	2.3	0		potas	
1.7	0.8	0	b-carotene, E, folate	potas	One of few good vegetable sources of vitamin E. A natural diuretic. Its glycosides may be anti-inflammatory and of use in rheumatoid arthritis. Asparagus contains purines, which may trigger gout.
2	1	0	K		Aubergines have a range of vitamins and minerals but none in rich quantities.
2.6	1.2	0	B6, E	potas	Very good source of vitamin E and monounsaturated fats, and contains many other vitamins and minerals.
1.7	0.4	0		potas, cop	

	food state	portion size	calories	k joules	total fat (g)	% poly	% mono	% sat	protein (g)	carbo (g)	starch (g)	sugars (g)	
⭐ **Beans** broad	shelled	100g	59	247	1	50	10	10	5.7	7.2	5.4	1.3	
Beans French		100g	24	99	0.5	60	tr	20	1.9	3.2	0.9	2.3	
Beans runner		100g	22	93	0.4	50	tr	25	1.6	3.2	0.4	2.8	
Beansprouts (mung)		50g serving	16	66	0.3	40	20	20	1.5	2	0.9	1.1	
Beetroot		100g	36	154	0.1	50	tr	tr	1.7	7.6	0.6	7	
⭐ **Broccoli** green		100g	33	138	0.9	56	20	22	4.4	1.8	0.1	1.5	
⭐ **Brussels sprouts**		100g	42	177	1.4	50	7	21	3.5	4.1	0.8	3.1	
Cabbage red		100g	21	89	9.3	67	tr	tr	1.1	3.7	0.1	3.3	
⭐ **Cabbage** Savoy		100g	27	114	0.5	60	tr	20	2.1	3.9	0.1	3.8	
Carrots old		100g	35	146	0.3	67	tr	33	0.6	7.9	0.3	7.4	
Cauliflower		100g	34	142	0.9	56	11	22	3.6	3	0.4	2.5	
Celeriac		100g	18	73	0.4	n/k	n/k	n/k	1.2	2.3	0.5	1.8	
Celery		100g	7	32	0.2	50	tr	tr	0.5	0.9	tr	0.9	
⭐ **Chillies** fresh		100g	20	83	0.6	n/k	n/k	n/k	2.9	0.7	tr	0.7	

total fibre (g)	soluble fibre (g)	chol (mg)	useful source of vitamins	good source of minerals	special health notes
6.1	1.4	0	b-carotene, nic ac, folate, pant ac, C	potas	Excellent source of fibre, including soluble fibre, which can help lower blood cholesterol, and a range of vitamins and minerals. Also contains flavonoid quercetin to help prevent CHD.
2.2	0.9	0	b-carotene, folate, C	potas	Reasonable source of the antioxidant vitamins beta-carotene and C, and a good source of fibre.
2	0.8	0	b-carotene, folate, C	potas	As French Beans.
0.8	0.3	0	folate, C		
1.9	0.9	0	folate	potas, manga	In some people, beetroot turns urine pink. Juice is said to be an aid to kidney function, but there is no scientific proof. The leafy tops are an excellent vegetable, containing calcium, beta-carotene and iron.
2.6	1.1	0	b-carotene, folate, C	potas	High in fibre, antioxidant vitamins beta-carotene and C, which help against heart disease, and rich in folate. Its phytochemicals (glucosinolates) have important properties, especially against cancer.
4.1	2.2	0	b-carotene, folate, C	potas	Excellent source of fibre, folate and vitamin C, and second-best source of the anti-carcinogenic glucosinolates (see Broccoli).
2.5	1.2	0	folate, C	potas	May be useful in fighting skin infections as thought to contain natural antiseptic properties.
3.1	1.7	0	b-carotene, folate, C	potas	The dark green leaves contain most of the vitamins and minerals while the pale centre leaves contain much less. Contains similar phytochemicals to broccoli and sprouts, which help to fight cancers.
2.4	1.4	0	b-carotene		Richest source of beta-carotene (more available when cooked) converting in body to vitamin A, lack of which is associated with poor night vision. Also an antioxidant, helping fight heart disease and cancer.
1.8	0.9	0	folate, C	potas	Another good source of the cancer-fighting glucosinolates (see Broccoli).
3.7	2.4	0	folate, C	potas	
1.1	0.5	0		potas	A phytochemical in celery lowers blood pressure by 13% and blood cholesterol by 7% — in rats! This has yet to be tested on humans, but Oriental medicine has long used celery to lower blood pressure.
n/k	n/k	0	C		Contain high levels of pain-killer and antioxidant capsaicin (see Red peppers). They also stimulate metabolic rate, seem to have a cholesterol-lowering effect, relieve congestion, and are an aid to digestion.

	food state	portion size	calories	k joules	total fat (g)	% poly	% mono	% sat	protein (g)	carbo (g)	starch (g)	sugars (g)	
Chinese leaves		100g	12	49	0.2	50	tr	tr	1	1.4	tr	1.4	
Courgettes		100g	18	74	0.4	50	tr	25	1.8	1.8	0.1	1.7	
Cucumber		100g	10	40	0.1	tr	tr	tr	0.7	1.5	0.1	1.4	
Fennel Florence		100g	12	50	0.2	tr	tr	tr	0.9	1.8	0.1	1.7	
⭐ **Garlic**		1 clove	3	12	0	0	0	0	0.2	0.5	0.4	0.1	
Ginger		1 small knob	2	10	0	0	0	0	0.1	0.5	0.3	0.2	
⭐ **Kale**		100g	33	140	1.6	56	6	13	3.4	1.4	0.1	1.3	
Leeks		100g	22	93	0.5	60	tr	20	1.6	2.9	0.3	2.2	
Lettuce Cos		100g	16	65	0.6	67	tr	17	1	1.7	tr	1.7	
Lettuce iceberg		100g	13	53	0.3	67	tr	tr	0.7	1.9	tr	1.9	
Mange-tout peas		100g	32	136	0.2	50	tr	tr	3.6	4.2	0.8	3.4	
Mushrooms		100g	13	55	0.5	60	tr	20	1.8	0.4	0.2	0.2	
Mustard and cress		1 container	5	22	0.2	50	50	0	0.6	0.2	tr	0.2	
Okra		100g	31	130	1	30	10	30	2.8	3	0.5	2.5	

total fibre (g)	soluble fibre (g)	chol (mg)	useful source of vitamins	good source of minerals	special health notes
1.2	0.6	0	folate, C	potas	Source of glucosinolates (see Broccoli), but not as rich as darker greens.
0.9	0.4	0			
0.6	0.2	0			Mildly diuretic. Some evidence that the phytochemicals in cucumber called sterols (mainly in the skin) can lower blood cholesterol.
2.4	1.1	0	b-carotene, folate	potas	
0.1	0.1	0			Contains allicin, which is antibiotic and antifungal, and possibly antiviral. Also contains sulphides, which may help prevent cancers, and an antioxidant that lowers blood cholesterol and prevents clotting.
n/k	n/k	0			A well-known anti-nausea remedy — ideal for travel and 'morning' sickness. Also stimulates circulation and aids digestion. An infusion of grated ginger is said to help cold and bronchial symptoms.
3.1	1.9	0	b-carotene, folate, C, E	potas, potas, cal, manga	Good source of all three of the vitamin antioxidants, beta-carotene, C and E, and rich in glucosinolates (see Broccoli) which help to fight cancers.
2.2	1.1	0	b-carotene, folate, C	potas	Mildly diuretic. Member of same family as onions and garlic and, as such, if eaten regularly may help to keep cholesterol levels low and the blood healthy.
1.2	0.6	0	b-carotene, folate	potas	Much richer source of fibre and potassium than pale lettuce, as well as a good source of beta-carotene.
0.6	0.3	0	folate	potas	Dark lettuce leaves contain useful amounts of beta-carotene but pale leaves don't. Most lettuce is rich in folates. All lettuce contains phytochemicals that act as a mild sedative.
2.3	1	0	b-carotene, C	potas	Excellent all-round vegetable, containing good amounts of many nutrients, including protein and soluble fibres.
1.1	0.2	0	B2, nic ac, folate, pant ac	potas, cop	Contains very little carbohydrate but high in protein and fibre. Dark-gilled and oriental mushrooms contain the phytochemicals lentinan and canthaxanthin, which help fight cancer.
0.4	0.2	0	carotenoids, C		Not normally eaten in enough quantity to provide many nutrients.
4	2.4	0	b-carotene	magnes, potas	Very high in soluble fibre, which can help to lower blood cholesterol.

	food state	portion size	calories	k joules	total fat (g)	% poly	% mono	% sat	protein (g)	carbo (g)	starch (g)	sugars (g)
★ **Onions** Spanish		100g	36	150	0.2	50	tr	tr	1.2	7.9	tr	5.6
Onions spring		100g	23	98	0.5	40	20	20	2	3	0.2	2.8
Parsnips		100g	64	271	1.1	18	45	18	1.8	13	6.2	5.7
★ **Peas** Fresh		100g	83	344	1.5	47	13	20	6.9	11	7	2.3
Peas frozen		100g	66	279	0.9	56	11	22	5.7	9.8	45	2.6
Peas canned		100g	80	339	0.9	44	11	22	5.3	14	6.3	3.9
Peppers green		100g	15	65	0.3	67	tr	33	0.8	2.6	0.1	2.4
★ **Peppers** red		100g	32	134	0.4	50	tr	25	1	6.4	0.1	6.1
Peppers yellow		100g	26	113	0.2	50	tr	tr	1.2	5.3	tr	5.1
Potatoes boiled		100g	72	306	0.1	100	0	0	1.8	17	16	0.7
Potatoes oven chips		100g	162	687	4.2	14	38	43	3.2	30	29	0.7
Potatoes chips	frozen, straight-cut, fried in corn oil	100g	273	1,145	14	52	25	19	4.1	36	35	0.7
Pumpkin		100g	13	55	0.2	tr	tr	50	0.7	2.2	0.3	1.7
Spinach fresh		100g	25	103	0.8	63	13	13	2.8	1.6	0.1	1.5

total fibre (g)	soluble fibre (g)	chol (mg)	useful source of vitamins	good source of minerals	special health notes
0.4	0.8	0			Onions are from same family as garlic, with several probable medicinal benefits. Many experts believe they can help lower blood cholesterol and blood pressure and 'thin' blood to minimize risk of clotting. Also contain flavonoids and sulphurs which may help fight cancers, and natural antibiotics for help with bronchitis, colds and flu, as well as quercetin, an antioxidant. The green portions of spring onions contain beta-carotene and folate.
1.5	n/k	0	C		
4.6	2.6	0	b-carotene, B1, nic ac, folate, C	potas, phos, iron	
4.7	1.3	0	b-carotene, B1, nic ac, folate, C	potas	Popular source of vitamin C, fibre and many other vitamins and minerals.
5.1	1.6	0	b-carotene, B1, nic ac, folate, C	potas	Freezing peas hardly alters their nutritional value at all. In fact, if frozen soon after picking, will probably contain more vitamin C than fresh peas.
5.1	1.4	0	b-carotene nic ac	potas	Canning diminishes the vitamin C in vegetables.
1.6	0.7	0	b-carotene, folate, C	potas	Green peppers are one of the best vegetable sources of vitamin C, the antioxidant action of which is thought improved by flavonoids found in peppers. Red peppers are much higher in beta-carotene than other colours and, again, very rich in vitamin C. They contain the natural pain-killer capsaicin, clinically proved to be effective when rubbed on joints as a cream; the same effect may be gained by eating peppers and may be useful against arthritis pain.
1.6	0.7	0	b-carotene, B6, C		
1.7	0.7	0	b-carotene, B6, C	potas	As for green peppers.
1.2	0.7	0	B6, C	potas, cop	Potatoes are one of the cheapest sources of vitamin C, potassium and fibre and, eaten in quantity (as is usual), provide many other vitamins and minerals too. Green bits on the skin are poisonous and should be removed. The skins contain the most fibre and the flesh just under the skin contains the most vitamin C. New potatoes contain much more vitamin C than old. Potatoes should be cooked in their skin or peeled just before cooking, and should never be left soaking in water, both of which lose vitamin C. Oven chips are healthiest when the oil they contain is sunflower oil. Check labels.
2	1.1	0	nic ac, B6, C	potas, cop	
2.4	1.3	0	nic ac, B6, C	potas, cop	
1	0.4	0	b-carotene, C		Orange-fleshed varieties contain the carotenoid phytoene which may help prevent some cancers.
2.1	0.8	0	b-carotene, folate, C, E	potas, cal	Oxalic acid content of leaves hinders absorption of iron and calcium. Contains large amounts of antioxidant beta-carotene and carotenoid lutein, which may be important in eye health. High in folate.

	food state	portion size	calories	k joules	total fat (g)	% poly	% mono	% sat	protein (g)	carbo (g)	starch (g)	sugars (g)	
⭐ **Spring greens**		100g	33	136	1	60	10	10	3	3.1	0.4	2.7	
⭐ **Squash** butternut		100g	36	155	0.1	tr	tr	tr	1.1	8.3	3.4	4.5	
Swede		100g	24	101	0.3	67	tr	tr	0.7	5	0.1	4.9	
Sweetcorn frozen kernels		100g	85	361	0.8	40	25	25	25	17	15	1.9	
Sweetcorn baby corn cobs		100g	24	101	0.4	n/k	n/k	n/k	2.5	2.7	0.8	1.9	
⭐ **Sweet potato** orange-fleshed		100g	87	372	0.3	33	tr	33	1.2	21	16	5.7	
⭐ **Tomatoes** fresh		100g	17	73	0.3	50	25	25	0.7	3.1	tr	3.1	
Tomatoes canned		100g	16	69	0.1	tr	tr	tr	1	3	0.2	2.8	
Turnips		100g	23	98	0.3	67	tr	tr	0.9	4.7	0.2	4.5	
⭐ **Watercress**		100g	22	94	1	40	10	30	3	0.4	tr	0.4	
⭐ **Adzuki beans**		50g dry weight	136	579	0.3	n/k	n/k	n/k	10	25	22	0.5	
Baked beans in tomato sauce		100g (5 tbsp)	81	345	0.6	50	25	25	4.8	15	9.3	5.8	
Baked beans in tomato sauce	low-salt low-sugar	100g (5 tbsp)	73	311	0.6	50	25	25	5.4	12	9.7	2.8	
Black-eye beans		50g dry weight	156	662	0.8	44	6	31	12	27	24	1.5	

total fibre (g)	soluble fibre (g)	chol (mg)	useful source of vitamins	good source of minerals	special health notes
3.4	1.7	0	b-carotene, folate, C	potas	See Kale or Cabbage.
1.6	0.7	0	b-carotene, C, E	potas	Orange-fleshed squashes are rich in carotenoids as well as the other antioxidants, vitamins C and E.
1.9	0.9	0	b-carotene, C		Member of the brassica family and contains the same glucosinolates which are thought to help fight cancers. Also contains the antioxidant vitamins beta-carotene and C, and is a good source of fibre.
2.1	n/k	0	folate, C	potas	High in fibre and vitamin C.
2	0.4	0	b-carotene, folate, C		
2.4	1.1	0	C, E	potas	The orange-fleshed kind is rich in beta-carotene, but the white-fleshed kind contains very little. Both are good sources of the other antioxidant vitamins C and E.
1	0.4	0	b-carotene, C, E	potas	Tomatoes are rich in lycopene, the antioxidant phytochemical which is important in helping to prevent heart disease and cancers. They also contain the antioxidants beta-carotene, vitamin C and vitamin E.
0.7	0.3	0	b-carotene, C, E	potas	Lycopene (see above) is more potent in cooked and canned tomatoes than in raw ones. Tomato purées, pastes and juices are all rich in lycopene.
2.4	0.9	0	C		Member of the brassica family and thus will contain a certain amount of glucosinolates (see Broccoli).
1.5	0.7	0	b-carotene, C, E	potas, cal, iron	Although rich in antioxidants and minerals, it is usually eaten in such small quantities. Contains phenethyl isothiocyanate which, in large amounts, fights lung cancer caused by tobacco.
5.6	1.3	0	nic ac	magnes, potas, iron, zn, cop, manga	Though the nutritional content of each pulse varies slightly, as a group they are, perhaps almost the perfect health food. They are low in fat (apart from soya beans, the fat of which is mostly unsaturated anyway) and cholesterol-free, high in protein, high in complex carbohydrate, high in fibre and most are particularly rich in soluble fibre, which helps to lower blood cholesterol levels. Most contribute valuable iron and B vitamins to the diet of people who don't eat meat, and valuable for people who eat little or no dairy produce. Regular pulse eaters will also get plenty of zinc and other vitamins and minerals present in pulses in smaller quantities than will show on this chart. They are also low on the Glycaemic Index. Soya beans are among the few plant sources of complete protein, containing all eight essential amino acids which make up the protein in our diets. Many health claims have been made for soya (e.g. protection against heart disease, cancer, menopausal symptoms and more), but the evidence is mostly inconclusive and more trials need
3.5	2.1	0	b-carotene, folate	magnes, potas, phos, iron, manga	
3.8	2.3	0	b-carotene, folate	cal, magnes, potas, phos, iron, manga	
4.1	1.5	0	folate	potas, phos manga, cop	

	food state	portion size	calories	k joules	total fat (g)	% poly	% mono	% sat	protein (g)	carbo (g)	starch (g)	sugars (g)	
⭐ **Broad beans** (dried)		50g dry weight	123	521	1	52	14	14	13	16	12	3	
Butter beans		50g dry weight	145	617	0.9	47	6	24	10	27	23	1.8	
⭐ **Chickpeas**		50g dry weight	160	678	2.7	50	20	9	11	25	22	1.3	
Chickpeas canned, drained		100g	115	487	2.9	45	24	10	7.2	16.1	7.6	0.2	
⭐ **Haricot beans**		50g dry weight	143	609	0.8	31	25	19	11	25	21	1.4	
Lentils red		50g dry weight	159	677	0.6	39	15	15	12	28	25	1.2	
⭐ **Lentils** brown and green		50g dry weight	149	632	0.9	42	16	11	12	24	22	0.6	
Red kidney beans		50g dry weight	133	567	0.7	57	7	14	11	22	19	1.3	
Red kidney beans canned, drained		100g	100	424	0.6	50	17	17	3.5	8.9	6.4	1.8	
⭐ **Soya beans**		50g dry weight	185	776	9.3	49	19	12	18	7.9	2.4	2.8	
Split peas		50g dry weight	164	698	1.2	50	13	17	22	29	27	0.9	
Quorn chunks		100g	86	362	3.3	n/k	n/k	19	12	2	tr	1.1	
Tofu standard		100g	73	304	4.2	48	19	12	8.1	0.7	0.3	0.3	
Vegeburger		one 50g	98	411	5.6	n/k	n/k	n/k	8.3	4	2.2	1.8	

total fibre (g)	soluble fibre (g)	chol (mg)	useful source of vitamins	good source of minerals	special health notes
16	3	0	b-carotene, folate	manga	to be done. Soya products are, however, useful for people with a cows' milk allergy. But for babies, a diet high in soya may not be a good idea (see page 35).
8	3.2	0		potas, manga, cop	Baked beans in tomato sauce contain lycopene and can contribute good quantities of calcium in quantities larger than the 100g portion stated.
5.3	1.6	0	folate, E	potas, iron, cop. manga	Pulses can be toxic if prepared and cooked incorrectly — soak them properly and discard the soaking water before boiling for 10 minutes and then cooking until tender.
2	0.7	0	E	manga	Beans canned in brine are nutritionally similar to dried pulses, except their sodium content will be higher. Baked beans in tomato sauce are also high in salt and sugar, unless the reduced-salt and -sugar brand is chosen.
8.5	4	0		magnes, potas, iron, manga	
2.5	0.6	0		potas, iron	
4.4	1	0	B6, folate	potas, iron, sel, manga	
7.8	3.5	0	folate	potas, iron, manga, cop	
3.1	1.5	0		potas, iron, manga	
7.8	3.4	0	B6, nic ac, folate, E	magnes, potas, phos, iron, cop, manga	
3.2	1.1	0	nic ac	manga	
4.8	0.8	0	B1	phos, zn, cop, manga	'Man-made' protein food, low in fat and high in fibre, made from a 'mycoprotein' derived from mushroom family. Useful protein and source of zinc for vegetarians trying to eat less dairy produce.
tr	n/k	0		cal	Made from soya beans, tofu contains all their health benefits (see Soya milk and Soya beans). Suitable protein food for vegans and a good alternative to dairy produce for vegetarians.
2.1	1	0	B1, nic ac, folate	potas, iron, manga	These nutrient notes are given for a typical burger. Different brands of vegetable burger vary in their nutrient composition, but all contain reasonably high amounts of fat.

Index

(For an index of recipes, see page 209)

Appendix

Alcoholics Anonymous
PO Box 1, Stonebow House, Stonebow, York YO1 7NJ; Helpline 0845 769 7555
www.alcoholics-anonymous.org.uk

Alzheimer's Society,
Gordon House, 10 Greencoat Place, London SW1P 1PH; 020 7306 0606
www.alzheimers.org.uk

Arthritic Association
l Upperton Gardens, Eastbourne, East Sussex BN21 2AA; 01323 416550
www.arthritisassociation.org.uk

Allergy UK
3 White Oak Square, London Road, Swanley, Kent BR8 7AG; 01322 619898
www.allergyuk.org

Asthma UK
Summit House, 70 Wilson St, London EC2A 2DB; 08457 010203
www.asthma.org.uk

British Dietetic Association
5th floor, Charles House, 148–149 Great Charles Street, Queensway, Birmingham B3 3HT; 0121 200 8080 www.bda.uk.com

British Heart Foundation
14 Fitzhardinge St, London W1H 6DH; 020 7935 0185 www.bhf.org.uk

British Nutrition Foundation
52–54 High Holborn, London WC1V 6RQ: 020 7404 6504
www.nutrition.org.uk

Cancer Research UK
PO Box 123, Lincoln's Inn Fields, London WC2A: 3PX 020 7121 6699
www.cancerresearchuk.org

Coeliac UK
Octagon Court, High Wycombe, Bucks HP11 2HS: 01494 437278
www.coeliac.co.uk

Department of Health
Richmond House, 79 Whitehall, London SW1A 2NS; 020 7210 4850
www.dh.gov.uk

Department for the Environment, Food and Rural Affairs (DEFRA)
Nobel House, 17 Smith Square, London SW1P 3JR; 08459 335577 www.defra.gov.uk

Diabetes UK
Macleod House, 10 Parkway, London, NW1 7AA; 020 7424 1000
www.diabetes.org.uk

Eating Disorders Association
103 Prince of Wales Road, Norwich, NR1 1DW; adult helpline 0845 634 1414
www.edauk.com

Food Commission
94 White Lion Street, London N1 9PF; 020 7837 2250 www.foodcomm.org.uk

Food Standards Agency
125 Kingsway, London, WC2B 6NH; 020 7276 8829 www.food.gov.uk

Foresight Preconception
178 Hawthorn Road, West Bognor, W Sussex PO21 2UY; 01243 868001
www.foresight-preconception.org.uk

Friends of the Earth
26–28 Underwood Street, London N1 7JQ; 020 7490 1555 www.foe.co.uk

IBS Network
Unit 5, 53 Mowbray Street, Sheffield S3 8EN; 0114 272 3253
www.ibsnetwork.org.uk

ME Association
4 Top Angel, Buckingham Industrial Park, Buckingham, Bucks MK18 1TH; 0870 444 1835
www.meassociation.org.uk

Migraine Action Association
Unit 6, Oakley Hay Lodge Business Park, Great Folds Road, Great Oakley, Northants NN18 9AS; 01536 461333
www.migraine.org.uk

National Association for Colitis and Crohn's Disease
4 Beaumont House, Sutton Road, St Albans, Herts AL1 5HH; 01727 844296 www.nacc.org.uk

National Asthma Campaign
Providence House, Providence place, London, N1 0NT. Nurses' helpline: 08457 010203. www.asthma.org.uk

National Osteoporosis Society
Camerton, Bath BA2 0PJ. 08454 1303076; www.nos.org.uk

Soil Association
Bristol House, 40–56 Victoria Street, Bristol, BS1 6BY; 0117 314 5000
www.soilassociation.org

Sustain
94 White Lion Street, London N1 9PF. 020 7837 1228. www.sustainweb.org

Vegetarian Society
Parkdale, Dunham Road, Altrincham, Cheshire WA 14 4QG
0161 925 2000; www.vegsoc.org

for up-to-date healthy eating advice or to contact **Judith Wills**, visit www.thedietdetective.net

The author would like to thank Lewis Esson for a mammoth editing task completed in his usual unflappable and professional way, also to Mary Evans, Vanessa Courtier, and all the team at Quadrille; Jane Turnbull and Tony Allen. Thanks also to the following for help with information, facts and figures in many subject areas: British Heart Foundation, British Medical Journal, Child Growth Foundation, Department of Health, Dunn Clinical Nutrition Centre, The Food Commission, The Lancet, DEFRA, The National Food Alliance, Rowett Research Institute, The Soil Association, US National Cancer Research Institute, World Cancer Research Fund.

All photographs by Gus Filgate except: pp8, 10, 38, 54, 68, 70, 73, 76, 80, 84, 158, 186, 206 — Martin Brigdale; pp161, 164-5, 168-9, 171, 173-5, 179-181, 183, 185, 188, 193, 195-7, 199, 201-3, 205 — Patrick MacLeavey. The publisher thanks the following for their permission to reproduce the following pictures: 160 The Image Bank/Steve Niedorf; 167 The Image Bank/Nicolas Russell; 170 Getty Images/Ken Fisher; 172 The Stock Market/N. Schafer; 176 Getty Images/Christopher Bissell; 182 Getty Images/Peter Correz; 198 Getty Images/Dale Durfee.